MANUAL OF GYNAECOLOGY

α – Fœto Protein

Normal Range   15/40

16/40   < 75

17/40   < 82

18/40   < 110

19/40   < 125.

PCO   LH : FSH   3 : 1

Published volumes in the Manuals series

Paediatric Gastroenterology *J. H. Tripp and D. C. A. Candy*
Renal Disease *C. B. Brown*
Haematology *A. S. J. Baughan, A. S. B. Hughes, K. G. Patterson and
L. Stirling*
Clinical Blood Transfusion *M. Brozovic and B. Brozovic*
Chest Medicine *J. E. Stark, J. M. Shneerson, T. Higenbottam and
C. D. R. Flower*

Forthcoming volumes in the Manuals series

Gastroenterology *B. T. Cooper and R. E. Berry*
Cardiology *K. Dawkins*
Infectious Diseases *J. A. Innes*
Rheumatology *J. M. H. Moll*
Neonatal Intensive Care *A. R. Wilkinson*
Neonatal Medicine *D. Harvey and M. Cummins*
Hospital Paediatrics *G. Hambleton*
Geriatric Medicine *A. N. Exton-Smith and T. Van der Cammen*

MANUAL OF GYNAECOLOGY

Thankam R Varma PhD MB BS FRCS(Ed) FRCOG
Consultant Gynaecologist, St George's Hospital, London

Churchill Livingstone ▦
EDINBURGH LONDON MELBOURNE AND NEW YORK 1986

CHURCHILL LIVINGSTONE
Medical Division of Longman Group Limited

Distributed in the United States of America by Churchill Livingstone Inc., 1560
Broadway, New York, N.Y. 10036, and by associated companies, branches and
representatives throughout the world.

First published 1986

ISBN 0 443 033064

British Library Cataloguing in Publication Data
Varma, Thankam R.
Manual of gynaecology.
1. Gynaecology
I. Title
618.1   RG101

Library of Congress Cataloging-in-Publication Data
Varma, Thankam R.
Manual of gynaecology.
(Manuals series)
Includes index.
1. Gynecology—Handbooks, manuals, etc. I. Title.
[DNLM: 1. Gynecology—handbooks.   WP 39 V316m]
RG110.V37 1986   618.1   85-30923

Printed in Great Britain by Bell and Bain Ltd., Glasgow

PREFACE

This book covers aspects of gynaecology mainly for the benefit of residents and postgraduates who wish to specialise in gynaecology. It is meant to aid them also in the day to day management of common gynaecological problems. Within the constraints of size and its synoptic nature it is as comprehensive and up to date as possible. It provides comprehensive details of pelvic anatomy, reproductive physiology and important gynaecological diseases.

Finally, I wish to express my deep gratitude to my husband, Dr Rama Varma, for his support and help in preparing this manuscript; and to acknowledge Mrs Doreen Gray, not only for typing the manuscript, but also for her patience with me over the past few months.

London, 1986   T. R. Varma

CONTENTS

1. ANATOMY OF THE REPRODUCTIVE SYSTEM

The female reproductive organs are divided into two groups, the external and internal.

EXTERNAL GENITALIA

Collectively known as the vulva. Divided into surface and deeper structures.

Surface structures

Mons pubis
- This is a fibrofatty cushion.
- Lying anterior and superior to symphysis pubis.
- Covered by hair; distribution is different in the two sexes.

Labia majora
- These are two longitudinal raised folds of adipose tissue.
- Covered by skin which is rather heavily pigmented.
- Extend from the mons pubis above to the perineum below.
- Possess both sweat and sebaceous glands.
- Fourchette connects the posterior ends.
- They are homologous with the scrotum in the male.
- They respond to ovarian steroid hormones.

Labia minora
- These lesser labial folds extend from the clitoris to about two-thirds of the distance towards the perineum.
- Smaller and delicate and enclosed by the labia majora.
- Anteriorly they subdivide, one fold covering the clitoris to form its prepuce, the other passing beneath the glans to form the frenulum clitoridis.
- The skin contains fewer sebaceous and sweat glands and is devoid of hair.
- They are richly vascular and plentifully supplied with nerve endings.
- They are homologous with the structures that form the penile urethra in the male.

Clitoris
- It is homologous with the male penis.
- Composed of a vascular plexus (erectile tissue).
- Consists of a glans, a corpus or body, and the crura.
- It is attached to the inferior ischiopubic rami.
- The glans is richly supplied with nerve endings and·is extremely sensitive.

Vestibule
- This is the area enclosed by the labia minora.
- Urethra and vagina open into it.
- Paired Bartholin's ducts and some of the Skene's ducts open into it.
- It represents the lower portion of the embryological urogenital sinus.
- In the virgin the vaginal orifice is partly occluded by the hymen.
- The hymen is a rigid membrane of firm connective tissue covered on both sides by stratified squamous epithelium.

Urethral meatus
- It is a small slit-like or triangular external orifice of the urethra.
- Small pit-like depressions on either side of the meatus contain mucous glands called the lesser glands of the vestibule.
- The para-urethral of Skene's ducts open just below the outer part of the meatus.
- The female urethra is lined proximally by a stratified transitional epithelium, and its distal portion is covered with stratified squamous epithelium.
- The canal is surrounded by a labyrinth of para-urethral glands, and homologous of the male prostate.

Paraurethral ducts (Skene's ducts)
- These ducts serve the paraurethral glands which have a lubricating function.
- Their small openings can be seen inside the lower urethra, below and beside the external urethral meatus.

Vaginal introitus
- The vagina opens into the lower part of the vestibule just below the urethra.
- The orifice is closed by the hymeneal membrane, which has one or two openings in it.
- During the reproductive phase the hymen is broken down and the lower vagina is visualised when the labia are parted.
- Remnants of the hymen are represented by the caranculae myrtiformes.

Perineum
— This is the area outlined by the vaginal fourchette anteriorly and the anus posteriorly.

Deeper structures

Perineal body
— Lying beside the introitus of the vagina is the bulb of the vestibule and its surrounding bulbocavernosus muscle.
— It extends anteriorly to the clitoris and is joined by the ischiocavernosus muscle which arises from the medial and inferior portion of the ischiopubic ramus.
— Posteriorly, the two bulbocavernosus muscles join the superficial and deep transverse perineal muscles and also the muscle forming the external anal sphincter to form the strong perineal body.

Vulvovaginal or Bartholin's glands
— These lie on either side, posterolateral to the vaginal orifice in relation to the posterior end of the labia majora.
— They measure approximately 8–10 mm in diameter.
— Not normally palpable.
— The duct of each gland is about 20 mm long, runs downwards and inwards to open immediately lateral to the hymen in the groove between its attached border and the labium minus.
— Orifice of the duct is not normally visible.
— The main duct of the gland is lined with stratified transitional epithelium.
— The acini are lined with a layer of cuboidal cells.
— Bartholin's glands are homologous to Cowper's (bulbourethral) glands in the male.

Urogenital diaphragm
— This is situated in the triangular area bounded by the transverse perinei muscles posteriorly and the inferior ischiopubic rami on each side.
— It is a triangular-shaped diaphragm which lies below the levator ani muscles and through which pass the urethra and vagina.
— It is composed of a superficial and a deep layer.
— The superficial perineal muscles are superficial to the urogenital diaphragm.
— The deeper perineal muscles with other important structures are situated in the space between the two layers.
— Above the triangular ligament are the muscles of the deep compartment which comprise the compressor urethrae anteriorly and the deep transverse perineal muscles posteriorly.

— Below the triangular ligament or diaphragm are the structures already mentioned.
— Posteriorly, in the space behind the transverse perineal muscles, is the ischiorectal fossa, composed of fibrofatty tissue.

INTERNAL GENITALIA

Vagina

— It is an elastic musculo-membranous canal.
— It connects the uterus to the vestibule.
— The anterior wall is 80–100 mm in length and the posterior wall is 120–140 mm in length.
— In the resting state the walls are opposed.
— In the erect position its direction is, in general upward and backward from its vulvar to its uterine end.
— Its upper end expands into the cup-shaped fornix into which the cervix uteri is fitted.
— The portions of the fornix in front of, behind and at the sides of the cervix are designated as the anterior, posterior and lateral fornices.
— Anteriorly the vagina is closely related to the base of the bladder and urethra.
— Posteriorly it is related to the pouch of Douglas, rectum and anal canal.
— The vagina passes through the pelvic diaphragm (levator hiatus) and below this it passes through the perineal diaphragm.
— In the virgin the mucous membrane of the vagina is thrown into folds (rugae).
— It is reddish pink and is lined with stratified squamous epithelium.
— Beneath the mucous membrane is the muscular coat, made up of an inner circular and an outer layer.
— The outermost layer is fibrous, derived from the pelvic connective tissue.
— The vagina has no glands, its moisture being chiefly provided by the secretion of cervical mucus and by vaginal transudation.
— The vaginal squamous epithelium responds to ovarian hormones, the cells become rich in glycogen, which provides a medium for the resident lactobacilli of Doderlein.
— As a result of the lactic acid production of these bacilli the pH of the vagina is normally acid (pH4–4.5).

— Passing downwards in the anterolateral aspect of the vaginal wall are the vestigial wolffian or mesonephric ducts (Gartner's ducts). They may enlarge and become cystic.

Uterus

— It is the centre-piece of the reproductive apparatus.
— Is composed of two functional elements: a lower cervix which functions at different times as a passage way, a barrier and a reservoir; and an upper body in which the fetus develops.

Cervix

— The cervix in the infant is twice as large as the uterine body, in the adult this is reversed.
— There is a vaginal and supravaginal component to the cervix.
— It is a strong pivotal point for uterine stability, being attached to the pelvic walls by radiating fascial condensations called ligaments: pubocervical anteriorly, uterosacral posteriorly and transverse cervical (Mackenrodt) laterally.
— It is 20–30 mm in length and is delineated inferiorly by the external os and superiorly by the internal cervical os.
— The mucous membrane covering the external or vaginal surface is of the stratified squamous variety.
— The cervical canal is lined with columnar epithelium, the cytoplasm of these cells is rich in mucin.
— Columnar epithelium often extends to cover the central part of the ectocervix, resulting in a bright red colour (erosion) due to the closeness of the capillary vessels which lie underneath.
— The openings of cervical glandular clefts may become blocked by overgrowth of squamous epithelium (metaplasia) or by inflammation; small retention cysts form and these are obvious on the surface as nabothian follicles.
— Muscular coat of the cervix is well developed in the region of the internal os, but becomes increasingly sparse at a lower level, with corresponding increase in the proportion of connective tissue.
— Gland-like vestiges of the mesonephric duct are occasionally observed deep in the cervical musculature.

Uterine body

— It is a hollow thick-walled muscular organ, the cavity being roughly triangular.
— It is covered externally by peritoneum except the lower part anteriorly, where the peritoneum is reflected on to the bladder.

— It is globular externally, flattened in the anteroposterior direction.
— It is both anteverted and anteflexed normally.
— In 20% of patients the uterus is retroverted.
— In the nulliparous woman it measures about 80–90 mm in length, 60 mm in its widest position and about 40 mm in thickness.
— The mucous membrane of the uterine body is the endometrium; it varies in thickness at different phases of the menstrual cycle.
— The stroma is a characteristic immature type of connective tissue, made up of a homogeneous mass of small cells with round or slightly oval nuclei.
— The endometrium is composed of columnar epithelium which dips into the submucosa in the form of branched tubular glands.
— Both the epithelium and the glands are responsive to the two ovarian hormones.
— An additional feature of the endometrium is the typical coiled artries which also are under hormonal influence.
— The myometrium is the middle muscular layer and is composed of several interlacing layers of smooth muscle. The content of the muscle in the cervix is about 10%.

Fallopian tubes

— These measure 100–140 mm in length and lie in the upper part of the broad ligament behind the round ligament.
— They are musculo-membranous canals which transport the ova from the ovaries to the uterus.
— Divisible into four parts.
— The interstitial portion is the narrow portion of the tube contained in the muscular wall of the uterus, which the tube penetrates to reach the uterine cavity.
— The isthmus is the narrow portion of the tube close to its insertion into the uterine cornu.
— The ampulla is the wider, roomier middle portion of the tube.
— The distal third or so is the fimbriated extremity, which is rather funnel-shaped, the small orifice being surrounded by a number of peaked fringes or fimbriae.
— Histologically, the tube consists of three coats: the serous coat, the muscular coat arranged in an inner circular and an outer longitudinal layer.
— The mucosa, or endosalpinx, is disposed in longitudinal folds or rugae, usually three or four in number at the isthmus.
— The lining epithelium is composed of a single layer of cells which undergoes definite cyclical changes.

Ovaries

— They are two ovoid bodies placed one on each side of the pelvis just below the tubes, the outer ends of which are curved over them in an arc-like fashion.
— They measure about 35 mm by 20 mm by 15 mm.
— The external surface of the ovary is of dull whitish opaque appearance.
— The ovary is attached to the uterus by a well-developed ovarian ligament, while the outer upper pole is suspended from the side of the pelvis by the infundibulopelvic ligament.
— The ovary is attached to the posterior surface of the broad ligament, at the line of the attachment in the hilum, through which blood vessels and nerves enter and leave the ovary.
— On section, the ovary is divisible into an outer cortex and a central portion or medulla.
— Covering the cortex is the so-called germinal epithelium, made up of a single layer of cuboidal epithelium.
— Beneath the epithelium is the cortical stroma, which shows a slightly condensed layer called the tunica albunginea.
— The stroma is made up of compactly placed spindle cell connective tissue cells, in which are seen the follicular elements and their derivatives.
— In the ovary of the young child the follicles are exceedingly numerous, being estimated at about 2 million in number in the ovary of the newborn child and progressively less numerous after puberty.
— The cortex of the ovary contains primordial and developing follicles and specialised connective tissue called theca.
— The inner medulla is mainly composed of loose connective tissue and blood vessels.

PELVIC MUSCULATURE

Pelvic floor or diaphragm

— This comprises various parts of the levator ani muscles.
  • These run on each side from the back of the symphysis pubis around the lateral pelvic wall, on the fascia over the obturator internus muscle to the ischial spine and the side of the coccyx.
  • Together with the special muscular bundle, the puborectalis which decussates or joins with its opposite number around the vagina and lower rectum.

— The urethra, vagina and rectum all pass through this muscular diaphragm.

— The muscles of the two sides slope downwards and forwards in the form of a gutter.

— Fibres decussate around the vagina and rectum and anchor these structures by further fibres attached to their outer coats.

— The puborectalis portion of the levator complex is important in helping to maintain closure of the outlet by drawing the different structures passing through it anteriorly towards the shelf formed by the anterior portion of the muscle and symphysis pubis.

Urogenital diaphragm

— It is a triangular-shaped diaphragm which lies below the levator muscles.

— The urethra and vagina pass through it.

— This is a dense fascial sheet which fills in the triangle formed by the pubic arch, the pubic rami and a line drawn between the two tuberosities.

— It is composed of a superficial and a deep layer.

— The superficial perineal muscles are placed superficial to the urogenital diaphragm.

— The deeper perineal muscles are situated in the space between the two layers.

Pelvic ligaments

Cervical ligaments

— The cervix is supported centrally in the pelvis by ligaments which radiate out to the lateral plevic wall.

— These lie below the level of the peritoneal reflections and are arranged in three main groups.

— Anteriorly are the pubocervical ligaments, posterolaterally are the uterosacral ligaments, and laterally are the cardinal or Mackenrodt ligaments.

Round and ovarian ligaments

— These two ligaments are really continuous, although this is not obvious clinically.

— They represent an embryonic structure called the gubernaculum which, in the male, is responsible for pulling the gonad into the scrotum.

— In the female, the gubernaculum crosses the Mallerian duct and fuses with it at the point where the uterus and fallopian tubes are delineated.

— Round ligaments contain muscle fibres and fibrous tissue.

— They have a minor supporting role for the uterus.
— They are important landmarks in pelvic surgery.

The infundibulopelvic ligament
— It is a fold of peritoneum which runs from the outer and posterior aspect of the broad ligament to the pelvic brim.
— It carries vessels and nerves to and from the parametrial structures, fallopian tubes and ovaries.

URINARY TRACT

The anatomy of that part of the urinary tract in the pelvis is of considerable significance in gynaecology in view of its close relationship to the structures of the genital tract.

Ureters

— The ureters are two muscular tubes measuring 250–300 mm in length extending from the renal pelvis above to the bladder below.
— They run downwards and slightly medially in front of the psoas major muscle in a retroperitoneal position.
— It crosses the brim of the pelvis at the bifurcation of the common iliac artery into its external and internal branches.
— Its normal diameter is approximately 3 mm. It shows some constriction at its junction with the renal pelvis, where it crosses the brim of the pelvis, and as it passes through the wall of the urinary bladder.
— In the pelvis the ureter passes posterolaterally until it reaches the level of the ischial spine, where it runs medially towards the base of the bladder.
— As it lies on the posterolateral pelvic wall, it is anterior to the internal iliac artery.
— As the ureter approaches the entrance into the bladder, it comes into close relationship with the uterine vessels, the artery passing immediately anterior to it. It lies approximately 10–20 mm from the lateral vaginal fornix.
— This close relationship to the uterine artery renders it liable to damage during procedures such as hysterectomy.

Bladder

— This muscular structure forms the reservoir for the collection of urine, and its capacity ranges up to 1000 ml.
— Posteriorly it lies in intimate relationship with the uterus, cervix and upper vagina.

— Anteriorly it lies behind the muscles of the lower abdominal wall and the symphysis pubis.

— Anteriorly the peritoneum is reflected off the abdominal wall on to the fundus of the bladder, and behind the fundus forms the uterovesical pouch.

— The uterovesical pouch does not cover the lower part of the uterus or the base of the bladder and is much shallower than the rectovaginal pouch posteriorly.

— There is a potential space between the bladder neck anteriorly and the symphysis pubis, which is known as the cave of Retzius.

— The bladder neck is supported by two strong ligaments which run from the back of the symphysis pubis and the fascia over the levator ani muscles to the neck of the bladder and to the cervix behind.

— This tissue forms the pubo-urethral and pubocervical ligaments and fascia.

Urethra

— The urethra is 30–40 mm in length.

— Throughout its length it is in close relationship with the anterior vaginal wall, from which it is separated by a facial septum.

— It ends at the external urethral meatus, which lies between the clitoris anteriorly and the vaginal introitus posteriorly.

— The bladder and the upper urethra are lined with transitional epithelium, and the lower urethra is lined with stratified squamous epithelium.

Blood supply

— The blood supply of the uterus is derived from the ovarian and uterine arteries.

— The ovarian artery arises from the abdominal aorta passing down behind the peritoneum to the infundibulopelvic ligament, enters the mesosalpinx to supply the tube and ovary, finally anastomosing with the uterine artery.

— The uterine artery arises from the anterior branch of the hypogastric artery, passing towards, the uterus through the parametrium.

— The uterine artery turns upwards about 15 mm or 20 mm lateral to the cervix, coursing upwards in an extremely tortuous fashion to anastamose with the ovarian and giving off many branches to the uterine wall.

— As it turns upwards at the level of the cervico vaginal juncture, it is in close relation to the ureter, which passes downwards and inwards behind the artery on its course to the bladder.

— The hypogastric artery provides most of the blood supply to the pelvic viscera and the pelvic musculature.

— The vagina is richly supplied with blood vessels, receiving branches from the uterine, vesical, middle rectal and internal pudendal arteries.

— Profuse networks of veins accompany these vessels.

— The vulva is supplied mainly by the internal pudendal artery, which is a branch of the internal iliac artery. It is in close relation to the pudendal nerve and passes forwards through the ischiorectal fossa.

— The veins correspond in a general way with the artery.

— The ovarian veins from the hilum of the ovary towards the vena cava form between the layers of the broad ligament a rich network called the pampiniform plexus.

— The ovarian vein on the right side empties into the inferior vena cava, on the left into the left renal vein.

— The uterine vein empties into the internal iliac vein.

Nerve supply

— The genital tract is supplied by branches of both autonomic and spinal nerve pathways.

— Various sympathetic and parasympathetic fibres of the autonomic system below the bifurcation of the aorta form the superior hypogastric plexus or presacral nerve, which is the chief supply of the uterus.

— As they pass caudal they form the ganglion of Frankenhaüser or uterovaginal plexus located near the base of the uterosacral ligaments.

— The ovary is supplied by branches of the renal and aortic plexuses which are located in the suspensory ligaments of the ovary.

— The pudendal nerve of the spinal nervous system is the primary source of motor and sensory activation of the lower genital tract.

— The pudendal nerve is derived from roots of the second, third and fourth sacral nerves.

— The branches from ilioinguinal, genitofemoral and cutaneous femoral nerves also supply the vulva.

Lymphatic drainage

Vulva

— The vulva is richly supplied with lymphatic vessels.
— These pass primarily to four main groups of lymph nodes, the superficial and deep, inguinal and femoral.
— These in turn drain to deeper nodes in the pelvis, particularly the obturator and iliac nodes.
— Contralateral spread occurs with lesions situated anteriorly in the vulva.

Cervix

— Lymphatic spread first involves a primary group of nodes: parametrial, paracervical, vesicovaginal, rectovaginal, hypogastric, obturator and external iliac.
— Secondary groups of nodes are sacral, common iliac, deep and superficial vaginal and para-aortic.

Uterus

— Lymphatic spread is mainly along the ovarian vessels to the para-aortic nodes.
— Pelvic lymph node involvement is not common, except when the tumour has spread to the cervix.
— Lymphatic spread from the fallopian tubes and ovaries is mainly into para-aortic nodes.

SUGGESTED READING

Williams P L, Warwick R (Eds) 1980 Gray's anatomy. 36th edn. Longman, London
Jones H W, Jones G S (Eds) 1980 Gynecology, 3rd edn, pt 1. Williams & Wilkins, Baltimore
Last R J 1978 Anatomy, regional and applied. 6th edn. Churchill Livingstone, Edinburgh
Mackay E V, Beischer N A, Cox L W, Wood C (eds) 1983 Illustrated textbook of gynaecology, pt 1. Saunders, Eastbourne

2. REPRODUCTIVE PHYSIOLOGY

INTRODUCTION

The reproductive era is ushered in by the menarche and terminated by the menopause. During this period there is a delicately balanced cyclic activity, the most prominent feature of which is the monthly menstrual flow. The structures participating in the reproductive cycle are the hypothalamus, pituitary gland, ovary and uterus. In each organ there is a fluctuating but interrelated activity with modifying effects from other organs and sites.

HYPOTHALMIC PITUITARY–GONADAL HORMONAL RELATIONSHIPS

— Sexual maturation is a gradual process which is dependent on development of the central nervous system.
— It involves the concentration of adrenergic and cholinergic neurotransmitters in the hypothalamus.
— This is accomplished by transmission of the neurotransmitters, norepinephrine, dopamine and/or serotonin from the site of origin, along nerve tracts which have their endings in the hypothalamus.
— The hypothalamus has non-myelinated nerve fibres with neurons originating in the hypothalamus.
— These are peptidergic neurons with the function of synthesising the characteristic hypothalamic peptides and the tuberohypophyseal dopamine system.
— The hypothalamus also has myelinated nerve fibres with cell bodies outside the hypothalamus and axons only within the hypothalamus.
— These are transmitting noradrenergic or serotonergic impulses to the peptidergic neurons for increase or decrease of synthesis of peptide hormones.
— GnRH (LRH) is the hypothalamic hormone which stimulates

synthesis and release of pituitary gonadotropins, FSH and LH.

— GnRH is a decapeptide; it is not species-specific and is active by all routes of administration.

— GnRH synthesis is apparently stimulated by norepinephrine and perhaps inhibited by serotonin.

— An axon-axonal stimulus from dopaminergic neurons in the hypothalamus may cause release or inhibition of release of GnRH into the pituitary portal vessels

— The GnRH release is pulsatile, apparently dependent on the catecholamine control stimulus.

— Modulation of hypothalamic function occurs in three ways: steroid, testosterone and pituitary feedback.

— Steroid feedback, the long loop, is illustrated by the positive and negative oestrogen feedback at the hypothalamic and pituitary levels.

— Testosterone feedback at the arcuate nucleus on the tonic GnRH control and inhibin, the protein hormone from the granulosa cells of the follicle, feeds back to inhibit FSH preferentially over LH.

— Pituitary feedback, the short loop, produces decreased GnRH by LH, by a stimulatory effect upon L-cystine arylamidase, an enzyme which destroys GnRH.

— The intrapituitary feedback involves desensitisation of GnRH receptors on the pituitary gonadotropins by GnRH itself.

— The functional hypothalamic unit requires peptidergic neurons which are programmed to synthesise hypothalamic hormones, neurotransmitters to regulate the synthesis by both stimulus and inhibition, and a third set of neurons with axon-axonal function to initiate the release of the hormones.

— LH and FSH are secreted by the pituitary in an episodic fashion related to episodic GnRH secretion.

— There is no GnRH surge in midcycle to account for the LH surge; rather it is related to a change in the pituitary release mechanism which in turn is related to the ovarian oestrogen.

Physiology of menstruation

— The control of reproductive function arises from a complex interplay involving the central nervous system, a number of hormones and all of the organs concerned.

— The first recognisable stimulus to ultimate ovarian activity is the production of effective amounts of gonadotropin-releasing factor (GnRF) by the arcuate nucleus in the hypothalamus and its passage to the anterior pituitary gland by the hypophyseal venous portal system.

— This decapeptide hormone is released in a circhorial (pulsatile) manner at approximately hourly intervals.
— It brings about the production of follicle-stimulating hormone (FSH) and luteinising hormone (LH) from the acidophil cells of the anterior lobe of the pituitary gland.
— The secretion of LH is much greater, so that GnRH is often called LH releasing factor or LRF.
— FSH begins the process of follicular maturation in the ovary, and this takes approximately 14 days in the human.
— Although a large number of follicles develop, one of these (the primary or graafian follicle) develops faster and is destined to ovulate, and the others undergo atresia.
— As the follicle grows, oestradiol is produced in increasing amounts, which suppresses FSH production by a process called negative feedback (i.e. inhibition) and this affects pituitary and hypothalamus (predominantly the latter).
— In response to FSH the theca cells in the stroma surrounding the follicle also develop and produce androgens, mainly androstenedione, which are taken up by the granulosa cells in the follicle and converted to oestrogens, mainly oestradiol.
— The rising oestradiol reaches a peak level about the twelfth day of the cycle.
— By a process termed positive feedback, the oestrogen peak sensitises the gonadotropic cells of the pituitary gland to the action of GnRF, the resulting LH surge acts as a trigger for further enlargement and then rupture of the dominant follicle, leading to ovulation.
— Prostaglandin is also involved in the final stages of maturation of the follicle and extrusion of the ovum.
— LH luteinises the granulosa cells in the ruptured follicle, they secrete progesterone, the follicle becomes corpus luteum and secretes oestrogen and progesterone for about 14 days.
— If the ovum becomes fertilised and implants in the endometrium, chorionic gonadotropin (HCG) is produced from the trophoblast, and this maintains corpus luteum function beyond its normal 14-day span.

The effect of hormones

— Progesterone is antagonistic to oestrogen, partly by reducing the number of oestrogen receptors in the cells and partly by interfering with the binding of the oestrogen-receptor complex to the nucleus.
— Oocyte maturation inhibitor (gonadocrinin) from the developing granulosa cells stops multiple egg development in a particular cycle.
— Luteinisation inhibitor and inhibin in the follicular fluid in

smaller follicle preferentially inhibits the secretion of FSH in relation to LH.

— Prostaglandins, secotonin, bradykinin produce local effects of a vascular or biochemical nature.

— Ovarian hormones, oestrogen and progesterone, act primarily on those structures involved in reproduction, uterus, cervix, vagina and breasts (Table 2.1, Fig. 2.1).

— Up to the time of ovulation the endometrial glands proliferate and under the influence of progesterone enter the secretory phase.

— If conception does not occur, withdrawal of the corpus luteum hormones leads to a spasm of arterioles in the basal layer of endometrium, and the resulting ischaemia results in the breakdown of the more superficial endometrial layer.

— The shedding of this layer and the accompanying bleeding constitute the phenomenon of menstruation which usually lasts about five days. The whole cycle lasts approximately 28 days.

— The life of the corpus luteum is probably inherently self-limited. Its hormones feed back to the hypothalamus and inhibit GnRF and also the pituitary gonadotropic hormones. Corpus luteum cells become refractory to gonadotropic stimulation about 10–11 days after ovulation. This results in regression, beginning at about day 26–27 of the cycle.

— As the levels of ovarian hormones fall, the hypothalamus secretes more GnRF and thus a new cycle is started. Oestrogen from the newly stimulated granulosa cells produces regeneration of the endometrium and cessation of bleeding.

— There is a continuous interplay of hormonal activity involving the hypothalamus, pituitary gland and ovary.

Table 2.1 Actions of female sex steroid hormones

Oestrogen
1. Oestrogen specifically binds to tissues of the reproductive tract and breast (epithelium, glands, stroma, smooth muscle and vessels) causing stimulation of growth and function. There is less pronounced effect on other tissues such as other epithelia, bone, connective tissue.
2. Feedback effects on the hypothalamic–pituitary system — inhibition of FSH release, stimulation of LH release.
3. Stimulation of prolactin secretion.
4. Increase in certain binding proteins in the plasma e.g. for testosterone, cortisol, thyroxine.
5. Antagonises certain androgen effects.

Progesterone
1. Progesterone specifically binds to tissues of the reproductive tract and breast, antagonising the effects of oestrogen and stimulating the accumulation and secretion of glycogen and other substances necessary for fertilisation and growth of the conceptus, and causing proliferation of the acinar system of the breast.
2. Feedback effects on the hypothalamic–pituitary system — inhibition of LH release.
3. Stimulates the production of prostaglandin in the endometrium.
4. Inhibits prolactin secretion.
5. Inhibits smooth muscle activity, particularly in the uterus.
6. Antagonises aldosterone, promoting sodium diuresis.

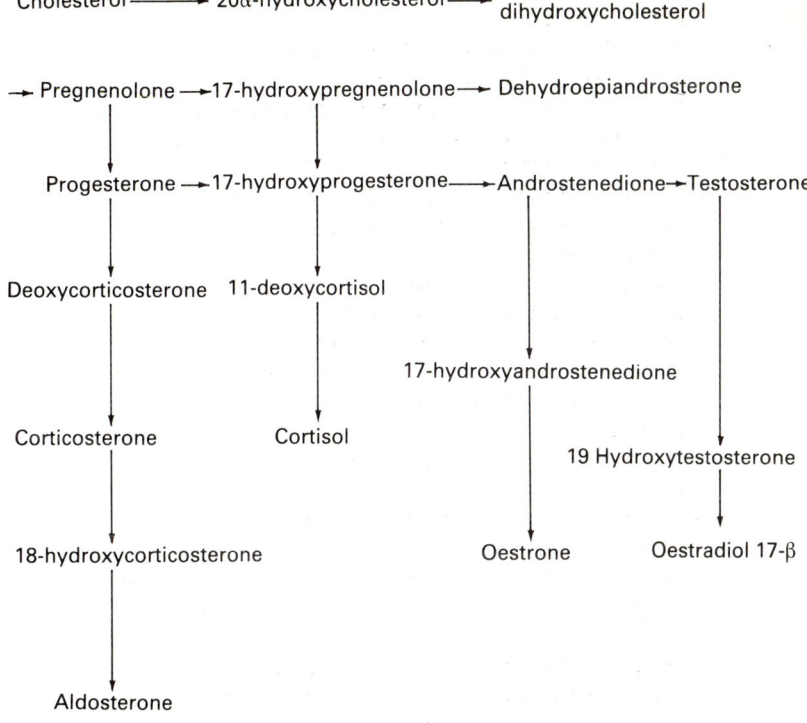

Fig. 2.1 Steroidogenesis in the ovary

— Hypothalamic and pituitary hormones are purely stimulatory in action.
— The ovarian hormones control the activity of the hypothalamic pituitary system by a complicated, poorly understood mechanism, which through most of the cycle is an inhibitory one (negative feedback).
— The exception occurs later in the follicular phase when the oestrogen feedback causes a surge of LH some 24 hours later and this triggers ovulation (positive feedback).

Development of ovarian follicle

There are four phases of development in the ovarian follicle: proliferative (days 1–9), preovulatory (days 10–12), ovulatory (usually 12–14) and luteal (days 14–28).

— The primordial follicle consists of an ovum surrounded by granulosa cells and theca cells. As some follicles enlarge, fluid appears between the granulosa cells and this coalesces to form a small cystic space. The granulosa cells are pushed

to the periphery, but attached to one side is the cumulus
oophorus containing the ovum.
— The follicle continues to enlarge, and the surface layers of
the ovary become very thin prior to ovulation.
— In the five days preceding ovulation, the dominant or
graafian follicle is seen to increase from about 12 mm to
22 mm (range 18–24 mm).
— There are smaller follicles, but they seldom reach a diameter
of more than 14 mm.
— It is thought that between 100 and 1000 follicles may begin
development each month.
— The remaining shell of the now empty follicle crumples, and
the wall thickens as the granulosa and theca cells multiply.
— Macroscopically the corpus luteum is seen as a yellow-red
projection on the surface, 10–20 mm in diameter. It can
usually be recognised on ultrasound examination.
— The corpus luteum reaches a peak at about 8–9 days and
thereafter the output of oestradiol and progesterone declines.
Oestrogen and prostaglandin are involved in this
regression.

Effect of ovarian steroids on target organs

Endometrium

— During the follicular phase the endometrium becomes thicker
due to proliferation of stroma and glands which regenerate
from the remaining basal one-third of the endometrium.
— Further thickening occurs during the secretory phase; the
glands have a dilated, scalloped appearance and are filled
with glycogen, which is secreted during this phase.
— The stroma becomes oedematous; capillary lakes form before
the breakdown at the end of the cycle.

Cervix

— The major change observed during the cycle is in the cervical
mucus.
— Under the influence of oestrogen in the proliferative phase,
the mucus increases in quantity, becomes clearer and less
viscous.
— The above changes are maximal soon after the midcycle
oestrogen peak which occurs at about day 12 or 13.
— Approximately 48 hours after ovulation, although relatively
high oestrogen levels are present, the mucus decreases
markedly in amount and becomes thick and turbid.
— The latter changes are due to high levels of progesterone
from the corpus luteum which counteracts the oestrogen
effect.

Vagina
— There is little clinical change observed in the vagina during the cycle.
— The vaginal cytology shows a predominance of superficial squames in the follicular phase and a predominance of intermediate navicular cells in the luteal phase.
— The accumulation of glycogen in the luteal phase is due to the effect of oestrogen.
— The high acidity of the vagina during the reproductive phase is due to Doderlein bacilli forming lactic acid from glycogen within vaginal squames.

Effects of other hormones on the hypothalamic–pituitary ovarian cycle

— Menstruation often becomes irregular or ceases altogether if the other endocrine glands are not functioning correctly.
— Hypo- and hyperthyroidism and diabetes mellitus may have an adverse effect on gonadotropic secretion.
— Hyperadrenalism, because of the large amounts of circulating androgens, usually causes amenorrhoea because of the steroid feedback on the hypothalamus.
— Prolactin is another hormone which, if present in excess, inhibits gonadotropins and causes amenorrhoea.

Normal pubertal development

Onset of puberty
— Several factors are involved, including genetic influence.
— The major factor is hormonal, namely the activity of the hypothalmic centre responsible for production of gonadotropin-releasing hormone (GnRH).
— Body weight has an important role. A minimum of 45 kg appears to be critical for hypothalamic gonadotropic function.
— There is build-up in the adrenergic and catecholamine transmission system in the brain until sufficient for GnRH release.
— This activity just prior to puberty occurs independently of gonad steroids (e.g. oestrogen). Prolactin shows an increase in pulsatile activity during sleep before that of LH, and this may be responsible for the increase in adrenocortical function between 8 and 12 years of age.
— The average age of onset of puberty is 10–11 years ± 2 years. The duration is normally 3–4 years.
— Breast development is usually the first observable sign in the female. The initial change is the formulation of a palpable

bud, which steadily becomes larger due to growth of the nipple, areola and underlying parenchyma.

— Growth of axillary and pubic hair is similar during puberty in the female and the male. It is related to secretion of androgens from the adrenal gland. In 10–15% of children it is the first sign of puberty.

— The growth spurt in the female occurs in the first year or so after the start of the puberty.

— The duration of growth spurt is 3–5 years and the mean increase is about 180–200 mm. Half of this is gained in the year of maximal increase.

— As a result of marked increase of gonadal steroids, oestrogen and testosterone, bone growth is halted towards the end of puberty.

— The onset of menstruation (menarche) usually occurs soon after the growth spurt starts to wane, usually between 12 and 14 years.

— Over the first 3–18 months the cycles are usually anovulatory, painless and perhaps irregular.

— With further maturation of the hypothalamic–pituitary ovarian function, a positive feedback response to the midcycle peak of oestrogen occurs, with consequent LH surge, ovulation occurs and corpus luteum develops.

— With increasing levels of oestrogen production, further development of the internal genitalia and external genitalia occurs.

Delayed puberty

— Delay in puberty is considered if none of the physical signs are evident by the age of 14 and menarche has not occurred by the age of 17.

— In idiopathic or constitutional delayed puberty there is an abnormal delay in the activating mechanism, but puberty eventually occurs with characteristic clinical features.

— It might occur in hypothalamic–pituitary gland pathology or in gonadal pathology.

— It can be delayed when there is general debility or in anorexia nervosa.

— Investigation should be initially clinical to check for signs of puberty.

— Later investigation is aimed to assess hypothalamic–pituitary-ovarian function.

— Patency of the lower genital tract should be checked (Table 2.2).

Precocious puberty

— Puberty begins before 9 years of age. Premature initiation of either sexual development and/or menstrual bleeding occurs (Table 2.3).

Table 2.2 Aetiological classification of delayed puberty

I. Lesions of central origin
  A. Functional and organic brain disease
    1. Traumatic, toxic and infectious lesions
      a. Encephalitis, epilepsy, hypothalamic tumours
    2. Neuroendocrinological dysfunction
      a. Neurotransmitter excess or deficiency
      b. Releasing hormone
      c. Feedback defects
    3. Ahumada-Del Castillo syndrome
    4. Isolated releasing hormone deficiencies
      a. Hypothalamic hypogonadism
    5. Kallmann's syndrome — hypogonadotropic hypogonadism with anosmia
  B. Psychogenic amenorrhoea
    1. Major and minor psychosis, emotional shock
    2. Anorexia nervosa
  C. Pituitary disturbances
    1. Tumours
      a. Non-functioning
      b. Functioning: prolactin, HCG, ACTH, TSH
    2. Congenital defects
      a. Isolated gonadotropin deficiency (pituitary hypogonadism)
    3. Empty sella syndrome
II. Lesions of intermediate origin
  A. Chronic illness
    1. Rheumatic fever, tuberculosis, childhood leukaemia
  B. Metabolic diseases
    1. Thyroid
    2. Diabetes mellitus (juvenile)
    3. Adrenal
      a. Congenital adrenal hyperplasia
      b. Cushing's syndrome
      c. Virilising tumour
  C. Nutritional disturbances
    1. Malnutrition
    2. Exogenous obesity
III. Lesions of peripheral region
  A. Ovarian causes
    1. Congenital developmental defects
      a. Ovarian dysgenesis
      b. True hermaphroditism
      c. Virilising or feminising male hermaphroditism
    2. Tumours
      a. Virilising and feminising tumours
    3. Insensitive ovary syndrome
  B. Vaginal and uterine defects
    1. Congenital defects
      a. Imperforate hymen, transverse vaginal septum
      b. Congenital absence of the vagina and uterus
      c. Congenital malformation of the uterus
IV. Physiological amenorrhoea — pregnancy

— Idiopathic precocity mimics normal puberty except for the earlier onset (true and complete precocious puberty).
— No pathology is detected and it is due to spontaneous and premature activation of the hypothalamic–pituitary system, resulting in total ovarian function with ovulation.
— Incomplete pseudoprecocious puberty occurs when causes act by either interfering with a mechanism which inhibits the

Table 2.3 Differential diagnosis of precocious puberty

I. Complete true precocious puberty
 A. Idiopathic or constitutional
 B. Neurogenic, cerebral lesions
  1. Tumours of hypothalamus, pineal or cortex: hamartoma, craniopharyngioma, glioma
  2. Infections: toxoplasmosis, encephalitis, meningitis
  3. Neurocutaneous syndrome: neurofibromatosis
  4. Developmental defects: tuberous sclerosis, microcephaly, aqueduct stenosis, craniostenosis
  5. Trauma
  6. Miscellaneous: Sturge-Weber syndrome, diffuse encephalopathy, idiopathic epilepsy
 C. McCune–Albright syndrome
 D. Juvenile primary hypothyroidism
 E. Silver syndrome (cranial–fascial disproportion, small stature, retarded bone age, increased gonadotropin level)
II. Incomplete or pseudo-precocious puberty
 A. Premature pubarche
 B. Premature thelarche
 C. Adrenal lesions: congenital adrenal hyperplasia Cushing's syndrome, tumours
 D. Ovarian tumours: oestrogen-producing (granulosa cell, theca cell, luteoma)
 E. Iatrogenic: androgen or oestrogen administration; administration of oral contraceptives
III. Extra-pituitary gonadotropin production
 A. Gonadotropin-secreting tumours (choriocarcinoma, teratoma, hepatoblastoma, dysgerminoma)
 B. Exogenous gonadotropin administration

hypothalamus (e.g. melatonin from the pineal) or acting in some way to stimulate the centre prematurely.

— In the McCune–Albright syndrome (polyostotic fibrous dysplasia), vaginal bleeding is usually the first sign. Café-au-lait spots on the skin which are seen on one or other side of the body are diagnostic.

— In feminising tumours, the raised oestrogen level from a granulosa or theca cell tumour of the ovary or rarely from the feminising tumour of the adrenal gland produces precocious development of puberty.

— General and neurological examination, including visual fields, head circumference, together with a pelvic assessment by recto-abdominal examination to detect ovarian tumour, is needed.

— Radiograph of longbones will detect polyostotic fibrous dysplasia.

— Skull radiology may be helpful if a cerebral cause is suspected.

Treatment

— For constitutional or cerebral precocious puberty or McCune–Albright syndrome, the usual treatment has been with oral cyproterone acetate (CPA)80–140 mg/m²/day, provided bone age is 11 years or less.

— Exogenous GnRH after a period of critical stimulation acts as an anti-gonadotropin and is useful later in addition to CPA.
— Medroxy progesterone acetate in doses of 100–200 mg i.m. weekly or bi-weekly is useful.
— Danazol 150–300 mg/m^2/day is also tried.
— The major concern is shortness of stature if the child is seen late in pubertal development.
— Accidental pregnancy may occur

The gynaecology of infancy and childhood

— Gynaecological problems are generally uncommon before the onset of puberty (Table 2.4).
— Anomalies of development, lower genital tract infection and new growths are the common problems.
— The most common symptoms will be puritis or soreness of the vulva, vulvo-vaginal discharge or bleeding and lower abdominal and pelvic pain.
— History of family and pregnancy, and ingestion of drugs in pregnancy, should be elicited.

Table 2.4 Gynaecological disorders of infancy and childhood

Condition	Features	Investigation	Management
Diaper rash, dermatitis	Red, oedematous, vesicular, pustular rash	—	More frequent changing, washing, calamine ointment/lotion. Secondary infection may need treatment
Vulvovaginitis	Vary according to aetiology	Hanging drop, cultures and smears	According to aetiology, hygiene usually needs improving
Pinworms (*Enterobius vermicularis*)	Vulvovaginitis, scratching effect	Perianal worms seen, sticky tape to perianal skin to pick up ova	Vanquin etc. by mouth to child and other family members
Labial adhesions	Unable to visualise introitus	—	Nightly application of 0.1% dienoestrol cream for 2 weeks. May need surgical separation
Foreign body in vagina	Offensive, purulent and often bloodstained discharge	Smears, cultures, vaginoscopy, rectal examination	Removal
Benign tumours of vagina	Usually cysts of Gartner's ducts	Needs the expertise of specialist	Excised if large
Malignant tumours of vagina and cervix	Usually bleeding from grape-like mesodermal mixed tumours	Needs the expertise of specialist	Usually radical therapy in a specialised unit
Tumours of ovary (usually germ cell or mesenchymal cell origin)	Pain, mass, pressure symptoms, vaginal bleeding if hormonally active	Needs the help of specialist	Cystectomy — oopherectomy, or more radical surgery depending on type

— External genitalia of the newborn are examined to exclude intersex states — in particular to determine the presence of an adequate vagina in the female.

— Clitoral enlargement can be caused by congenital adrenal hyperplasia or an intersex state.

— Excess androgen in the mother, either endogenous (ovarian/adrenal hyperplasis or tumour) or exogenous (androgen/progestin medication), is rare.

— In childhood the problems are mainly related to the child's abnormal behaviour or untoward symptoms or physical appearance.

— Thorough general examination including height, weight, development of secondary sexual characteristics and assessment of mental development, rectal examination and examination of pelvic organs under anaesthesia are necessary.

— The site and patency of the anal canal should be checked.

SUGGESTED READING

Bahr J M, Nalbandov A V 1980 Neural relationships of the hypothalamus. In: Gold J J, Iosimovich J B (eds) Gynecologic endocrinology, 3rd edn. Harper & Row, New York, p 18

Flickinger G L 1980 Hormone action and receptors. In: Gold J J, Iosimovich J B (eds) Gynecologic endocrinology, 3rd edn. Harper & Row, New York, p 93

Jones H W, Jones G S 1980 Gynecology. Williams & Wilkins, Baltimore/London, p 9

Mackay E V, Beischer N A, Cox L W, Wood C 1983 Illustrated textbook of gynaecology. Saunders, Philadelphia, p 51

Nikitowitch W M B 1980 Hypothalamic–pituitary–ovarian axis. In: Gold J J, Iosimovich J B (eds) Gynecologic endocrinology, 3rd edn. Harper & Row, New York, p 3

1978 Neuro-endocrinology of reproduction. In: Tyson J E (ed) Clinics in obstetrics and gynaecology, vol 5. Saunders, Philadelphia

Schwartz N B, McCormack C E 1980 Newer concepts of gonadtrophin and steroid feedback control mechanism. In: Gold J J, Iosimovich J B (eds) Gynecologic endocrinology, 3rd edn. Harper & Row, New York, p 31

Speroff L, Glass R H, Kase N G 1984 Neuro-endocrinology, 3rd edn. Williams & Wilkins, Baltimore/London, p 41

Speroff L, Glass R H, Kase N G 1984 Regulations of the menstrual cycle, 3rd edn. Williams & Wilkins, Baltimore/London, p 75

3. DEVELOPMENT AND ANOMALIES OF THE UROGENITAL SYSTEM

INTRODUCTION

Urogenital differentiation in the embryo is a rather complex process involving genetic and hormonal factors.

Since the urological and genital tracts develop in close relationship, structural errors in either system may be associated with errors in the other.

GONADAL DEVELOPMENT

— See Table 3.1.
— The first phase of sexual development is genetic sex determination.
— This is determined by whether the X-bearing ovum is fertilised by a sperm bearing an X or Y chromosome.
— The XX combination will cause a female differentiation of the gonad and XY a male differentiation.
— The germ cells can be identified very early in fetal life — ini

Table 3.1 Sexual development timing and differentiation

	Duration of gestation/age	Female
Genetic	Conception	XX H–Y Ag$^-$
Gonad	Week 6–7	Cortical development → ovary develops
Internal genitalia	Week 10–12	Development of müllerian ducts — differentiate into fallopian tubes, ovaries and upper $\frac{3}{4}$ of vagina
External genitalia	Week 10–12	Genital tubercle → clitoris Labioscrotal folds become labia majora Urethral folds become labia minora
Sex	Decided at birth	Vagina is normal ($\geq$ 30 mm) Clitoris $\leq$ 10 mm Separate labia
Hormonal sex	Puberty	Cyclic centre in hypothalamus → activate → ovaries → oestrogen and progesterone
Secondary sexual characteristics	Puberty	Breast development Body configuration

tially in the endoderm of the yolk sac, then in the gut and its mesentery.
— Around week 5 of gestation, these germ cells migrate to the urogenital ridges which have already formed on the dorsal body wall, lateral to the attachment of the gut mesentery.
— A primitive undifferentiated gonad forms with a cortex and a medulla.
— The upper parts of the urinary and genital systems develop from the urogenital ridges.
— By week 7, differentiation into an ovary (46XX) or a testis (46XY) occurs.
— This step is determined by the H–Y antigen, production of which is mediated by a gene locus on the short arm of the Y chromosome close to the centromere

Ovary

— Early meiotic (chromosome reduction) divisions occur 12–16 weeks after fertilisation, characterising the transition of oogonia into oocytes.
— Primitive granulosa cells surround the ova, forming primordial follicles, which are separated by mesenchymal cells.
— This development corresponds with the first appearance of follicle-stimulating hormone from the pituitary gland.
— By about week 20 of fetal life the ovary contains approximately 6–7 million ova.
— At birth the ovary contains approximately 2 million ova.
— Cortical stroma develops from the interfollicular mesenchyme.
— The inner medullary region consists of loose fibro-elastic connective tissue containing the blood vessels, lymphatics and nerves.

Duct development

— The tubules of the primitive pronephros and mesonephros atrophy in both sexes. In the female the mesonephric duct undergoes atrophy.
— In adult life, the mesonephric tubular remnants maintain a juxtaposition to the ovary as they lie in the broad ligament. They are known as the epoophoron above the ovary and paroophoron beside it.
— The mesonephric (Gartner's) duct decends on the anterolateral aspect of the cervix and vagina.
— The fallopian tubes, uterus and upper two-thirds of the vagina are developed from the müllerian ducts and the lower third of the vagina forms from the urogenital sinus.

— The müllerian ducts form by an invagination of the surface of the genital ridge at about week 6.
— They are initially lateral to both the gonad and mesonephric system at about week 10. During development they swing medially to unite in the midline.
— The upper unfused parts become the fallopian tubes, the lowerfused parts become the uterus and upper two-thirds of the vagina.
— The urogenital ridge has a mesentery and this becomes the broad ligament, with extension anterolaterally over the round ligament and posterolaterally over the infundibulopelvic ligament.
— The gubernaculum is attached to the lower pole of the gonad and is crossed by the müllerian ducts.
— The utero-ovarian ligament is a remnant of the gubernaculum and is continued as the round ligament.
— The round ligament runs out into the inguinal canal and thence to the labium majus.

External genitalia

— Early in embryo life, both the allantois and the lower end of the hind gut communicate with the cloaca.
— At about week 7, the urorectal septum divides the cloaca to form the rectum and anal canal posteriorly and the urogenital sinus anteriorly which forms the future bladder, urethra and lower vagina. The septum forms the perineum.
— The müllerian system grows downwards to the urogenital sinus forming the müllerian tubercle and, by hollowing, forms the upper two-thirds of the vagina.
— The essential primordia for the external genitalia are the genital tubercle, which forms the clitoris, and the labio-scrotal folds which form the labia majora.
— The urethral ridges remain open to form the labia minora.
— Skene's glands and Bartholin's glands develop as buds from the urogenital sinus.
— The female urethra is homologous with the prostatic urethra and Skene's glands correspond to the prostate gland.

ANOMALIES OF SEXUAL DEVELOPMENT (Table 3.2)

— Development along the female line is the basic mechanism in sexual development.
— It is important to recognise anomalous sexual development at an early age, to ensure that the sex of rearing is appropriate to future sexual functioning and reproductive potential.

Table 3.2 Origin and developmental anomalies of the genital tract

Structure	Origin	Normal development	Abnormalities
Hymen	Urogenital sinus membrane	Breaks down	Imperforate → amenorrhoea → haematocolpos → haematometra
Lower one-fourth of vagina	Urogenital sinus	Meets Mulllerian bulbs and forms vagina	Aplasia. Hypoplasia May have haematocolpos and haematometra
Upper three-quarters of vagina	Lower end of müllerian ducts	Fusion septum breaks down	Artificial vagina will be needed. Uterus is usually absent
Uterus	Middle part of müllerian ducts	Fusion and the septum breaks down	Absence Lack of fusion Septum and rudimentary horn surgery may be needed
Fallopian tubes	Upper part of müllerian ducts	Remains separate	Absence Hypoplastic
Ovary	Yolk sac Genital ridge	Cortical development ova and theca develops	Absence or hypoplasia
Labia minora	Urethral ridge	Forms the boundaries of vestibule	Anomalous persistence or closure
Labia majora	Labioscrotal folds	Remain separate Cover the vestibule	May be fused

— Investigations are directed towards establishing genetic sex and the state of the internal genitalia.

— Sex of rearing will usually be obvious from the functional state of the external genitalia which will often dictate a female choice.

Mechanism

— Even if there is no gonad, the müllerian duct structures will form fallopian tubes, uterus and vagina, and the wolffian duct structures will atrophy.

— The urethral groove will persist, the labioscrotal folds will not fuse and the phallus will not grow.

— Female differentiation of the brain (cyclic gonadotropin secretion, prolactin response to oestrogen) does not require hormone stimulus, whereas male differentiation requires androgen stimulus during fetal and post-natal life.

— A normal male gonad is required to suppress the müllerian system and to stimulate the wolffian system.

— Most cases of genital ambiguity will involve an excess of androgen in the gonadal female or an insufficiency in the gonadal male.

— Excess of androgens in the female is usually due to an

enzymatic defect in the adrenal gland, or rarely an androgen-producing tumour in the adrenal or ovary.
— Androgen insufficiency in the male is more complex. The gonad is either poorly developed or may be due to an enzymatic block in the production of testosterone, or testosterone may not affect target tissue because of partial or total enzyme receptor block.
— In most cases the basic cause is a genetic or chromosomal defect with or without an accompanying hormonal abnormality.

CLINICAL SYNDROMES

Turner's syndrome (gonadal dysgenesis)

— Occurs in 1 in 2500 female babies.
— Abnormality is loss of one of the X chromosomes from the nucleus.
— It can occur in either pure or mosaic form.
— In pure form (XO) there is a genetic material which produces gonadal failure, short stature, congenital lymphoedema, webbing of the neck, increased carrying angle of the arm and coarctation of the aorta.
— Children appear as normal female, but at puberty sexual infantilism persists, with absence of growth spurt.
— On investigation there is negative sex chromatin 45 XO karyotype, low oestrogen and high gonadotropin levels.
— Mosaicism in Turner's syndrome can occur only after fertilisation. One of the cells, at a variable time during embryogenesis, receives the normal complement XX, whereas the other loses one of the sex chromosomes — an XO results.
— This will produce the XX/XO pattern. The degree of abnormality produced will depend on the relative proportions of the normal (XX) and abnormal (XO) lines in those tissues of the body where they have an important regulating effect.
— Thus an XX/XO female may have few or no stigmata of the syndrome because of the preponderance of the XX line.
— If the XX line is predominant, she will menstruate and develop normal secondary sexual characteristics as a result of oestrogen production from the ovary.
— The ovaries soon stop working and secondary amenorrhoea from ovarian failure occurs in the late twenties or early thirties.
— If the XO cell is significant, premature atrophy of the gonad occurs even in fetal life.

— When XY/XO (male Turner's syndrome) exists, the testicular tissue will be formed and testosterone is secreted as in a normal male.

— Inadequate secretion of testosterone does not suppress the natural female development.

— When there is a testis on one side and a streak gonad on the other, it produces mixed gonadal dysgenesis.

— Dysgenetic gonad-containing Y chromosome is at high risk of becoming malignant and should be removed.

— The other risk is masculinisation of the children reared as female at puberty.

— They will need hormone replacement therapy which should be started at the time of expected puberty to allow secondary sexual development.

H–Y antigen disorders

— Testicular development requires the translation of genetic sex (XY) into gonadal sex (the testes).

— The H–Y antigen on the short arm of the Y chromosome is believed to be largely responsible for this.

— If Y chromosomes do not possess H–Y antigen, such patients cannot develop testes and without an XX chromosome they cannot develop ovaries from the primitive gonad.

— If H–Y antigen is present on one of the female X chromosomes, a normal male will result, the second X chromosome from the father with the translocated H–Y antigen acting like a Y.

Klinefelter's syndrome

— This anomaly occurs in approximately 1:200 newborn infants.

— There is defect in meiotic (reduction) division of sperm and ovum, but in this condition there is an additional sex chromosome, an XX ovum uniting with a Y sperm or an X ovum uniting with an XY sperm.

— Testis develops and functions sufficiently to suppress the müllerian system and to organise male external genitalia, though there is poor development of the seminiferous tubules.

— Testis may remain undescended and the volume may not exceed 4 ml.

— Subjects tend to be eunuchoid and tall, with sparse hair and sometimes breast enlargement.

— Sexual ability is often impaired and sterility is usual.

— Mosaic patterns can exist if chromosome aberrations take place after fertilisation.

— No treatment is available to improve fertility.
— With every addition of chromosomal material there is further deterioration in gonadal and often mental and/or physical function.

True hermaphroditism

— Rare outside the Bantu race.
— It should be remembered in the differential diagnosis of intersex states.
— Clinical features depend on the presence of testicular and ovarian tissue.
— The gonadal tissue may be in the form of an ovotestis or a separate ovary and testis.
— There is ambiguous development of external genitalia.
— 50–66% of such patients have an XX karyotype as determined on lymphocytes.
— Sex of the rearing depends on the state of the external genitalia.
— Female sex is usually chosen unless the penile size appears adequate.
— Since müllerian duct development is often present, menstrual function and, rarely, pregnancy can occur in those raised as females.
— Testicular tissues should be removed from those reared as female.

Agonadism

— There is failure of the gonadal analgen to form in the yolk sac and migrate to the genital ridge area.
— These subjects can be genetically female or male.
— Usually all develop as females without the presence of either müllerian or wolffian duct structures or the somatic stigmata of the XO individual.
— They tend to be tall and eunuchoid in appearance because the bone epiphyses are not closed at puberty by the gonadal sex hormones.
— Secondary sexual characteristics remain infantile.
— Neither XY nor the XX subjects will have even a streak gonad, so there is no risk of malignancy.

HORMONE DISTURBANCE

Congenital adrenal hyperplasia

— It is an autosomal recessive condition.
— Absence of one of the three enzymes involved in the biosynthetic pathway from acetate to cholesterol to cortisol is responsible for this problem.
— There is an excess of androgenic precursors and a vicious cycle of excessive stimulation of the adrenal gland by ACTH because of the absence, or lack, of cortisol feedback inhibition.
— The most common defect is in the 21-hydroxylase enzyme, which can also produce salt-losing status.
— The most severe form of salt wasting occurs with the 3-beta-OH-dehydrogenase deficiency.
— The 11-beta-hydroxylase deficiency can be associated with hypertension due to salt retention.
— The baby may be severely androgenised at birth with closure of the labioserotal folds and enlargement of the clitoris or phallus.
— Plasma 17-hydroxyprogesterone and urinary 17-ketosteroids are elevated.
— Therapy involves adequate cortisol replacement for life, supplemented by mineralocorticoids if necessary.
— Plastic surgery may be necessary to reduce the size of the phallus and open the fused labioscrotal folds.

Other androgen excess state

— In utero the female fetus may be exposed to androgens from ovarian or adrenal tumours.
— Ovarian virilising tumour (arrhenoblastoma or Leydig's cell type) or adrenal hyperplasia or tumour are the sources of androgen in postnatal life.
— Synthetic progestins and androgens in pregnancy can produce masculinisation of the female fetus.

Androgen insensitivity syndrome (testicular feminisation)

— The genetic sex is normal, XY, thus testes develop normally and the müllerian system is inhibited.
— The problem is at the level of target tissues.
— There is lack of receptor in the target cell for testosterone.
— The testosterone fails to reach the nucleus and set in train

such events as closure of the labioscrotal folds and penile growth.
— At birth the part of the vagina that forms from the urogenital sinus is usually present.
— There is failure of menarche.
— Oestrogen is secreted by the testes and, unopposed by the testosterone at receptor, secondary sex changes such as breast development will be seen.
— Hair remains sparse because of the receptor defect.
— Testes may be inguinal and may be associated with hernia.
— The wolffian ducts, testosterone-dependent, fail to develop.
— Invariably the appearance and sex of rearing will be female.
— Testes are retained until puberty to allow normal development and then removed because of the risk of malignancy.
— Cyclic oestrogen/progestin replacement therapy will be required.
— Because of the familial nature of the condition, close female relatives should be checked.
— Negative sex chromatin and XY karyotype, elevated plasma testosterone are the characteristic findings.

Testicular enzyme defect

— There are a variety of autosomal defects which can result in a failure of one or more of the enzymes responsible for the production of testosterone by the testes (desmolase, dehydrogenase, hydroxylase, reductase).
— Sufficient testosterone is usually produced in the fetus to suppress the müllerian ducts and induce the wolffian ducts.
— Full masculinisation of the external genitalia may not occur and thus an ambiguous state can arise.
— Condition may resemble androgen insensitivity.
— Oestrogen and testosterone synthesis are blocked so there is no development of secondary sex characteristics.

Alpha-reductase deficit

— This enzyme is responsible for conversion of testosterone to the active dihydrotestosterone in certain target cells (external genitalia, skin).
— Testosterone is the main hormone involved in stimulating the wolffian duct system and is responsible for the change in the male at puberty.
— Dihydrotestosterone is responsible for fusion of the labioscrotal folds in the fetus, and at puberty for stimulation of the prostate and peripheral target tissues.

— Children with deficient alpha-reductase will appear more female than male at birth due to the failure of the labioscrotal folds to fuse, but will be male in orientation.
— At puberty a strongly masculine development occurs because of testosterone effects.

Miscellaneous

— Failure of testosterone production may also arise from the disorders such as Leydig's cell agenesis and deficient Leydig's cell receptor for luteinising hormone.
— Secondary failure will result from lack of LH production from the pituitary gland.

OTHER ANOMALIES

Internal genitalia

— A range of malformations can occur in the müllerian system in the absence of any specific anomaly in the process of sexual differentiation.
— Abnormality may be due to problems of fusion or formation.

Abnormalities of fusion

— Lower halves of the müllerian system fail to unite, producing a dual system.
— The whole tract may be duplicated, producing a duplicate uterus, cervix and vagina.
— Lesser degrees will manifest as bicornuate uterus, septate or subseptate uterus.

Abnormalities of formation

— Any part of either müllerian duct may fail to develop.
— One side may be totally absent, leaving a uterus and one fallopian tube (unicornuate uterus).
— There may be abnormalities of the renal tract, along with the abnormalities of the müllerian duct on the same side.
— Malformations of the upper two-thirds of the müllerian ducts are rarely diagnosed before reproductive life.
— They can be a cause of dysmenorrhoea, menstrual disorders and infertility.
— When the vagina is absent, usually the uterus is also absent. Treatment is aimed to restore coital function. Some form of surgery is necessary (Macindoe or Williams).

External genitalia

— Clitoral anomalies are unusual. Most cases of abnormal clitoris are due to an intersex state.

— The lower urogenital–rectal structures develop in a close relationship.

— Failure of the urogenital septum to separate the urogenital sinus and rectum will result in rectocloacal fistula.

— Failure of the müllerian ducts to invade the septum will result in the absence of a vagina.

— Failure of the cloacal membrane will result in an imperforate anus or imperforate hymen.

— Failure of the ventral body wall to close will result in ectopic vesicae, rectovaginal or rectovestibular fistulae.

— They all need surgical correction.

SUGGESTED READING

Beazley J M 1974 Congenital malformations of the genital tract. In: Dewhurst J (ed) Paediatric and adolescent gynaecology clinics in obstetrics and gynaecology, vol 1. No 3. Saunders, London, p 571

Dewhurst J (ed) 1981 Integrated obstetrics and gynaecology for postgraduates, 3rd edn. Blackwell, Oxford

Jewelewicz R 1980 Normal growth and development of the female. In: Gold J J, Josimovich J J (eds) Gynecologic endocrinology, 3rd edn. Harper & Row, New York, p 14

Richardson G S 1980 Hormonal physiology of the ovary. In: Gold J J, Josimovich J J (eds) Gynecologic endocrinology, 3rd edn. Harper & Row, New York, p 123

Simpson J L 1980 Abnormalities of sexual development of function. In: Gold J J, Josimovich J J (eds) Gynecologic endocrinology, 3rd edn. Harper & Row, New York, p 515

4. DISEASES OF THE VULVA

BENIGN DISORDERS OF THE VULVA

Introduction

- The vulva is a relatively common site of involvement by a variety of inflammatory and dystrophic skin disorders.
- Introduction of new techniques such as colposcopy and drill biopsy has improved diagnosis and management.
- Common benign disorders of the vulva are:
  - Pruritus vulvae
  - Dermatoses — oedema
    - intertrigo
    - eczema and seborrhoeic dermatitis
    - psoriasis
    - lichenification
  - Bullous lesions
  - Ulcerative lesions
  - Sexually transmitted diseases
  - Vulval dystrophy

Pruritus vulvae

- Common complaint.
- Approximately 10% of women attending gynaecology clinics have this problem.
- Mucocutaneous functional areas of the body, such as the vulva, are well endowed with nerve endings and the itch potential is correspondingly high.

Aetiology

- Infections — local
  - fungal
  - tinea cruris
  - viral
  - parasitic
  - sexually transmitted
- Local dermatological conditions.
- Atrophic dermatoses of the vulva.

— Neoplasm.
— Drug sensitivity.
— Miscellaneous.
— General causes:
  • Part of generalised dermatosis
  • Part of general medical disorder
— Psychosomatic

Local infection

Fungal infection–Candida
— Incidence is rising.
— Caused by *Candida albicans* (95%) *Candida glabrato* 5%.
— *Candida albicans* is not normally present in the vagina.
— Carried in the gastro-intestinal tract and/or the mouth.

Clinical features
— Intense pruritus, soreness, worse at night.
— Thick white discharge (like curdled milk), adherent to the vaginal skin.
— Erythema of the vagina, labia minora and sometimes perianal area.
— Vagina is frequently infected via the perineum but minor trauma (e.g. coitus) facilitates infection.

Predisposing factors
— Pregnancy — commonest infection is in pregnancy. 15–20% of women may be affected.
— Menstrual cycle — commonly occurs towards the end of the cycle.
— Medical disorders — diabetes mellitus and sometimes iron-deficiency anaemia.
— Drugs:
  • Oestrogen-containing oral contraceptives
  • Broad-spectrum antibiotics
  • Corticosteroids
  • Immunosuppressive agents
— Clothing — occlusive tight nylon underwear.

Diagnosis
— Clinical features — examination of vagina and vulva.
— Microscopy of discharge suspended in a drop of normal saline — mycelial filaments and spores will be visible.
— Culture — on glucose agar of swabs obtained in Stuart's transport medium.

Treatment
— Fungicidal drugs:
  • Nystatin or one of the imidazoles (miconazole, clotrimazole or econazole — vaginally) effective in 80%
  • Ketoconazole (Nizoral) is a new agent for oral administration in recurrent resistant infection

— One per cent aqueous gentian violet paint helps in resistant infection.

— Avoid combined antifungal and antiprotozoal drugs.

— Genital hygiene — bland soap and water.

— Clothing — clean, loose-fitting underclothes.

Other infections

— Tinea cruris infection.

— Viral infection:
- Herpes genitalis
- Genital warts
- Molluscum contagiosum

— Parasitic infestation:
- Scabies
- Pediculosis pubis
- Thread worms
- *Trichomonas*

— Sexually transmitted diseases:
- *N. gonorrhoeae*
- *C. trachomatis*
- *M. hominis*
- *U. urealyticum*
- Granuloma venereum
- Lymphogranuloma venereum
- Chancroid

Local dermatological conditions

— Contact dermatitis (allergic or irritant).

— Lichen simplex.

— Seborrhoeic dermatitis.

— Psoriasis.

Atrophic dermatoses of the vulva

— Lichen sclerosus et atrophicus.

— Primary atrophy.

— Lichen planus.

— Leukoplakia.

Tumours

— Pre-malignant (Bowen's disease, Paget's disease).

— Squamous cell carcinoma.

Drug reaction or sensitivity

Miscellaneous

— Foreign bodies.

— Poor hygiene.

General causes

— Part of generalised dermatosis

— Part of general medical disorder:
- Diabetes mellitus

- Liver disease
- Thyroid disease
- Crohn's disease
- Chronic renal failure
- Polycythaemia
- Chronic lymphatic leukaemia
— Psychogenic causes

Diagnosis

History

— Duration.
— Site intensity.
— Pattern of occurrence.
— Vaginal discharge.
— Medications.
— Other skin problems.
— Hygiene.
— Psychosomatic disturbance

Examination

— Look for generalised skin disorders and metabolic disturbance.
— Examination of the vulva/vagina — e.g. fungal disease.
— Condylomata acuminata are easy to recognise.
— Skin changes from rubbing, scratching and local drug application

Investigation

— Look for causative organisms:
  - Trichomonas
  - Fungal
  - Thread worms
— Microbiology.
— Serology.
— Skin sensitivity tests.
— Glucose tolerance tests.
— Full blood examination.
— Renal, liver and thyroid function.
— Biopsy of the vulva

Treatment

— Remove the cause, if possible.
— Identify and avoid sensitising chemicals, drugs, food.
— Antibiotic and other drug therapy should be re-assessed.
— Improve general and local hygiene.
— Recommend loose-fitting cotton underwear.
— To stop stratching:
  - Soothing lotions
  - 2 per cent testosterone propionate cream

- 1 per cent hydrocortisone or 0.1% triamcinolone cream is useful in early phase
- There is danger in long-term use of fluorinated steroids
- Soft zinc cream with 1% crude coal tar is protective and soothing
- Local anaesthetic cream should be avoided.
- Oral anti-pruritic drugs may be tried
- Inveterate scratchers may need anxiolytic drugs, sedation, padded gloves
- Subcutaneous alcohol injection may be helpful.
- Psychotherapy
- Local oestrogen preparation may be useful in post-menopausal women. Usually not helpful in pruritus

Dermatoses

Oedema

— Usually secondary to an inflammatory process.
— Urticarial manifestation of allergy.
— Lymphoedema from lymphatic obstruction (filariasis).

Intertrigo

— Commonly seen in the interlabial and intercrural folds.
— Seen in obese patients due to combination of warmth, moisture and chafing.
— Bacterial and monilial infections are common.

Management

— The patient should reduce weight.
— Recommend loose cotton underwear
— Keep the vulva dry.
— Swab for examination and culture.
— Exclude diabetes.
— Soothing antiseptic lotion.
— Appropriate treatment of infection.

Eczema and seborrhoeic dermatitis

— Usually primary irritant or allergic contact dermatitis.
— Seen in obese patients in the folds of the genital area.
— Treat the cause if found. Antibiotic corticosteroid cream.
— Avoid irritants such as deodorant sprays, detergents, disinfectants.
— Saline sitz bath is useful.

Psoriasis

— Chronic non-tender lesions.
— Seen in other parts of the body.
— High concentration steroid cream is effective.
— Coal-tar preparations are of value.

Lichenification
- Is the result of rubbing.
- Area appears white, thickened and leathery.
- Fissuring and shallow ulceration may follow intense scratching.
- If in doubt — swab, scraping of the skin and biopsy of the affected area.
- Treatment of infection if present, and pruritus, is essential.

Bullous lesions

Epidermolysis bullosa
- Hereditary disorder.
- Affects other mucous membranes (oropharynx and conjunctiva).
- Vesicles and bullae on slight trauma.

Pemphigus
- Occurs in middle age. Jewish people are more susceptible.
- Blisters arise in normal skin and rupture.
- Develops in crops or continuous succession — purulent.
- High-strength steroid cream is useful.
- Treat infection if present.

Ulcerative lesions

Behçet's syndrome
- Common in males.
- Affects vulva and the mouth of females.
- Ulcers vary in size, last for weeks — pain is less acute.
- There may be associated iritis with hypopyon and the patient may develop arthralgia, thromboplebitis, neurological abnormalities.

Aphthous ulcers
- As in the mouth, may occur in the vulva
- Painful — have yellow base and a bright red margin.
- Seen in labia minora.
- Heal quickly without scarring.

Herpes simplex
- Produces acute inflammation.
- Caused by the herpes simplex virus 2 (HSV2).
- HSV 1 is also involved — related to more frequent oral–genital sex practice.
- Incubation period 3–7 days, may be up to several weeks.
- Produces burning, itching, hyperaesthesia.
- Labial and perianal skin may be involved.
- Tender papules appear, then vesicles, which break down to form shallow, very painful ulcers.

— Inguinal lymph nodes are often enlarged.
— Dyspareunia is intense.
— Dysuria may be present if lesion is near the urethral meatus. May develop retention of urine.
— Herpes simplex infections, of the oral cavity or lower genital tract, are emerging as a major problem.
— Virus has a high infectivity — about 80% of susceptible females who have sexual contact with an infected male will become infected.
— Virus persists in the body.
— It is 5–10 times more common than primary syphilis.
— Immunity usually develops after one or two attacks.

Diagnosis

— History, examination of crops of vesicles or shallow ulcers.
— Stained smear.
— Swabs in the virology transport medium and held at 4 °C or below, pending transport to the virology laboratory.

Treatment

— Prophylaxis if male partner had it.
— Ice applied to the lesion.
— Soothing local creams and analgesics (not cortisone-based).
— Analgesics (2% lidocaine) may be used.
— Idoxuridine is a topical anti-viral applied every 5 minutes for 30 minutes, then very half to 4 hours. It is relatively ineffective for type 2 genital herpes. Better results are achieved with 20 per cent or more dissolved in dimethyl sulphoxide.
— Acyclovir in a 3% ointment is useful
— A 10% silver nitrate solution applied to ulcer expedites healing.
— Laser therapy is effective.
— Saline sitz bath, solution or compress of 4% zinc sulphate in water or normal saline gives relief of pain.
— Providone-iodine (Betadine) is useful for control of secondary infection.
— A condom plus a chemical barrier contraceptive may help if attacks appear to be coitally related.

Sexually transmitted diseases

Introduction

— The classical sexually transmitted diseases are: gonorrhoea, syphilis, chancroid, lymphogranuloma vernereum and granuloma inguinale.
— Gonorrhoea continues to be a relatively common problem.
— Syphilis is largely controlled; other conditions are relatively

uncommon and mostly confined to tropical and under-developed areas.

— Trichomonads, herpes simplex, papilloma viruses, chlamydia, mycoplasma and gardenerella vaginalis are now considered to be sexually transmitted infections. Less common agents are group B streptococci, cytomegalovirus, actinomycosis, hepatitis B virus and schistosoma. The genital area may be host to scabies and lice (Table 4.1).

Fungal infection (see p. 37)

Trichomonas vulvovaginitis

— This flagellated protozoon is thought to originate in the bowel.
— Relatively common in the female after the onset of sexual activity.
— Discharge is profuse, thin grey to yellow-green in colour, a frothy discharge.
— Infection is usually associated with normal or increased oestrogen levels — worse after coitus and menses.

Diagnosis

— History — examination.
— Microscopic examination of discharge mixed with saline shows the moving flagellated protozoa.
— Culture — charcoal swab placed in Stuart medium.

Treatment

— Metronidazole (600–1000 mg/day) for 4–7 days for the patient and partner. (Nausea and alcohol intolerance are side-effects.)
— Tinidazole (Fasigyn) — 2 g for a day.

Herpes simplex (see p. 41)

Papilloma virus — condylomata acuminata

— This genital wart virus is a variety of the papilloma virus.

Table 4.1 Organisms

Group	Common	Less common
Fungi	*Candida*	
	Tinea	
Protozoa	*Trichomonas*	Entamoeba
		Giardia
Viruses	Herpes simplex	Hepatitis B
	Papilloma	Cytomegalovirus
		Molluscum contagiosum
Bacteria	*Chlamydia*	Group B streptococci
	Mycoplasma	*Donovania granulomatis*
	Gardnerella	*Haemophilus ducreyi*
	Gonococcus	Shigella
Spirochaetes	*Treponema pallidum*	
Parasites	Pediculosis pubis	
	Sarcoptes scabiei	

— Identified as intranuclear particle.
— Incubation period can be weeks to months.
— Infectivity is highest soon after the development of lesion.
— Transmission is usually venereal.

Clinical features

— Initial lesion is usually a single, small, warty growth. Seedling lesions soon appear.
— Growth is luxuriant in moister areas. It is soft and friable.
— Ulceration and secondary infection can occur.
— It can involve external genitalia and perianal region and vagina.
— Histological features comprise a thick papillary squamous epithelium with thickening and elongation of the rete pegs acanthosis, parakeratosis K, with fine dermal projections which are oedematous and infiltrated with chronic inflammatory cells.

Diagnosis

— Characteristic appearance.
— Macroscopical and microscopical.
— D.D. from other sexually transmitted diseases.

Treatment

— 20% podophyllum resin.
— Cautery, laser, cryotherapy.
— Surgical excision in some cases.
— Careful history of sexual contacts and education in relation to sexual hygiene.

Gonorrhoea

— Highly contagious disease.
— Affects mucosal and glandular structure.
— May effect the rectum and oropharynx.
— Incubation period is usually 3–7 days, but may be 1–28 days in some.
— Incidence is 1 in 250. Factors contributing to its high prevalence include a rapid incubation period, high infectivity, low immunity, asymptomatic carriers and an increasing rate of casual sexual encounters.

Clinical features

— Endocervicitis results in purulent vaginal discharge.
— Urethritis causes dysuria.
— Bartholin's glands can be swollen and tender.
— Ascending infection produces salpingitis.

Diagnosis

— History — examination.
— Swabs from the endocervix, urethral meatus, orifices of Bartholin's gland.

— Sometimes rectal — microscopy and culture.
— Serology to exclude syphilis is mandatory.

Treatment

— In acute uncomplicated cases, aqueous procaine penicillin G, 4.8 million units.
— Oral probenecid 1 g is given half an hour before penicillin to delay its renal excretion.
— Ampicillin 3.5 g or amoxycillin 3 g are also effective.
— Cephalosporin derivatives which are lactamase-resistant will cure more than 95% of patients.
— If patient is sensitive to penicillin or the organism is resistant to this drug, tetracyclines 1 g followed by 500 mg q.i.d. for 5 days or twice daily doxycline or septrin (trimethoprim/sulpha methoxazole) for 5 days may be used.
— Condoms provide satisfactory protection from gonorrhoea if used intelligently.
— Adequate drug regimen, routine bacteriological follow-up, systematic contact tracing and testing of patients with resistant disease for penicillinase-producing organisms.
— Approximately 5% of males and 50% of females with gonorrhoea are asymptomatic or virtually so, and these individuals contribute to the spread of the disease.

Granuloma inguinale

Clinical features

— Begins as a painless nodule, which breaks down into an ulcer, which soon extends in a destructive manner to involve the vulva and perianal areas.
— Lymphatic spread occurs to the inguinal nodes.
— Discharge, swelling, ulceration and dyspareunia are the usual clinical features.
— Causative organism is *Donovania granulomatis*, a bacterial organism related to the *Klebsiella* group.
— Characteristic intracellular Donovan bodies are found on microscopic examination of the exudate or crushed tissue smears.
— Granuloma inguinale is moderately contagious and auto-innoculable secondary infection is usual.
— Common in the tropics and sub-tropical zones.
— Heat, humidity and poor hygiene are predisposing factors.

Differential diagnosis

— Lymphogranuloma venereum.
— Syphilis.
— Condylomata acuminata.
— Carcinoma.
— Conditions leading to vulval oedema

Treatment
- Tetracycline, 1–2 g daily for 2–3 weeks.
- During pregnancy erythromycin in the same dose is given.

Lymphogranuloma venereum

Clinical features
- Initial lesion is a small papule or vesicle which appears 1–2 weeks after contact.
- Lesions breaks down in 1–2 weeks to produce a painless ulcer.
- 2–3 weeks later inguinal adenitis develops.
  - Nodes are multiple, matted and adherent to skin which is inflamed and breaks down into multiple sinuses.
- Sometimes proctocolitis, rectal stricture, intestinal obstruction and pelvic lymphadenitis may develop.
- Perianal or rectovaginal fistulae are rare complications.
- Elephantiasis of vulva may develop from lymphatic blockage.
- Disease is caused by a member of the Chlamydia group of organisms.
- Disease responds to usual antibiotics, but damage to lymphatic system may persist.

Diagnosis
- Serological tests are of most value (micro-immuno fluorescence).
- The complement fixation test is more easily quantitated to assess the effect of treatment.

Treatment
- Tetracycline and erythromycin are effective.
- Sulphisoxazole 1 g q.i.d. for 21 days is an alternative.
- Abscess needs drainage.

Chancroid

Clinical features
- Causative organism is *Haemophilus ducreyi*, a small gram-negative organism.
- Produces a soft chancre which is painful, should be differentiated from chancre of syphilis.
- Regional lymph adenitis develops in 1–2 weeks, usually few glands are involved, but often undergoes suppuration.

Diagnosis
- Aspiration of the pus allows laboratory confirmation.

Treatment
- Sulphisoxazole, amoxicillin and clavulanic acid are useful.

Syphilis
- Formerly the dominant venereal disease.
- Incidence reduced by routine serological testing in all

pregnant women, lack of acquired resistance of the organism to penicillin, and a long incubation period which allows contact tracing.
— Incidence is 1 in 1000–5000.
— Higher in poor urban communities and in male homosexuals.

Clinical features
— There are four classical stages of syphilis.
— Incubation period is 10–80 days.
— *Primary lesion* is a painless papule in the mucosa of the lower genital tract, could be in the mouth or ano-rectal region.
— After one week it becomes chancre solitary — non-tender indurated ulcer. It heals in 2–6 weeks, one or two lymph nodes are enlarged. If not treated, secondary syphilis appears in a further 6 weeks to 6 months.
— *Secondary syphilis.* Skin rash, painless shallow mucosal ulceration. Condylomata lata are flat wart-like growths on the skin of the external genitalia and perianal region. There are non-specific symptoms such as myalgia, headache and lymphadenopathy.
— *Further late stages* are characterised by progressive, often silent, pathological changes with the formation of gumma (painless tumour). There is interference with functions of the cardiovascular, neurological, osseous and hepatic systems.

Diagnosis
— Dark field examination and direct fluorescence microscopy of materials from suspicious lesions in early phases. The characteristic *Treponema pallidum* is visualised.
— In secondary and later stages serological methods are most reliable.
— Examination of material from mucosal ulcers may show the characteristic spirochaetes.
— Condylomata lata are the most highly infective of the syphilitic lesions, serous exudate teems with the spirochaetes.
— In late syphilis, serological reactivity may be lost.
— In pregnancy, false positive reagin tests are more common: (VDRL and RPR) which detect antibodies not specific for the treponema, fluorescent treponemal antibody absorption test (FTA–ABS) or treponema immobilisation test (TPI) are more specific.

Treatment
— For primary and secondary syphilis, Benzathine penicillin G 2–4 million units in 2 doses at different sites and repeated after one week, coupled with probenecid 500 mg t.d.s.
— Tetracycline and erythromycin are alternatives, 500 mg orally 4 times daily for 15 days.

— Serological studies should be done at 1, 3, 6 and 12 months.
— VDRL test usually reverts to negative within 2 years if treatment is adequate.
— For later stages referral to a specialist, and/or a longer course of penicillin is required.

Swellings of and around the vulva

— Trauma causing a haematoma.
— Infections (see above).
— Uterovaginal prolapse.
— Cysts — sebaceous, inclusion dermoid, wolffian duct remnants, endometrioma.
— Varicose veins.
— Enlargement of Bartholin's glands. Bartholin's glands, being at the vaginal introitus, are relatively prone to infection by gonococcus and by general organisms — streptococci, staphylococci, coliforms, anaerobes.
— Initial infection often causes fibrosis and narrowing of the distal part of the duct, and this gives rise to cyst formation in the duct, stasis of secretions and chronic infection.

Clinical features and diagnosis

Acute bartholinitis

— Marked pain and tenderness in the introital area are characteristic features.
— Abscess develops in most cases.
— Labium majus is reddened, swollen and tender.
— Gland punctum may exude a small amount of pus.
— Classical site and features.
— Differentiate from infected sebaceous cyst.

Chronic bartholinitis

— A small, slightly tender lump.
— Palpated with the index finger in the vagina and the thumb on the perineum.
— Seldom causes symptoms until it gets infected.

Treatment

— In the acute phase: rest, antibiotics depending on the possible organism — cotrimoxazole or penicillin and metronidazole or clindamycin.
— Analgesic is often needed.
— If there is abscess, it is marsupialised under anaesthesia, followed by saline sitz bath to keep it clean. If it is a chronic cyst, marsupialisation. Surgical excision is rarely necessary.

Other swelling

— Urethral and paraurethral conditions — urethral prolapse, diverticulum or caruncle, Skene's and paraurethral glands.
— Inguinal hernia or hydrocele of the canal of Nuck.
— Tumours — benign and malignant.

Vulval dystrophy

Classification
— Hyperplastic dystrophies
a. without atypia
b. with atypia
— Atrophic dystrophies
— Mixed dystropies (lichen sclerosis with foci of epithelial hyperplasia)
a. without atypia
b. with atypia

Vulvar atypias
— Dysplasia, atypical hyperplasia (mild, moderate, severe)
a. without dystrophy
b. with dystrophy
— Squamous cell carcinoma in situ
— Paget's disease of the vulva
— These lesions are chronic, associated with pruritus and have histo-architectural changes in the epidermis and subjacent dermis.
— There are two main entities, hypertrophic and atrophic.
— Single biopsy may show a mixture of dystrophic and atrophic lesions.
— In atrophic dystrophy, there is loss of rete pegs, thinning of the epithelium and hyalinisation of the dermis.
— In hypertrophic dystrophy, there is thickening of the epithelial layer, increased mitotic activity of basal layer, thickening of the prickle cell layer with enlargement and deepening of the rete pegs (acanthosis), and an accumulation of keratin on the surface (hyperkeratosis) is seen. There is a variable degree of chronic inflammation in the underlying dermis.

The four main groups are senile atrophy, primary vulvar atrophy, lichen sclerosus and leukoplakia.

Senile atrophy
— Occurs in elderly women.
— Never complicated by leukoplakia.
— Histology shows general atrophy of epidermis and dermis.
— Often causes no symptoms.
— Marked vulval shrinkage may be seen.
— Periodic course of oestrogen may help.
— Kraurosis is a general descriptive term for marked vulval shrinkage and may be the end result of a number of conditions, lichen sclerosis being one and senile atrophy being another.

Primary vulvar atrophy
— May occur in less elderly.

— Can be accompanied by leukoplakia.
— There is thinning and fibrosis of the vulvar skin.
— Shrinkage and contracture are common.

Lichen sclerosus

— Relatively common.
— May occur in middle ages.
— Aetiology is unknown.
— Affects vulval and perianal area.
— Begins with irregular flat-topped small white papules, often having a central keratotic plug.
— Main clinical symptoms are pruritus (80–90%) and dyspareunia when atrophic changes supervene.

Diagnosis
Chronic pruritus — distribution of lesion, biopsy of the lesion to exclude epithelial atypia.

Histology
— Thinning of epidermis, with hyperkeratosis. Absence of dermis papillae and elastic tissue, hyaline replacement of the collagen fibres with lymphocytic infiltration.
— Colposcopy and the application of 1% toluidine blue to delineate suspicious sites for biopsy may be advocated.

Treatment
2% testosterone propionate cream 2–3 times a day for 6–8 weeks. 1% hydrocortisone or 0.1% triamcinolone cream may be used.

Leukoplakia (hyperkeratosis)

— Characterised by elevated thickened patch of white skin or mucosa.
— Intense pruritus is not uncommon.
— Usually seen in older women.
— Labia majora, minora, clitoris, perineum and perianal region natal cleft are commonly affected.

Histology
Epidermis is thickened, marked increase in keratin, hypertrophy of basal cell layers with irregular enlargement of interpapillary downgrowth; dermis has oedema, absence of elastic tissue, lymphocytic infiltration.

Differential diagnosis
Lichen simplex and planus, psoriasis, fungal infection, primary atrophy, lichen sclerosus, intra-epithelial carcinoma, invasive carcinoma.
— Approximately 10% of women with leukoplakia will develop carcinoma of the vulva.

Management
— Exclude deficiencies of iron, riboflavin, vitamin B12 and folica acid.
— Allergies — clothing, cosmetics, toilet preparations.
— Generalised dermatosis.

— Diabetes mellitus.
— Fungal infection.
— Biopsy of vulva.
— Toluidine blue 1% aqueous solution applied to vulva free of lubrication and powder, after 2 minutes washed with 1% aqueous acetic acid; parakeratotic areas will be stained blue.
— Colposcopy could be used.
— Relief of pruritus and soreness.
— Severe hyperkeratosis with fissuring of the skin can be softened by 2% salicylic acid ointment.
— Pruritus often responds to hydrocortisone cream or topical corticosteroids in difficult cases.
— Alcohol injection may help.
— Skinning vulvectomy and skingraft may be tried in the younger patient.
— Vulvectomy should be considered when there is epithelial atypia.
— Laser therapy.
— Condition can recur.

NEOPLASMS OF THE VULVA

Benign neoplasms

— Condylomata acuminata
— Papilloma
— Naevus
— Hidradenoma
— Bartholin gland adenoma
— Neurofibroma and fibrolipoma.

Condylomata acuminata

— Occur in the vulva and around the anus.
— They are generalised excrescences without pedicles.
— Genital wart virus is a variety of the papilloma virus.
— Transmission is venereal.
— Diagnosis is made on characteristic appearance.
— Treatment 20–25% podophyllum resin, cautery or laser.

Papilloma

— Similar in appearance to condylomata.
— May be large and pedunculated.
— Brown in colour with irregular surface.
— Basal cell lesion may be locally recurrent.

Naevus

— Composed of nests of melanocytes.

Table 4.2 Management of suspected vulval neoplasia (summary)

Evaluation	— Cytology — colposcopy Collins test. P^{32} uptake.
Biopsy	— Directed by above. Local or excision biopsy
Selective treatment	—
Benign dystrophy	— Medical therapy
Intra-epithelial cancer	— Local excision Cryotherapy Laser therapy Superficial skinning and graft Simple vulvectomy
Invasion to 3–5 mm depth	— Wide local excision Simple vulvectomy Radical vulvectomy depending on depth, anaplasia, vessel and lymphatic invasion
Invasion to 6+ mm	— Radical vulvectomy with block dissection of nodes
Long-term follow-up	

- Naevi are common on all parts of body (15) more prone to malignant change when situated on the vulva.
- There are two types: in the *junctional*, the pigment cell clusters are situated in deeper layers of epidermis; in the *intradermal lesion*, the cell clusters are below the basement membrane. in a *compound* naevus, they occur at both levels.
- Treatment is removal of the naevus.

Hidradenoma
- Sweat gland tumour, rare and often not diagnosed before excision.
- Usually forms a painless nodule on the labium majus.
- Patient is in the second half of the reproductive phase.
- Treatment is excision.

Bartholin's gland adenoma
- Characteristic site is the posterior aspect of the labium majus.
- Rare, and needs to be differentiated from adenocarcinoma.
- Surgical removal is the treatment of choice.

Neurofibroma and fibrolipoma
- Rare, can attain large size.
- Treatment is excision.

Malignant tumours

- Pre-invasive — hypertrophic vulval dystrophy
    - Bowen's disease
    - Paget's disease
- Invasive cancer — squamous cell carcinoma
    - melanoma
    - adenocarcinoma
    - sarcoma

Pre-invasive cancer

— Hypertrophic vulval dystrophy (10%) and lichen sclerosis (1%) may develop malignant lesions.

— Intra-epithelial carcinoma of the vulva (Bowen's disease), (Paget's disease).

— Recent studies with electron microscopy, immunohistochemistry, and microspectrophotometric methods have localised virus particles compatible with the papilloma virus in condylomata and intra-epithelial neoplasia.

— Patients are older and give a history of condylomata of the vulva often or more years.

— Virus is causative or associated, is obscure.

— Papovavirus has a definite place in this condition.

Bowen's disease

— Well-defined reddish brown moist papular or plaque-like lesions. Incidence is increasing.

— Pruritus is a common clinical feature.

— Usually occurs in middle-aged to elderly women.

— May have co-existent leukoplakia.

— May become invasive carcinoma.

— There is associated similar lesion in the vagina and cervix following colposcopically directed biopsy.

Histology

— Shows hyperkeratosis — parakeratosis, acanthosis; cells are pleomorphic with mitotic figures.

— Basement membrane is intact.

— Dermis shows chronic inflammatory changes with lymphocytic infiltration.

Paget's disease

— Extra-mammary Paget's disease is comparable to intraductal carcinoma of the breast because the apocrine sweat glands are also involved.

— Reddened, sharply demarcated, slightly elevated lesion.

— Characteristic large pale vacuolated cells in the epidermis.

— There may be an underlying apocrine gland cancer.

Clinical features of Paget's disease

— Average age is usually between 45 and 50.

— Significant numbers of cases occur in women aged under 40.

— May present with pruritus and vulval dystrophy.

— 20% are asymptomatic and seen on routine examination.

— Red velvety appearance.

— Past history of pre-invasive and invasive cancer higher in the birth canal is not unusual (20–30%).

Diagnosis of pre-invasive carcinoma

— Biopsy — colposcopy may be used, and Collin's test, which depends on staining of dysplastic nuclei by toluidine blue dye

1% and resistance to decolourisation by acetic acid (1–2%) applied a minute or so later.

— Administration of radioactive phosphorous (p^{32}) to the patient, followed by counting the beta emission from the vulval skin in vivo or in vitro (biopsy specimen) was used to diagnose pre-invasive lesions of vulva.

— Examination for co-existent lesion in the vagina and cervix.

Management of pre-invasive carcinoma (see Table 4.2)

— Definitive treatment is a simple vulvectomy. Paget's disease requires wide excision because recurrence is common.

— With modern colposcopic techniques and the use of toluidine blue dye, diagnosis could be made more accurately and more localised. Superficial excision is preferred by some to a simple vulvectomy, which is a sexually mutilating procedure.

— A single, small distinct and demarcated lesion can be locally excised.

— Subcutaneous injection of absolute alcohol is tried to relieve itching.

— Local 5% fluorouracil cream may be used, but results are disappointing.

— Laser treatment may be tried.

— If lesions are extensive, multifocal and associated with dystrophy or there is Paget's disease, a more widespread but still superficial skinning may be done, with skin grafting in younger patients.

— Frozen section from the margin of the resection is done to ensure complete removal.

Factors to be considered in planning treatment

— The certainty of the diagnosis. Benign and invasive lesions may co-exist.

— Age of the patient and sexual activity.

— Size and location of the lesion.

— Condition of the rest of the vulva.

— Motivation and facility for follow-up.

Carcinoma of the vulva

Introduction

— Makes up 3–4% of gynaecological cancers.

— Often preceded by pathological changes in the vulval skin.

— Tumour is of the squamous type in 90–95%.

— Patient tends to be elderly, the peak incidence being in the seventh or eighth decade.

— Increasing number of early lesions occur in younger women.

— Symptoms occur relatively early; patients seek advice late.

Incidence

— 2–3 new cases each year per 100 000 people.

— Vulval cancer makes up 3–4% of genital tract cancer.
— The types and incidence of primary invasive tumours:
  • Squamous cell carcinoma   85–90
— Verrucous carcinoma
  • Melanoma   3–5%
  • Sarcoma   <2%
  • Basal cell carcinoma   1%
  • Bartholin's gland tumour   1%
  • Adenocarcinoma   <1%
  • Unidentified/undifferentiated   5%

Classification

Stage 0 Intra-epithelial carcinoma. Bowen's disease, Paget's disease. Hyperplastic vulval dystrophy with atypia.

Stage 1 Lesion <20 mm — no suspicious groin nodes (15% show node involvement on pathological study).

Stage 2 Lesion >20 mm — no suspicious groin nodes (30% show node involvement on pathological study).

Stage 3 Lesion extending beyond the vulva and/or suspicious or positive groin nodes (50% show node involvement on pathological study).

Stage 4 Fixed groin nodes and/or distant spread.

TNM classification (figo).

Primary tumour (T)

T1 — Tumour confined to the vulva <20 mm in diameter.

T2 — Tumour confined to the vulva >20 mm in diameter.

T3 — Tumour of any size with adjacent spread to the urethra and/or vagina and/or anus.

T4 — Tumour of any size infiltrating the bladder (including the upper part of the urethra) mucosa and/or the rectal mucosa and/or fixed to the bone.

Regional lymph nodes (N)

N0 — Nodes not palpable.

N1 — Nodes palpable in either groin, not enlarged, mobile (not clinically suspicious of malignancy).

N2 — Nodes palpable in either one or both groins, enlarged firm and mobile (clinically suspicious of malignancy).

N3 — Fixed or ulcerated nodes.

Distant metastases (M)

M0   — No clinical metastasis.

M1a — Palpable deep pelvic lymph nodes.

M1b — Other distant metastasis.

Staging (figo).

Stage 0   Carcinoma in situ, e.g. Bowen's disease non-invasive Paget's disease.

Stage I T1 N0 M0 Tumour confined to the vulva, 20 mm or less in

	T1 N1 M0	diameter. Nodes are not palpable or are palpable in either groin, not enlarged mobile, not suspicious of malignancy.
Stage II	T2 N0 M0	Tumour confined to the vulva, more than 20 mm in
	T2 N1 M0	diameter. Nodes are not palpable; if palpable they are in the groin, not enlarged mobile, not suspicious of malignancy.
Stage III	T3 N0 M0	Tumour of any size with (1) adjacent spread to the
	T3 N1 M0	urethra and any or all parts of the vagina, the
	T3 N2 M0	perineum and the anus, and/or (2) nodes palpable in
	T1 N2 M0	either groin or both groins, enlarged, firm, mobile,
	T2 N2 M0	suspicious of malignancy.
Stage IV	T1 N3 M0	Tumour of any size (1) infiltrating the bladder
	T2 N3 M0	mucosa or rectal mucosa, or both, including the
	T3 N3 M0	upper part of the urethral mucosa and/or (2) fixed to
	T4 N3 M0	the bone or other distant metastasis.
	T4 N0 M0	
	T4 N1 M0	
	T4 N2 M0	
	M1 A	
	M1 B	

Invasive carcinoma

— No satisfactory screening programme.
— 50% of carcinoma of vulva is preceded by vulval dystrophy.
— Venereal diseases, especially syphilis, have some aetiological relationship.
— Herpes and papovavirus infection also have some association.
— Early lesion is a small nodule in the anterior half of the vulva.
— Ulcer or papillary lesions develop.
— Site of origin:
  • Labia minora and vulvovaginal ring   40–45%
  • Labia majora   34–40%
  • Clitoris   10–15%
  • Perineum and anus   3%
  • Bartholin's gland   1%
  • Multiple lesion   10–20%
— Spread to draining lymph nodes occurs early.
  • 5–10% with lesions <20 mm
  • 30–40% lesions >40 mm
  • 50+ — >70–80 mm
  • Ulcerated lesions have higher incidence of node involvement
  • Node involvement is rare in micro-invasive lesions (≤ 3 mm depth)
  • Lesions close to the midline spread to the nodes on both sides

Clinical features
- Pruritus, lump, ulcer, vulval swelling may be present.
- Bleeding, pain, discharge.
- Urethral meatus involvement produces urological symptoms.
- Stenosis of urethra, vagina and anus may occur with advanced lesions.
- Enlargement of inguinal lymph nodes.

Diagnosis
- Under local or general anaesthesia — biopsy of lesion and careful examination to delineate the extent of the lesion; cervix, vagina, urethral meatus and anus are inspected.
- Most squamous cell carcinomas of the vulva are well differentiated.
- Cells are large with many abnormal and pleomorphic forms.
- 'Pearls' of well-differentiated squamous epithelium are often evident.
- Primary route of spread is lymphatic.
- (Superficial and deep inguinal group, deep femoral group. External iliac group. Obturator nodes, common iliac and para-aortic in late advanced cases.)
- Inguinal nodes are inspected: 56–75% of patients with enlarged nodes are positive, non-suspicious nodes contain cancer in 20–30%.

Differential diagnosis
- Benign causes of an ulcer herpes simplex, syphilis, chancroid, lymphogranuloma venereum).
- Benign mass (papilloma, condyloma).
- Surface nodule (Bartholin's cyst, benign connective tissue tumours).

Management
- Patient orientation:
  - Diagnosis, surgical procedure, the extent of the tissue to be excised, post-operative course should be discussed with patient
- Patient appraisal:
  - Mental and physical well-being is assessed
  - Cardiovascular, renal, pulmonary systems are evaluated, since patients are often elderly
  - Exclude diabetes mellitus
  - Treat local and systemic infections
  - Correct anaemia if present

Definitive treatment
- Radical vulvectomy — best undertaken in adequately equipped centres by experienced and trained gynaecologists in oncological surgery.

— Radical vulvectomy and bilateral lymph-adenectomy (but not routinely of the pelvic nodes).
— Outer limit of the incision includes the mons pubis and up to the labiocrural folds crossing the perineum above the anus.
— Inner incision follows the hymeneal ring and leaves a small amount of skin around the urethral meatus. The depth is limited by the deep fascia.
— Inguinal lymph adenectomy is carried out before excision of the vulva to reduce the risk of infection. It is done either as a first-stage or second-stage procedure.
— Pelvic nodes are removed if clitoris is involved or femoral (deep) node is involved, or lesion is melanoma.
— If patients are elderly and are poor risks, wide local excision is done.
— Basal cell carcinoma is treated by wide local excision. Same applies to verrucous carcinoma unless there is invasion of blood vessels.
— Radiotherapy — vulva tolerates radiotherapy poorly. Patients unfit or refusing surgery may be given this treatment. May be useful for potential or actual spread to the skin of the lower abdomen and inguinal areas. Palliative treatment may be given for the relief of pain.
— Cryosurgery can be used as a palliative measure.
— Chemotherapy may be used in few cases.

Post-operative problems
— Infection, lymph cyst, lymphoedema.
— Neocrosis of skin edges is common.
— Prophylactic antimicrobial therapy and measures to prevent thrombo-embolic disease are necessary.
— Skin grafting may be necessary.
— Prevention of bedsores is important.
— Inguinal and femoral hernia.

Prognosis
— Depends on lymph node involvement and the size of the tumour.
— Overall 5 years survival rate is approximately 50–60% (lesions >30 mm and positive nodes are unfavourable factors).
— 85–90% will survive if nodes are clear. Half this number survive if nodes are positive.
— Local recurrence is more frequent when the urethra, lower vagina and anal regions are involved.
— Multiple lesions carry poor prognosis.
— Melanomas rarely survive if lesions are larger than 20 mm and/or nodes are positive.

— Long-term complications — leg oedema, urinary problems, vaginal prolapse.
— Recurrence — 40% in the inguinal area, 60% in the vulval area.
— Child-bearing and sexual function can be normal for those who survive.

Advanced vulvar cancer
— Will need extensive surgical procedures.
— Exenteration surgery is usually needed.
— External irradiation may be tried; complications are higher.

Other cancers of the vulva

Basal cell carcinoma
— Extends locally to the surface of the skin.
— Usual site is labia majora.
— Presents as an ulcer.
— Local excision is the treatment of choice.

Melanoma
— Arises from pigmented naevi containing a junctional component.
— Prophylactic removal of pigmented naevi is recommended.
— Malignant melanomas produce few symptoms, hence the diagnosis is made late.
— Treatment is by radical vulvectomy and bilateral inguinal and, if necessary, pelvic lymphadenectomy.
— Prognosis is poor due to haematogenous spread to distant parts of body, including lungs and brain.

Sarcoma
— Rare and tends to occur in the younger age group, those of about 40 years.
— Treatment is by extensive local excision.
— Distant metastasis is common.
— Prognosis is poor.

Bartholin's gland tumours
— Rare lesions
— Could be adenocarcinoma (45%)
— Squamous carcinoma (39%)
— Sarcoma (3%)
— Melanoma (1%)
— Some are undifferentiated (2%)
— Diagnosis is made too late.
— Treatment is by extensive local excision, with inguinal and possible pelvic lymphadenectomy.
— Carries very poor prognosis.

Carcinoma of the urethra
- — Very rare (<1% of vulval cancers).
- — Lesion in the lower half is usually squamous.
- — Lesion in the upper half is transitional or adenocarcinoma.
- — Symptoms are usually urological (dysuria, retention, incontinence).
- — Differential diagnosis — urethral caruncle, papilloma.
- — Diagnosis is made — biopsy.
- — Exclude vaginal, cervical and uterine body cancer.
- — Treatment — small distal lesion.
  - • May be treated by surgery (radical vulvectomy and bilateral lymph adenectomy)
  - • Radioactive needle implants (radium or caesium) may be used
  - • Upper and larger lesions — anterior exenteration, radical radiotherapy may be used. Groin nodes need to be removed surgically as primary or second-stage procedure
- — Five year survival rate is 20–55% (upper lesions are less favourable).

SUGGESTED READING

Delgado G 1983 Cancer of the vulva. In: Studd J (ed) Progress in obstetrics and gynaecology, vol 3. Churchill Livingstone, Edinburgh, p 187

Douglas C P 1983 Vulval dystrophy. In: Studd J (ed) Progress in obstetrics and gynaecology, vol 3. Churchill Livingstone, Edinburgh, p 190

Lavery H A 1984 Sexually transmitted diseases of the vulva. In: Studd J (ed) Progress in obstetrics and gynaecology, vol 4. Churchill Livingstone, Edinburgh, p 351

Mackay E V, Beischer N A, Cox L W, Wood C 1983 Illustrated textbook of gynaecology. Saunders, Philadelphia

5. DISEASES OF THE VAGINA

BENIGN CONDITIONS OF THE VAGINA

Introduction

— Commonest disorder of the vagina is infection.
— Trichomonas and monilial infections are the most common vaginal infections.
— Wide range of pathogens are involved and they are directly or indirectly related to sexual activity.
— Benign and malignant growths are rare.

Vaginal discharge

— It is one of the most common gynaecological complaints.
— It may be physiological or pathological.

Physiological causes

— The vaginal fluid is a transudate along with desquamated cells, some polymorphs and bacterial flora, predominantly large gram-positive bacilli, lactobacilli.
— Cervical mucus and secretions from Skene's and Bartholin's glands contribute to the vaginal fluid.
— It is highly acidic and the pH varies with age.
— The natural defence mechanism of the lower genital tract is provided by:
  • Apposition of the labia and the vaginal walls
  • Secretion by the apocrine glands
  • Stratified epithelium
  • Vaginal flora
  • Vaginal fluid acidity
  • Bactericidal effects of cervical mucus
— Defence mechanism may be adversely affected by:
  • Age — infection is more likely during childhood and after the menopause
  • Menstrual flow is alkaline and less effective against infection

- During pregnancy and puerperium the pH is alkaline, which encourages infection
- Oestrogen-containing oral contraceptives increases the pH of vaginal fluid
- Foreign bodies in the vagina are a focus for infection
- Cervical ectropion (cervical erosion) raises the pH of vaginal fluid, which upsets the defensive mechanism

Pathological causes

— Infection:
  - *Candida*
  - *Trichomonas*
  - *Haemophilus vaginalis*
  - *Gardnevalla vaginalis*
  - Gram-negative and positive organisms
  - *Listeria monocytogenes*
  - Gonococcal vulvovaginitis

Management

— Investigation:
  - Cervical, vaginal and urethral swabs for culture and sensitivity
  - Direct microscopy of the discharge
— Treatment:
  - Depends on the cause of infection
  - Vaginal pessary
  - Oral medication
  - Partner may need treatment
  - Oestrogen — oral or topical
  - Ectropion may need cryocautery
  - Remove the foreign body and possibly prescribe antibiotics

Congenital disorders of the vagina

— They are rare.
— Congenital duplication causes little disturbance in the function.
— Vaginal agenesis is rare, but poses serious problems, since menstruation, coital function and fertility are affected.
  - In rare cases there is a functioning uterus present with vaginal agenesis.
  - Condition is treated by creating a vagina.
  - Optimum time to perform the surgery will depend on when coital function is planned.
— Imperforate hymen causes primary amenorrhoea.
  - Causes vaginal discomfort due to retained menstrual blood distending the vagina
  - May cause pressure symptoms
  - In late stages, abdominal swelling and pain
  - Condition is treated by incision of the membrane

Vaginal adenosis

— Patients' mother gives history of taking diethyl stilboestrol during the first trimester of pregnancy.
— In this condition there is a failure of squamous epithelial development in the vagina, particularly in its upper third.
— Columnar epithelium similar to that lining the endocervix is seen lining the vagina.
— There may be associated abnormalities in the upper vagina, cervix and body of the uterus which might affect fertility and coital function.
— Often produces mucous discharge.
— Malignant change can develop in a very few patients.
— It is called clear-cell carcinoma if the malignant change takes place in the area of adenosis, and squamous cell carcinoma if it involves the area of squamous metaplasia.

Cystic swelling

Gartner's duct cyst

— This arises in the remnant of the mesonephric ducts which run down from a para-ovarian position to lie in the anterolateral aspect of the vaginal wall.
— Seldom causes symptoms.
— Usually identified on routine examination.
— If it causes difficulty in coitus, it needs excision.

Inclusion cyst

— This occurs at the lower end of the vagina, usually on the posterior surface.
— Arises from inclusion beneath the surface of tags of mucosa resulting from perineal laceration or from imperfect surgical repair of the perineum.
— Usually causes few symptoms.
— Treatment is excision.

Bartholin's gland duct cyst

— It causes minimal symptoms.
— Usually follows a previous episode of infection.
— Cyst bulges into the lower part of the vagina.
— May get infected and become painful.
— Treatment is marsupialisation.
— Very rarely may need excision if the problem becomes chronic and recurrent.

Endometriotic cyst

— Common site is posterior wall behind the cervix.
— May appear as a blue area.
— May present as subepilthelial nodularity or as an irregular haemorrhagic mass.

— Biopsy is done to confirm the diagnosis.
— Treatment can be surgical (excision) or medical (suppression of menstruation).

Tumours of the vagina

— May be benign:
  - Fibromyoma
  - Very rare
  - Treatment is surgery
— Malignant tumour may be primary or secondary.

CARCINOMA OF THE VAGINA

— Primary carcinoma of the vagina is one of the least common of the genital tract malignancies.
— Majority are squamous cell carcinomas (95%).
— Commonly presents in women aged 60 years or more.
— Vagina is frequently involved in cancer arising from lower bowel, lower urinary tract, vulva and cervix.
— Vaginal metastasis is not uncommon from tumours arising from the uterus, ovary and other distant organs such as kidneys.
— Vaginal adenosis may be a predisposing factor, and the age groups involved are mainly the late teens and twenties.

Incidence

— Primary carcinoma comprises 1–2% of gynaecological neoplasms.
— Secondary carcinoma is more common.
— Primary malignant tumours of vagina:
  - Squamous cell carcinoma
  - Adenocarcinoma
  - Sarcoma
— Secondary malignant tumours of vagina:
  - Cervical
  - Endometrial
  - Vulval
  - Ovarian
  - Myometrial
  - Choriocarcinoma
  - Others

Staging

- Stage 0 — Pre-invasive.
- Stage 1 — Limited to the vaginal wall.
- Stage 2 — Outside the vagina but does not extend to pelvic side walls.
- Stage 3 — Extension to the pelvic side walls.
- Stage 4 — Extension beyond the true pelvis, or to bladder and/or rectum.

Aetiology and pathology

- Primary carcinoma is usually of squamous cell origin.
- Occurs in older women in their sixties.
- Carcinoma arising from ulceration from a pessary sited in the posterior fornix.
- Intra-epithelial neoplasia and carcinoma may develop from vaginal adenosis.
- Adenocarcinoma is rare and may arise from adenosis (clear-cell carcinoma) or from mesonephric remnants.
- Rhabdomyosarcoma is rare and unusual; it occurs in infancy and childhood and arises from the upper vagina or cervix.
- Malignant melanoma and sarcoma are rare (1%).
- Spread occurs very early, tumours in the lower third of the vagina spread to inguinal nodes, upper half drain to pelvic nodes.
- Lesions are moderately well differentiated.

Diagnosis and clinical features

Pre-invasive and micro-invasive lesions

- Usually asymptomatic.
- May give history of previous treatment of pre-invasive or invasive carcinoma.
- Patient may complain of watery discharge or post-coital bleeding.
- Diagnosis is usually made on routine cytology.
- Colposcopic appearance may be similar to cervical lesion.
- Clinical examination may show leukoplakic areas or red velvety areas.
- Majority of lesions occur in the upper third of the vagina.
- Schiller's test and/or colposcopy and biopsy will confirm the diagnosis.

Invasive lesions

- May have vaginal discharge and irregular bleeding.
- May have post-coital bleeding.

— Extension to bladder, urethra and lower bowel is more common, and symptoms referable to such spread can occur.
— Inguinal glands may be palpable.
— Clinical examination may reveal a papillomatous or ulcerative lesion in the vagina.
— Combined rectovaginal examination may confirm the induration and extent of the lesion.
— Biopsy from the margin of the lesion will confirm the diagnosis.
— Colposcopy and Schiller's test may be useful.
— Patients are usually post-menopausal.
— Adenocarcinoma associated with vaginal adenosis is a disease of younger age groups.

Treatment

— Pre-invasive cancer is usually treated by:
  • Local radiotherapy
  • Partial or complete vaginectomy
  • A course of 5FU (5% ointment) may be tried initially.
  • Laser therapy may be used
— Invasive cancer is usually treated by:
  • Radiotherapy (external beam followed by intracavity or interstitial radium or caesium therapy) is tried to preserve vaginal function
  • Total vaginectomy is a difficult procedure and rarely warranted
— Exenteration may be necessary because of lesion extending into lower urinary tract and lower bowel.
— Partial or total vaginectomy may be done if growth is confined to vagina and is still superficial, followed by split skin or myocutaneous graft.
— A Wertheim-type procedure is useful for cancers of the upper vagina.
— If the growth involves the lower third of the vagina, a radical vulvectomy procedure is indicated.
— For sarcoma, surgery and chemotherapy may be useful.
— Adenocarcinoma is rare, and is seen in younger women.
— Adenocarcinoma is treated by radical hysterectomy, vaginectomy and pelvic lymphadenectomy and/or radiotherapy.
— Local radiotherapy may be used in young women with a small localised lesion.
— Metastatic carcinoma (secondary carcinoma) is more common, secondary to uterus, ovary, cervix, vulva, urethra, bladder, rectum, colon and hypernephroma.

— Treatment is directed towards the primary and secondary and is palliative.

Prognosis

— Five-year survival is 35–45%.
  - Stage 1 — 85%
  - Stage 2 — 50–60%
  - Stage 3 — 40%
  - Stage 4 — 0%

SUGGESTED READING

Emens J M 1983 The diagnosis and treatment of vaginitis and vaginal discharge. In: Studd J (ed) Progress in obstetrics and gynaecology, vol 3. Churchill Livingstone, Edinburgh, p 213

Robboy S J 1981 Diethyl stilboestrol exposure in human offspring. In: Studd J (ed) Progress in obstetrics and gynaecology, vol 1. Churchill Livingstone, Edinburgh, p 199

Stafl A, Wilkinson H J 1979 Cervical and vaginal intra-epithelial neoplasia. In: Stallworthy J, Bourne G (eds) Recent advances in obstetrics and gynaecology, vol 13. p 257

Tindall V R 1976 The treatment of cancer of the vagina. In: Langley F A (ed) Clinics in obstetrics and gynaecology, vol 3. Saunders, Philadelphia, p 243

Wade-Evans T 1976 The aetiology and pathology of cancer of the vagina. In: Langley, F A (ed) Clinics in obstetrics and gynaecology, vol 3. Saunders, Philadelphia, p 229

6. DISEASES OF THE CERVIX

BENIGN DISORDERS OF THE CERVIX

Introduction

— Although the cervix is anatomically part of the uterus, it does display a significant degree of individuality in terms of anatomy, biology and pathology.

— The cervical epithelium undergoes dynamic change during the woman's reproductive phase as a result of exposure of the everted endocervical columnar cells to the acid vaginal milieu and the subsequent induced metaplasia.

— Introduction of colposcopy to view the cervix has helped to understand changes taking place in the cervical epithelium.

— The cervical mucus has a very important role in maintaining fertility.

— The cervix is subject to a variety of infectious agents, mainly as a result of sexual activity.

Congenital anomalies

— As a result of the formation of the reproductive tract from the paired müllerian ducts, duplication of varying degree may be seen.

— Complete duplication seldom produces problems.

— However, some types of malformation may cause dysmenorrhoea, infertility, abortion and certain obstetrical complications.

Erosion — now known as eversion

— Eversion or ectropion is an area of columnar epithelium which has extended beyond its normal boundaries.
  • It may arise as a result of the squamocolumnar junction lying on what should be the ectocervix (congenital).
  • Secondary to oestrogen-containing oral contraceptives.

- May be due to childbirth — the squamocolumnar junction is normally sited, but the parous cervix is patulous and sometimes may give a false impression of ectropion when a bivalve speculum is used.

Pathophysiology
- The cervix is a meeting place of a single layer of mucin-secreting columnar cells, which is largely confined to the endocervix, and a stratifield squamous layer, which is largely confined to the ectocervix.
- In the woman's childbearing period, under the influence of oestrogen the cervix becomes everted.
- The columnar epithelium, exposed to the acid vaginal milieu, converts to a native-type squamous layer. The process is termed metaplasia.
- The area in which the metaplastic change occurs is called the transformation zone.
- While this metaplastic change takes place, the epithelium is exposed to a number of potentially noxious agents such as micro-organisms and chemicals.
- Subsequent outcomes are cervicitis and malignant changes.
- There is no need for treatment of asymptomatic and uncomplicated ectropion.
- Ectropion (eversion) may produce vaginal discharge of the non-infective type.
- The area covered by columnar epithelium may increase with parity and use of the contraceptive pill, and may sometimes cause post-coital bleeding.
- Usually regresses after the age of 40 years.
- For symptomatic ectropion, the treatment is cryocautery, provided the cervical cytology and/or colposcopic examination are normal.

Infections

Acute cervicitis

Aetiology
- Gonococcal infection.
- *Chlamydia trachomatis.*
- Herpes virus.
- Papilloma virus.
- Other micro-organisms.

Clinical features
- Cervix may look inflamed, congested and reddened.
- There may be purulent discharge from the external os.
- Main symptom is discharge, which may be yellow or yellowish-white in colour.

— There may be deep pelvic discomfort, dyspareunia and menstrual discomfort.
— If it is gonococcal infection, there may be symptoms related to urethritis.
— Acute cervicitis is seldom seen as an isolated condition.
— Usually seen as part of an acute infection involving the genital tract as a whole, including the fallopian tubes, which may produce systemic symptoms.

Diagnosis

— Inspection of the cervix.
— Gram-staining of the cervical discharge may show intracellular diplococci.
— Culture may identify the specific organism, together with a variety of bacteria which are common inhabitants of the cervix.

Treatment

— Depends on the nature of the infection and state of the cervix and the remaining genital tract.
— For acute infection associated with gonococcal infection, the treatment is antibiotics, usually penicillin.

Chronic cervicitis

— It is a common gynaecological lesion.
— A common cause of vaginal discharge.
— It is often the aftermath of childbirth damage or previous acute infection.
— Cervix is usually normal in appearance on its vaginal surface, but the endocervix is thickened and produces a mucopurulent discharge.
— It can cause chronic pelvic pain, dyspareunia and menstrual problems.

Diagnosis

— Appearance of the cervix.
— Culture, sensitivity and microscopy may be helpful.
— Colposcopy and cytology will be necessary to exclude malignancy or premalignant conditions.

Treatment

— If it is associated with symptoms, the choice of treatment is cryotherapy, cauterisation and conisation.
— Cryotherapy involves the destruction of cervical epithelium by freezing using refrigerants such as nitrous oxide.
— Electrocautery or hot cautery has long been an effective method of therapy, but recently it has been replaced by cryotherapy.
— Conisation may be needed when there is extensive endocervicitis with profuse mucopurulent discharge.

Non-bacterial infections

Herpes simplex virus
— Can affect the cervix.
— Produces oedema, vesicles, ulcers and, in extreme cases, granulomatous lesions.
— Clinical manifestation of the lesion in the cervix is self-limited and lasts for 2–3 weeks.
— Diagnosis is based on the history, cultures, and the appearance of the lesions.
— Genital herpetic infection is sexually transmitted.
— The diagnosis of lower genital tract herpes is important during pregnancy because of the risk of infection to the child if vaginal delivery is allowed.
— There is some association between herpes infection and malignant disease of the cervix.

Chlamydia trachomatis
— This micro-organism is isolated from the cervix in 12–31% of women.
— It is often associated with vaginal discharge.
— Cervix may look inflamed and reddened.
— Chlamydia trachomatis can produce salpingitis.
— Hence, sexual partners need treatment when the diagnosis is made by culture.
— It is usually sensitive to tetracycline and trimethoprim sulphamethoxazole.

Mycoplasma hominis
— Has been implicated in genital infection.
— There is no specific clinical manifestation of mycoplasmic infection of the cervix.

Syphilis
— Is largely a disease of the past.
— In the cervix it presents as a primary lesion.
— Produces few symptoms, and the discharge is infective.

Tuberculosis
— It is an uncommon lesion.
— Usually it is secondary to infection in the tubes and uterus.
— Very rarely contracted through coitus.
— Presents either as a hyperplastic or ulcerative lesion.
— Can be mistaken for carcinoma.
— Microscopy, biopsy, lesions in other parts of the body confirm the diagnosis.
— Treatment is specific antituberculous treatment.

Cervical stenosis

— Stenosis of the cervical canal with obstruction of the uterine drainage may occur with atrophic change with age, scarring from trauma or surgery.
— As a result, haematometra or pyometra develop.
— Cervical stenosis due to atrophy in old age produces few problems because the endometrium is inactive.
— However, if there is associated malignancy, then it can produce symptoms.
— In the presence of pyometra in old age, malignancy of the uterine body or endocervix should be ruled out.
— Treatment is drainage and antibiotics, if malignancy is excluded.
— Recurrent pyometra needs hysterectomy.
— Cervical stenosis may also occur after lacerations, cone biopsy, cryotherapy or cervical cauterisation.
— In menstruating women the main symptom is dysmenorrhoea, or amenorrhoea due to occlusion of the cervix, when no external bleeding occurs.
— Treatment is dilatation of the cervix.

Benign tumours

Endocervical polyp

— Cervical polyps are generally pedunculated tumours arising from the intracervical mucosa.
— May sometimes arise from the vaginal surface of the cervix.
— Like their endometrial counterpart, these are quite common.
— They are rounded or elongated and attached to the endocervix by a stalk.
— The most common type is adenomatous with endocervical-type glandular elements set in a vascular stroma (90%).
— They are usually cherry red in colour and velvety in appearance.
— Other tissues such as fibrous or vascular may predominate, and variable degrees of inflammatory change may be present.
— In rare cases a fibromyomatous polyp may arise from the cervix.

Clinical features

— Polyps may be single or multiple.
— Usually they are small and single.
— Usual age group is 40–60 years, and 60% or more cases occur in the post-menopausal age group.
— Condition is usually asymptomatic and seen on routine examination.

— Larger polyp may cause intermenstrual bleeding or post-coital or post-menopausal bleeding.
— Diagnosis is made on seeing the characteristic appearance.

Treatment

— Removal of the polyp is a simple procedure.
— It involves twisting the pedicle, removing the polyp and cauterising the base of the pedicle.
— Histological examination is essential because of malignant change in rare cases.
— Curettage of the endometrial cavity is done to exclude polyps in the uterine cavity; in rare cases adenocarcinoma of the uterus may co-exist.
— If the pedicle is thick, it may need ligation.

Papillomas

— There are two types: the true squamous cell papilloma and the condyloma acuminatum.
— It is difficult to distinguish between the two.
— The condyloma is often flatter on the cervix.
— Papillomas usually exhibit characteristic changes on cytology and colposcopy.
— Similar lesions are often present in the vagina or in the vulva.

Leiomyoma

— These smooth-muscle tumours are similar to those described in the uterus.
— They can be big and may produce pressure symptoms.
— They may also produce complications in pregnancy and labour, and caesarean section is often needed.
— Treatment is surgery.

CARCINOMA OF THE CERVIX

Introduction

— The use of cytology and colposcopy over the past three decades or so has helped us to understand the natural history of cervical carcinoma better than any other tumour.
— Mostly carcinomas arise from the squamous cell in the transformation zone of the cervix.
— Early pre-invasive or micro-invasive stage can be identified by cytology, colposcopy and biopsy, and these lesions are curable.

Incidence

— Carcinoma of the cervix, preinvasive and invasive, is the
  most common malignant tumour of the genital tract, though
  more women die annually from ovarian cancer.
— It accounts for 50–60% of the total genital tract neoplasia.
— The disease causes the death of approximately 1% of women.
— Depending on the women's socio-economic and cultural
  status, 5–75 new cases per 100,000 population may develop
  carcinoma of cervix per year.
— In the age group of 30–39 years, invasive cervical cancer will
  account for 50% of the total malignancy seen.

Aetiology and pathogenesis

— In almost 95% of cases the tumour is of squamous origin and
  arises in the transformation zone of the cervix.
— In the remaining 5% it arises from the glandular element in
  the cervical canal.
— The transformation zone results from oestrogen stimulation
  which causes the single-layer endocervical columnar
  epithelium to become everted and thus exposed to the acid
  pH of the vagina.
— The alteration of the pH causes the columnar epithelium to
  undergo metaplasia to the more protective squamous type.
— During this process the epithelium is susceptible to mutagenic
  agents such as virus, sperm and smegma, and becomes
  dysplastic (exhibits disordered growth).
— Times of intense oestrogen stimulus include the neonatal
  period, adolescence and pregnancy; after menopause, the
  squamocolumnar junction is usually inside the endocervix.
— Similar eversion results from lateral laceration of the cervix
  during labour.
— Cervical cancer is more common in those whose coital
  activity and childbearing start early.
— There is also an association with lower socio-economic status.
— Correlation is strong between multiplicity of sexual partners
  and both intra-epithelial and invasive carcinoma of the
  cervix.
— There is some correlation between the use of oral
  contraceptives and smoking and neoplasia in the cervix.
— Barrier contraceptive methods are thought to have a
  protective effect.
— Herpes simplex virus (HVS) type II and the papova (wart)
  virus have been incriminated with cervical neoplasia.
— Distinct racial differences exist. The disease is twenty times
  higher in Puerto Ricans than in Jews.

— The peak age incidence of pre-invasive cancer occurs in the 30s, and invasive cancer in the late 40s to early 50s.

Staging of carcinoma of the cervix (FIGO, 1976)

Clinical staging

Stage ∅   Intra-epithelial neoplasia (CIN).

Stage I   Invasive carcinoma confined to the cervix; extension to the body is disregarded.

Ia   No lesion visible at clinical examination, but stromal invasion >3 mm (micro-invasive carcinoma).

Ib   All other stage I lesions.

Stage IIa   Extends to the vagina but not the lower third. No parametrial involvement.

IIb   Parametrial involvement but not up to the pelvic wall.

Stage III   The carcinoma extends to the pelvic side wall and/or the lower one-third of the vagina is involved. Presence of hydronephrosis and non-functioning kidney.

Stage IIIa   No extension to the pelvic wall, involves lower one-third of the vagina.

IIIb   Parametrial involvement up to the pelvic wall. No cancer-free space — may cause hydronephrosis and non-functioning kidney.

Stage IV   Extends beyond the true pelvis. Involvement of bladder and rectal mucosa (bullous oedema is excluded).

IVa   Spread to adjacent organ.

IVb   Spread to distant organ.

Pre-invasive cancer (CIN)

— Cytology and colposcopy have enabled us to diagnose cervical neoplasia before it becomes invasive.

— Regular cytological examination at intervals of 1–2 years for life beginning at the age of first coitus may help to diagnose cervical neoplasia in early stages.

— Colposcopy is required when cytology is abnormal to select the areas for biopsy or to determine the need for cone biopsy.

Diagnosis

— Cytology.
— Colposcopy.
— Schiller test.
— Cone biopsy.

Cytological screening (Fig. 6.1)

— Specimens for cervical and vaginal cytology are usually taken with a wooden or plastic Ayre spatula.

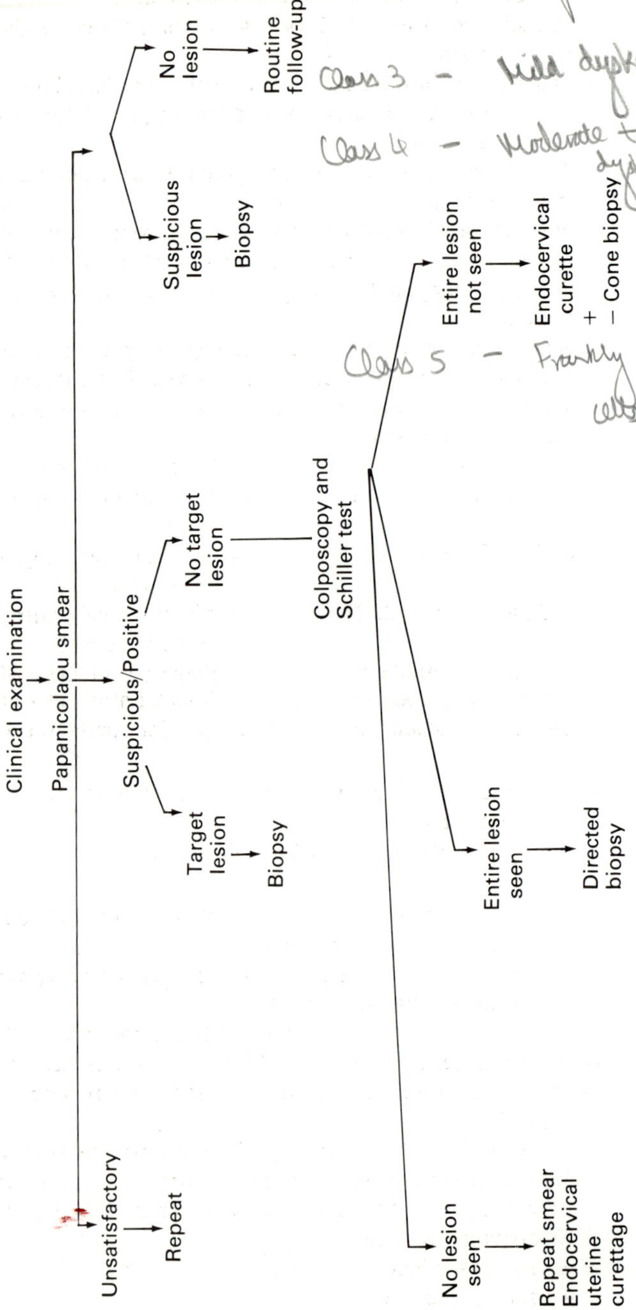

smear

Class 1 — Normal

Class 2 — Inflammatory changes

Class 3 — Mild dyskaryosis

Class 4 — Moderate to severe dyskaryosis

Class 5 — Frankly malignant cells.

Fig. 6.1 Cervical cytology flowchart

— The days of menstrual loss are best avoided.
— The slide must not be allowed to dry in air because the cells become distorted.
— Fixation is in alcohol and ether or with a wax-based resin.
— All smears must be accompanied by adequate information about the patient.
— All women, regardless of age, should be screened regularly from the onset of sexual activity.
— For reasons of economics and cost-effectiveness the policy is to take a cervical smear at 25 years or when women attend family planning, antenatal, gynaecology and venereal disease clinics.
— Sexually active people need screening irrespective of age.
— The first smear should be repeated a year later, thereafter at intervals of 3–5 years if the initial two smears are normal.
— Classification of smears:
  • Class I or grade I   — No abnormal cells
  • Class II or grade II   — Abnormal cells, probably benign
  • Class III or grade III   — Abnormal cells suggestive of neoplasia
  • Class IV or grade IV   — Abnormal cells with grossly dyskaryotic cells
  • Class V or grade V   — Frankly malignant cells
— A smear with too little or too much material is not suitable.
— Blood and inflammatory exudate make interpretation difficult.

Incidence

— Incidence of positive smears varies according to the population studied.
  • Usual incidence ranges 2.5–10 per 1000

Problems

— Cervical cytology programme falls short of the ideal because not all cancers exfoliate abnormal cells, the lesion may be endocervical, deep in glands covered with normal epithelium or not the exfoliating type.
— Faulty technique may miss the exfoliated abnormal cells.
— Abnormal cells may be missed by the inexperienced screener.
— The above causes produce false negative report; rate ranges 5–30+%.
— Some cancers progress rapidly in the interval between visits.
— In view of the possibility of false negative results, the initial screening should be followed by another in 6–12 months.
— High-risk groups are:
  • First coitus before 18 years
  • Multiple partners
  • Lower socio-economic status

— Abnormal smear should be followed up by colposcopic examination by an experienced and skilled person.
— In the post-menopausal group, annual screening of the genital tract, ovaries and breasts should be encouraged.

Cytological changes in cervical intra-epithelial lesions

— The terms dysplasia and carcinoma in situ are histological diagnoses.
— In smears, abnormal cells described as dyskaryotic.
— The features of dyskaryosis are mostly in the nucleus:
  • Enlargement and hyperchromasia
  • Uneven chromatin distribution
  • Irregular nuclear membrane
  • Multinucleation
— The three grades of severity are:
  • Superficial cell (mild) — have the above nuclear abnormalities with abundant cytoplasm and angular cell borders
  • Intermediate cell (moderate) — have larger nucleus in proportion to the whole cell, but occupying less than 50% of the cell
  • Parabasal cell (severe) — have very large nucleus occupying more than 50% of the cell; cells have round or oval border
— Smears from the dysplastic epithelium usually contain cells with various degrees of dyskaryosis.
— Parabasal cell dyskaryosis is seen in a smear from a cervix showing CIN III.
— Smears from invasive carcinoma are often bizarre, and cytological characteristics are not specific.
— False-negative smears are defined as those reported as normal when the cervix has a neoplastic lesion of the cervix:
  • Due to an error in taking the smear
  • Smear is too thin or too thick
  • Smear is contaminated with blood and inflammatory exudate
  • Smear is allowed to dry before fixation
  • Misinterpretation by the cytologist
  • The lesion is too small, so few cells exfoliate
— Endocervical sampling and a separate smear may improve the reliability of initial screening.
— False-positive smears are those in which abnormal cells are seen and cervix fails to reveal any abnormal lesion.
  • Errors in the laboratory are possible
  • Positive smear should be repeated before any surgery
  • May be due to lesions higher in the cervical canal which could be missed by colposcopy and cone biopsy

Colposcopy

— See Figure 6.2.
— When the cervical smear is abnormal, it should be followed by colposcopic examination.
— Colposcopy can identify the affected areas, and biopsies can be properly directed.
— The technique involves:
  • Inspection of the unprepared cervix
  • Inspection after the application of normal saline
  • After 3% acetic acid with or without the use of green filter for display of the angio-architecture
  • Inspection after the application of Lugol's iodine (Schiller test)
— Detection of dysplasia and early cancer depends on three factors:
  • Tint and opacity — related to nuclear size and density in the epithelial cells — acetic acid draws water from the cells, and dysplastic areas are revealed as white opaque patches
  • Vascular pattern — there is increase in blood vessels followed by distortion due to enhanced metabolic requirements of the cancer cells — revealed as 'punctation' or 'mosaic' structure. Later vessels exhibit irregular calibre, corkscrew formation and increase in intercapillary distance

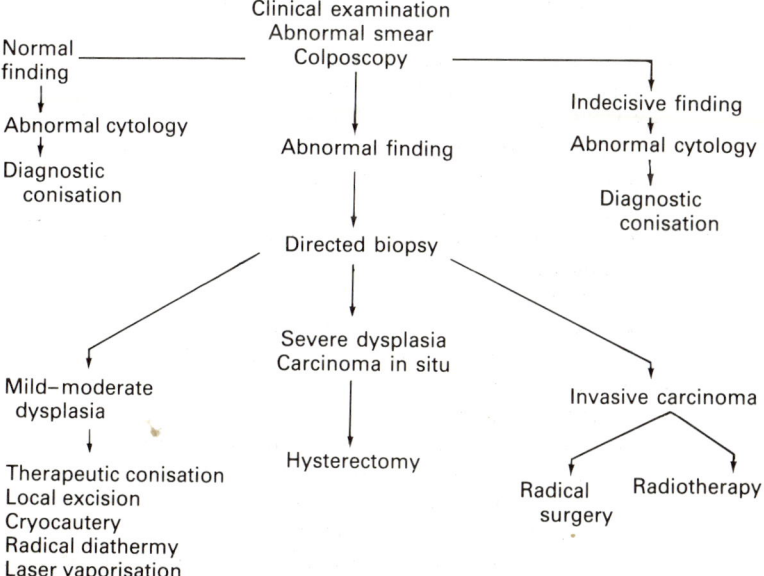

Fig. 6.2 Colposcopy flowchart

- • Surface elevation is seen as the neoplastic process progresses, showing a raised and irregular surface
- — Immature metaplasia and papilloma virus infection show colposcopic picture similar to CIN and need careful evaluation.
- — The advantages are: the lesions are clearly demarcated, so accurate biopsy is possible; their site, size and biological potential can be assessed; minimum curative treatment can be employed; and follow-up examination is better if treatment has been conservative.
- — The disadvantages are: colposcopy needs skilled staff and expensive equipment; the transformation zone is not always clear and visible, as in post-menopausal women and in women who have had cervical surgery.
- — Colposcopy is useful for evaluation of abnormal cytology during pregnancy.
- — If the squamocolumnar junction is higher up in the cervical canal, or the examination is unsatisfactory, endocervical curettage should be done.
- — If the above procedure is not helpful, a cone biopsy should be done.

Schiller test

- — This is of ancillary rather than diagnostic value.
- — Based on the mahogany brown stain of the squamous epithelial cells containing glycogen with Schiller iodine reagent.
- — Dysplastic areas and cancer take up the iodine only partially or not at all.
- — The disadvantages are: everted normal columnar epithelium which is common in the reproductive phase does not take up the iodine; epithelium with loss of surface cells also shows no stain; and the false positive rate is very high (30–40%).
- — Many neoplastic lesions with more differentiation may have enough glycogen in the cells to stain brown, and this increases the false negative rate (40–50%).
- — The advantages are: helpful if colposcopy is not available in defining the area for biopsy and in delineating the limits for cone biopsy.

Cone biopsy

- — Used if colposcopy is not available.
- — Accurate histopathological examination is possible.
- — Indicated if the transformation zone is not seen and the whole lesion is not visualised colposcopically due to extension higher up in the cervical canal.
- — Curettage of the endocervical canal is not helpful.

Pathology

— WHO classification is mild, moderate and severe dysplasia.
— Now the new classification is CIN grades I, II, III.
— Dysplasia:
  - A lesion in which part of the thickness of the epithelium is replaced by cells showing varying degrees of atypia.
  - Dysplastic changes can occur in the squamous epithelium of the portio and in the metaplastic epithelium of the endocervical mucosa
  - Changes may be seen in the cervical glands
  - This lesion may be seen in association with carcinoma in situ or invasive cervical carcinoma
  - Dysplasia is divided into three groups according to the degree of cellular atypia and epithelial architecture:
  - Mild dysplasia — the loss of polarity and regular stratification is minimal, the nuclei are enlarged, irregular and stained dark, mitosis is seen, occasionally abnormal and confined to the lower third of the epithelium, cytoplasm is preserved, and keratinisation is a common feature
  - Moderate dysplasia — the changes are intermediate between mild and severe dysplasia
  - Severe dysplasia — atypia is a pronounced loss of polarity, crowded cells have large darkly stained nuclei, mitosis is more common, abnormal cells are seen right through the thickness of the epithelium, the superficial cells show a degree of maturation
— Carcinoma in situ is a lesion in which all, or most, of the epithelium shows the cellular features of carcinoma.
  - Small hyperchromatic nuclei are surrounded by scanty cytoplasm with little squamous differentiation
  - Orderly stratification is absent
  - Cellular polarity is often vertical or diagonal rather than horizontal
  - Normal and abnormal mitosis is seen throughout the epithelium
  - Flattened parakeratotic cells may be present on the surface
  - The lesion often involves the cervical glands
— CIN terminology has been introduced to comply with the modern belief that severe dysplasia and carcinoma in situ are of equally sinister importance:
  - CIN I   — mild to moderate dysplasia
  - CIN II — moderate dysplasia
  - CIN III — severe dysplasia and carcinoma in situ

Management of the abnormal cytological cervical smear

— Ideally, all patients should have colposcopic assessment of the cervix.
— If colposcopy is not available and cytology is positive, cone biopsy following Schiller's iodine test should be done.
— If cytology is suspicious and there is no clinical evidence of invasive carcinoma, then the cytology should be repeated in 3 months, during which time any infection or inflammatory condition should be treated.
— If the second cytology is suspicious, then a cone biopsy should be performed.
— If colposcopy is available, colposcopically directed biopsy should be done.
— If it shows that the lesion is intra-epithelial in nature, then identify the extent of the lesion and remove it by surgery or destruction.
— Carcinoma in situ is usually treated in a relatively short period of time.
— In a younger patient with a minor·degree of dysplasia, treatment is delayed until her family is complete.
— A non-intervention policy could be adopted if the patient is very young and sexually active with positive cytology, if she is seen regularly by an expert colposcopist.
— With the introduction of destructive methods of treatment there is no need to withhold treatment as in the case of surgery.

Treatment of CIN

— Conservative, and observation.
— Cone biopsy.
— Local excision.
— Hysterectomy.
— Destructive therapy.

CIN — 1

— 85% of such lesions will regress and disappear.
— Patient is observed, with regular 6 monthly cytology and colposcopy.
— 15% may progress and will need treatment.

CIN — II, III.

— Need treatment and further follow-up using cytology and colposcopy.

Cone biopsy

— The aim of cone biopsy is two-fold: diagnostic and also therapeutic.
— Colposcopically directed cone biopsy tended to be smaller, had fewer complications and was therapeutic.

— In the absence of colposcopy, the Schiller test is used prior to cone biopsy.
— It is desirable to leave intact as much of the endocervical canal, for the following reasons:
  • Haemorrhage is rarely a problem.
  • Future fertility is not impaired.
  • The internal os is left intact.
  • Nulliparous patients and patients desirous of further children should be offered less extensive tissue removal.
— If the lesion is small and completely visible, it can be removed by a small cone or ring biopsy which removes the lower third of the endocervical canal.
— If the lesion extends beyond the limit of colposcopic vision, then the whole endocervical canal needs removal.
— Patients with persistent positive cytology with normal colposcopic appearance of cervix and lower endocervical canal need cone biopsy which includes the endocervical canal.
— In 4% of patients colposcopy shows the lesion involves the upper vagina. It then needs excision of the abnormal vaginal epithelium and amputation of the cervix.
— The above condition may be treated by abdominal or vaginal hysterectomy with a cuff of vagina after excluding invasive carcinoma by colposcopically directed biopsy.
— The complications following cone biopsy are:
  • Haemorrhage
  • Infection
  • Cervical stenosis — haematometra
  • Cervical incompetence
  • Subfertility or infertility
  • If invasive carcinoma is present and the cone has cut through the lesion, the dissemination is enhanced.
— The results of properly planned therapeutic cone biopsy are excellent, but the patient needs regular cytological and colposcopic follow-up.
— The development of subsequent invasive carcinoma is very rare.

Local excision
— Lesion is very small and removable.
— Can be removed by one or more punch biopsy.
— Or can be removed by incision under general anaesthesia.
— Good results are achieved if this is done by an expert using colposcopy.

Hysterectomy
— This is indicated when abnormal cytology and abnormal colposcopic finding following conisation persists, though such residual lesions can be dealt with by local excision, by repeat

conisation or by local destruction if childbearing function is necessary, or if the patient is young.
— If the lesion involves the upper vagina, it can be treated by local destructive therapy.
— If there is a co-existing condition such as fibroid, menorrhagia, prolapse or adnexal lesions, it is mandatory to exclude invasive carcinoma first.
— If the patient has completed her family, if follow-up is difficult and if she requests sterilisation, she may be offered hysterectomy, provided that invasive carcinoma is excluded.

Destructive therapy
— Patient with pre-malignant disease of the cervix can be treated safely by destruction, provided:
  • Patient is examined and assessed by an expert colposcopist.
  • The lesion is clearly seen in its entirety.
  • Invasive carcinoma is excluded by colposcopically directed biopsies by a colposcopist.
  • The destructive procedure is carried out by the colposcopist.
  • There is facility for adequate cytology and/or colposcopy follow-up.
— The methods available for destructive treatment are:
  • Cryocautery
  • Electrocautery
  • Electrodiathermy
  • CO_2 laser
— They destroy selective areas of cervical epithelium which will be replaced by normal squamous epithelium.

Cryocautery
— Destroys tissue by freezing.
— It is useful for small areas of mild to moderate dysplasia.
— There is some concern about the ability of this technique to destroy adequately which depends on the tissue destruction to about 3 mm or 4 mm below the surface epithelium.
— It may not destroy the lesion involving the glands and clefts in the endocervix.
— New regenerating epithelium may cover the residual disease until it becomes invasive.
— The advantage is that it can be used with minimal discomfort as an outpatient procedure.
— Healing is rapid; complications are minimal.
— The endocervical canal undergoes minimal stenosis, and fertility is not impaired.

Electrocautery
— Can be performed in the outpatient clinic.

— It is not possible to destroy tissue beyond a depth of 2 mm or 3 mm.
— If the lesion is small and totally visible and it shows mild to moderate dysplasia, this method could be used.
— Follow-up is essential.

Electrodiathermy

— Destroys tissue much more effectively than cryo- or electrocautery.
— Heat generated can produce intense pain, and patient will need general or regional anaesthesia.
— Should be done under colposcopic control.
— Used only when the lesion is completely visible.
— Using this technique it is possible to destroy cervical tissue up to a depth of 10 mm.
— Fibrosis is more common, but fertility is usually not affected.

Carbon dioxide laser

— CO_2 laser most widely used in gynaecology produces energy at a wavelength of 10.6 microns which is the infrared portion of the spectrum and invisible to the human eye.
— This energy, by a system of mirrors and lenses, can be focused to a specific spot 1.5 mm to 2.0 mm in diameter and at its focal point releases an enormous amount of energy.
— The tissue at the focal point of the laser is vaporised at the speed of light.
— The laser is attached to a colposcope.
— The area to be destroyed is under direct vision of the person performing the laser surgery.
— The main advantage of the laser is that almost all patients with cervical and upper vaginal lesions can be treated without analgesia or anaesthesia.
— Healing is usually rapid, starting within 10 to 12 days.
— There is usually no need for antibiotics or antiseptics, post-operatively.
— Destruction must be in a depth of 5 mm to 7 mm to achieve a high rate of cure (94%).
— 3% to 4% of patients with pre-malignant disease of the cervix will have vaginal involvement, and laser treatment has an important place if the patient is young or nulliparous or both.

Diethyl stilboestrol syndrome (DES)

— Diagnosed in the offspring of mothers taking the above drug during pregnancy.
— It is known as vaginal/cervical adenosis, because of the presence of excessive columnar epithelium in the ectocervix extending into the fornices and vagina.

— DES probably prevents the formation or upward extension of squamous epithelium.
— The incidence of adenosis in exposed females is in the range of 30–95%:
  • Depending on thoroughness of the examination
  • Use of colposcopy
  • Duration of therapy to mother
  • Time in pregnancy (if it was started before or after the 10th week)
— A similar lesion, usually less florid, is seen in 3–5% of non-DES-exposed females.
— Lesion is confined to upper vagina in 90–95% of cases. extends to the middle third in 5–10% and to the lower third in only 1%.
— It is rare to see adenocarcinoma of the clear cell type or carcinoma arising from the metaplastic squamous epithelium.
— Anatomic malformation of the upper vagina, cervix and uterus, hooded cervix, pseudopolyps of the cervix and ridge formation are also seen in this condition.
— Offsprings of mothers exposed to DES need careful follow-up using colposcopy and cytology.
— Colposcopically directed biopies should be taken if there are suspicious areas.
— Cervical/vaginal adenosis usually pursues a benign course, transforming via metaplasia to normal squamous epithelium.
— Risk of developing intra-epithelial neoplasia is slightly higher than normal.

INVASIVE CANCER OF THE CERVIX

Introduction

— Carcinoma of the cervix is the most common malignant tumour of the genital tract, although more women die annually from ovarian cancer.
— The incidence of invasion cancer is lower than that of pre-invasive cancer and depends on the cytological screening in that particular community.

Natural history and pathology

— May be seen from the age of 20 years onwards.
— Peak incidence is 45–55 years.
— More common in multiparous women.
— More common in women with multiple partners.

— More common in women from the lower socio-economic
  groups.
— Jewish women are relatively immune to this disease.
— Tumour may be exophytic, ulcerative or endocervical.
— In 95% it is squamous cell carcinoma and in 5% it is
  adenocarcinoma.
— Direct spread occurs mostly along the lymphatic/vascular
  channels that run in the cardinal and uterosacral ligaments.
— Extension to the vagina is common, but involvement of
  bladder and rectum occurs later.
— Spread by blood is relatively uncommon and is reflected in
  metastasis in bone, brain and lung.
— Lymph node involvement increases in parallel with the stage
  of the disease.
— Lymphatic spread first involves primary nodes:
  • Parametrial
  • Paracervical
  • Vesicovaginal
  • Rectovaginal
  • Hypogastric
  • Obturator
  • External iliac
— Secondary nodes are involved later:
  • Common iliac
  • Sacral
  • Vaginal
  • Para-aortic
  • Inguinal
— Parametrial spread causes obstruction of the ureters; many
  deaths occur due to uraemia.
— Obstruction to the cervical canal results in pyometra.

Squamous cell carcinoma

— Histology confirms the cell characteristics:
  • Loss of stratification
  • Various degrees of immaturity
  • Lack of differentiation
  • Pleomorphism of cells and nuclei
  • Hyperchromatic nuclei
  • Abundant and atypical mitosis
  • Giant cell formation
— The architecture also shows changes:
  • Malignant epithelium has broken through the basement
    membrane
  • The stromal penetration is more than 3 mm
  • Infiltration of the stroma by lymphocytes and polymorphs

Clinical features
- May be asymptomatic and detected by routine cervical smear or examination.
- Intermenstrual, post-menopausal or post-coital bleeding are the most common presenting symptoms.
- Vaginal discharge, water or bloodstained, is less frequent and occurs later.
- Pain in the pelvis or back occurs in late stages, associated with parametrial involvement.
- Pain radiating to the thigh and leg is due to involvement of sciatic plexus.
- Bone pain occurs very late in the disease due to metastasis.
- Bladder symptoms, dysuria, frequency, haematuria occur later.
- Bowel symptoms such as pain on defecation, constipation/diarrhoea, indicate stage IV.
- Fistulae of either of these two organs occur at a more advanced stage.
- If the lesion is entirely in the endocervical canal, it is often not seen on clinical examination.
- On examination the cervix may appear normal or hard with granular erosion which bleeds to the touch, or ulcerated lesion is visible.

Diagnosis
- Usually obvious unless the lesion is in the cervical canal or is small.
- Involved area is raised irregular, ulcerated, infected and reddened, bleeds on touch.
- Feels harder than normal.
- May be very friable if growth is rapid.
- Combined rectovaginal examination will confirm parametrial and uterosacral involvement.
- Biopsy will confirm the diagnosis.
- Wedge, punch, cone biopsy and cervical curettage may be necessary if lesion is early or occult.

Prognosis
- Major factor affecting prognosis is stage.
- Rate of tumour growth, metastatic tendency.
- General condition of the patient.
- Infection in the pelvis.
- Size of the tumour.
- Degree of differentiation.

Management
- Managed by a team consisting of gynaecologist, radiotherapist and histopathologist.
- Full assessment of the patient.

— Biopsy and clinicopathological assessment.
— Patient and her nearest relation are counselled.
— Pre-therapy assessment includes:
  - Cardiovascular
  - Haematological
  - Pulmonary
  - Renal function assessment
  - Chest X-ray and excretion urography
  - Nutritional status of the patient
  - Psychological stability
  - Presence of metastatic disease is sought
  - Value of lymphography remains controversial
  - Pelvic examination under anaesthesia to assess the staging
  - Dilatation and fractional curettage
  - Cervical biopsy
  - Cystoscopy
  - Associated diseases will need stabilisation
  - Anaemia and infection need treatment

Treatment of micro-invasive carcinoma

— Micro-invasive lesion is defined as one in which the carcinoma invades the stroma in one or more places to a depth of 3 mm or more below the basement membrane in which blood vessels and lymphatics are not seen to be involved.
— Management may be conservative as for intra-epithelial carcinoma.
— This lesion comprises approximately 5% of invasive lesions.
— It is usually asymptomatic.
— Often identified when patient is investigated for positive cytology.
— Diagnosis is made on histopathology, provided the biopsy of tissue taken is 6 mm in depth.
— It may be difficult to distinguish extensive gland or cleft involvement from stromal invasion.
— If clumps of tumour cells can be seen in capillary-like spaces, more extensive treatment is necessary.
— If the cone biopsy confirms the margins are free and stromal invasion is less than 3 mm and there is no involvement of lymphatics and blood vessels, and the patient is young and nulliparous, she is advised to complete the family. Close follow-up examinations are important.
— Adequate cone biopsy is mandatory for diagnostic and therapeutic purposes if the lesion is suspected to be micro-invasive. Further treatment will depend on whether micro-

D

invasion is associated with extension into lymphatics and blood vessels and if childbearing function is necessary.
— Micro-invasion with lymphatic and blood vessel involvement is treated as stage Ib.
— If childbearing function is completed and only micro-invasion is seen on cone biopsy, total hysterectomy only is necessary — vaginal cuff is removed if there is extension into vagina.
— Lymph node spread and death ocurs in 1–2%.
— Ectocervix and upper vagina is involved in 3–5%.
— Careful colposcopy and biopsy prior to decision of definitive surgery.
— If more than 3 mm invasion, radical treatment is necessary if the lymphatics are involved.
— If cone margin is free and childbearing is essential, careful cytological and colposcopic follow-up is necessary and when childbearing is completed a hysterectomy is advisable.
— If cone margin is not free and lesion is micro-invasive only, reconisation is essential if childbearing is essential; if not, a hysterectomy is advisable.

Treatment of invasive carcinoma stage I and II

— The basic treatment is radiotherapy.
— Surgery is reserved for carefully selected cases.

Surgery

— Surgery is indicated for:
  • Growth confined to the cervix
  • Minimal extension beyond the cervix
  • Associated pelvic pathology such as ovarian tumour, fibroid, pelvic infection
  • Adenocarcinoma
  • Pregnancy
  • Younger patients
  • If radiation cannot be applied accurately due to obliteration of cervical canal and narrowing of the upper vagina
— Wertheim radical hysterectomy is the ideal surgery.
— Surgery involves removal of the uterus, cervix, upper one-third to one-half of the vagina, parocolpos, parametria and all the pelvic lymph nodes.
— It is not necessary to remove the healthy ovaries, particularly in younger women.
— The Schauta radical vaginal hysterectomy is an alternative.

Advantages

— Cervix and uterus are excised and no recurrence of tumour is then possible

- Treatment is less prolonged
- Ovaries could be conserved in the younger age group
- Complications of radiotherapy are avoided
- Infection is not a problem for surgery
- Better long-term state of the pelvic tissue
- Accurate assessment of tumour including the lymphatic spread is a great advantage.

Disadvantages
- Only selected patients benefit
- It can be equally or more hazardous than radiotherapy
- Urinary and rectal fistulae are more common
- Prolonged bladder dysfunction is not uncommon
- Vagina is often shortened, which is a disadvantage in the sexually active young person.

Complications
- Immediate problems are anaesthetic problems, haemorrhage, shock, sepsis and thrombo-embolic problems
- Long-term problems are ureteric and rectal fistulae, bladder dysfunction and retention, and lymphocyst.

Radical radiotherapy
- Radiotherapy comprises a combination of intracavity radium, radon or caesium 137 using uterine tube, upper vaginal ovoids and super-voltage therapy using telecobalt or linear accelerator or betatron.
- The tumour and paracervical spread are treated with intra-uterine and intravaginal radium or caesium 137.
- The pelvic lymph nodes and their lymphatics are dealt with mainly by external irradiation.
- Using caesium, the aim is to deliver a strong cancerocidal dose to the tumour mass (6000–8000 roentgens (R) and at point A, 20 mm lateral to the midline, 20 mm above the lateral fornix in the same sagittal plane as the uterus.
- Point B is 50 mm away from the midline at the same level and plane as the above and receives 25% of the dosage according to the inverse square law.
- External irradiation by linear accelerator should deliver 5000–7500 R to the pelvic nodes and side wall.
- There is considerable variation in policies and regimen, but the overall aim is the same.
- Hyperbaric oxygen improves local tumour control and surival of patients with carcinoma of cervix, particularly if the tumour is bulky.

Complications
- Post-treatment ischaemia of the pelvis involving the vagina, causing sexual dysfunction (85%).

- Vaginal stenosis can be reduced to 30% if vaginal oestrogen therapy is used from completion of therapy.
- Irradiation affects bladder — frequency and dysuria is common, bladder mucosa may develop, ulcer and rarely vesicovaginal fistula develop after 6 months or more.
- Intestinal complications may arise, varying from proctitis, constipation/diarrhoea and rectal fistulae.
- Early reactions are malaise, nausea, anorexia and diarrhoea; these usually subside.

Combined radiotherapy and surgery

- Three radium/caesium insertions can be carried out on days 0, 7 and 21.
- Radical Wertheim hysterectomy is performed 4 to 6 weeks after the insertion of radium or caesium.
- 2–4 weeks later, external radiation is given to lateral pelvic wall and lymph nodes.
- If invasive carcinoma is diagnosed following cone biopsy, it is advisable to wait for 6 weeks before surgery or radiotherapy is given to avoid higher incidence of complications.

Results

- Comparable results are obtained with radiotherapy and surgery.
- Five-year survival for stage I is 85–90%, and for stage II 70–75%.

Treatment of carcinoma of the cervix stages III and IV

- Choice is radiotherapy.
- Pelvic exenteration is applicable when radiotherapy is unlikely to be effective or radiotherapy has not been effective.
- Anterior exenteration is indicated if the bladder is involved — radical hysterectomy, lymph adenectomy and removal of bladder and construction of ileal bladder or implant ureter in the rectum.
- Posterior exenteration is indicated if the rectum is involved, which includes removal of the rectum and radical hysterectomy with lymph adenectomy.
- Total exenteration is indicated when bladder and rectum are involved.
- Extensive surgery is worthwhile only if there is some expectation of useful life.
- Not undertaken if there are extrapelvic metastases.
- Terminal colostomy and ileal loop bladder are to be preferred to a 'wet' colostomy.
- Five-year survival for stage III is 30–40% and for stage IV is around 10%.

Special problems

Pregnancy

— Incidence of carcinoma in pregnancy is 1 in 5000 pregnancies and about 0.5% of cancer of the cervix.

— Poses problems, especially if fetus is nearing viability (24–28 weeks).

— It is advisable to avoid terminating the pregnancy by dilatation of cervix and vaginal termination.

— Fetus is disregarded prior to 24 weeks and the disease is treated unless mother has refused.

— In the first trimester, alternatives are primary surgery and irradiation followed by surgery.

— In the second trimester up to 24 weeks, large size of the uterus renders irradiation more difficult. Wertheim's hysterectomy, followed by super-voltage therapy to the pelvis if necessary, if favoured.

— From 24 to 28 weeks onwards caesarean section, initially followed by radiotherapy, is the choice of treatment.

Stump carcinoma

— Lesion occurs in the cervix following sub-total hysterectomy.

— It is very rare.

— If the cancer appears within 12 months of the hysterectomy, the disease was most probably present at the time of surgery and carries a poor prognosis.

— After one year it is probably coincidental.

— Treatment can be surgery or radiotherapy.

— Laparoscopy first to exclude bowel adherent to the vault of vagina which probably contra-indicates radiotherapy.

Recurrent carcinoma of the cervix

— Usually recurs within 18 months.

— Main sites are:

- Deep pelvis

- Distant spread } common sites

- Lateral pelvis
- Bladder or rectum } less frequent
- Central pelvis

Signs and symptoms

— Renewed vaginal bleeding

— Pain

— Weight loss

— Urological symptoms

— Evidence of urinary tract obstruction

Treatment

— Radiotherapy, if it was not given before

— Exenteration surgery

— Palliative surgery
— Symptomatic treatment

Causes of death in cancer of the cervix
— Uraemia
— Cachexia
— Haemorrhage
— Complication of treatment

Adenocarcinoma of the cervix

— This tumour is rare.
— Tumours seem to grow and spread in a manner similar to squamous carcinoma.
— They generally respond to surgery and to radiotherapy.
— Treatment is in general as for squamous carcinoma.

Follow-up

— Detection of persistent or recurrent disease after primary treatment is very important.
— Follow-up is carried out by the specialist interested in oncology and radiotherapist together.
— Positive smear may identify the lesion if it is in the cervix or vault.
— Recurrence is frequently in the parametrial tissue, cardinal and uterosacral ligament.
— Patient is seen 2–3-monthly in the first year, 3-monthly in the second year, 4-monthly in the third year and 6-monthly until the fifth year, and annually thereafter.
— Chest radiotherapy and excretion urography are done when indicated.
— In persistent or recurrent disease, the treatment will depend on site and extent of the disease, previous treatment and general condition of the treatment.
— Disease outside the pelvis in the lung and bone, hydronephrosis, leg oedema and sciatic pain are ominous signs.
— In rare cases, a new primary tumour may arise in the irradiated field.
— Dysplastic cells from the vault warrant colposcopy and biopsy.

Sarcoma botryoides

— Rare tumour, usually occurs in childhood.
— It may appear like a grape or simple polyp.

— It is probably a mixed mesodermal tumour, but histological appearance is variable.

— Prognosis was poor in the past, but the introduction of triple chemotherapy (vincristine, actinomycin D and cyclophosphamide), radiotherapy and then extended hysterectomy and vaginectomy followed by further year of chemotherapy appear to be promising.

SUGGESTED READING

Burghardt E 1976 Premalignant conditions of the cervix. In: Langley F A (ed) Clinics in obstetrics and gynaecology, vol 3. Saunders, Philadelphia, p 257

Burghardt E 1984 Microinvasive carcinoma in gynaecological pathology. In: Fox H (ed) Clinics in obstetrics and gynaecology, vol 2. Saunders, Philadelphia, p 239

Coppleson M (ed) 1981 Gynecologic oncology: fundamental principles of clinical practice, vol 1. Churchill Livingstone, Edinburgh

Dewhurst J (ed) 1981. Integrated obstetrics and gynaecology for postgraduates, 3rd edn. Blackwell, Oxford

Duncan I 1981 The management of stage I carcinoma of the cervix. In: Studd J (ed) Progress in obstetrics and gynaecology, vol 1. Churchill Livingstone, Edinburgh, p 217

Jordan J A 1976 The diagnosis and management of premalignant conditions of the cervix. In: Langley F A (ed) Clinics in obstetrics and gynaecology, vol 3. Saunders, Philadelphia, p 295

Jordan J A 1980 The modern treatment of premalignant disease of the cervix. In: Controversies in gynaecological oncology. Proceedings of scientific meeting of the RCOG. Jordan J A, Singer A (eds) p 25

Jordan J A, Sharp F, Singer A (eds) 1981 Pre-clinical neoplasia of the cervix. Proceedings of the ninth study group of the RCOG.

Jordan J A 1982 The management of pre-malignant condition of the cervix. In: Studd J (ed) Progress in obstetrics and gynaecology, vol 2. Churchill Livingstone, Edinburgh, p 153

Stafl A (ed) 1983 Diagnosis and treatment of intra-epithelial cervical neoplasia. In: Clinical obstetrics and gynecology, vol 26. Harper & Row, New York, p 925

7. MALIGNANT DISEASE OF THE UTERUS

CARCINOMA OF THE ENDOMETRIUM AND SARCOMA OF THE UTERUS

Introduction

— For the past three decades, the incidence of carcinoma of the endometrium has increased and now almost equals that of carcinoma of the cervix.
— Of the over 50 million women over 35 years of age, about 700 000 will eventually develop endometrial carcinoma.
— Greater longevity, a high-fat diet, post-menopausal unopposed oestrogen replacement therapy have some association with the increase in the number of cases.
— It is the disease of mature women: most cases are diagnosed in the 50–65-year age group.
— Uterine sarcomas form a mixed group of tumours arising, at least in part, in mesodermal elements of the endometrium and myometrium.
— Sarcomas are rare but highly malignant and spread through the bloodstream.
— Presentation is similar to carcinoma, and difficult to diagnose early, since sarcomas are located deeply.

Carcinoma of the endometrium

— Incidence is approximately 20–30 per 100 000 new cases per year.
— Incidence increases as age advances, 40–50 per year at age 50.
— In developed countries with greater longevity the incidence may be 1 in 100.
— In some countries the ratio of the cancer of the body to that of the cervix is 1:1.
— Six per cent of the cancers in the female are accounted for by cancer of the body of the uterus and 6% by cancer of the cervix.

— The incidence is low before the age of 40 years, then rises until the age of 55 years, and then falls slightly.
— A greater proportion of women with endometrial carcinoma are post-menopausal than in carcinoma of the cervix.

Aetiology

Hyperoestrogenic status

— Conditions causing high oestrogen levels, such as feminising tumours of the ovary, polycystic ovarian disease, anovulatory status and unopposed oestrogen replacement therapy, are associated with increased incidence of endometrial cancer.
— Raised levels of oestrone or oestradiol are found in patients with endometrial carcinoma and hyperplasia.
— Endometrial carcinoma is rare in women without ovaries.
— There is a significant association with nulliparity and low parity, and this may be due to anovulatory cycles in some.

Obesity

— Androgen precursors from the adrenal gland are converted to oestrone in body fat.
— The rate of conversion is increased in obese women and after the menopause.
— Diabetic and hypertensive patients often fall into this category.

Pathogenesis

— Progesterone receptors in the breast respond much more readily after the stimulus of a pregnancy and lactation.
— Similar effects possibly apply to progesterone receptors in the endometrium, so that less progesterone is needed to offset the cell proliferative effect of oestrogen.
— Basement membrane in the epithelium of the endometrial gland is lacking; pre-invasion and the concept of invasion do not have the same significance.
— Consequently, cellular details are more important in the diagnosis of carcinoma of the endometrium.
— The relative infrequency before the menopause (20%) may be related in part to the monthly shedding of the endometrium.
— The carcinoma may arise in an area of endometrial hyperplasia; it then extends superficially and inwards to the deeper endometrium and myometrium.
— Lesion may be polypoid initially and often confined to the fundus; occasionally it may be diffuse and involve the whole endometrium.
— In rare cases a fungating adenocarcinomatous polyp may protrude through the cervix.
— Majority of lesions are adenocarcinomas.

— Some may show benign squamous metaplasia and are termed adeno-acanthomas.
— Adenosquamous lesions show malignant change in the squamous element (20%), are poorly differentiated and rapidly growing, and show deep myometrial invasion and early metastasis.
— In general, both lymphatic and blood spread can occur.
— A significant number are well differentiated, slow-growing, predictable type and have a better prognosis.
— Spread down to the cervix and deep into the myometrium significantly alters the prognosis and management.
— Majority of cases present with stage I disease.
— Passage of tumour cells along the tubal lumen into the peritoneal cavity is common.
— Vaginal metastasis is seen at follow-up if radiotherapy is not given.
— Lymphatic spread is mainly along the ovarian vessels to the para-aortic nodes.
— Pelvic lymph nodes are not involved unless the growth spreads to the cervix.
— The carcinoma rarely involves the inguinal lymph nodes via the round ligament.
— Spread may occur to pelvic structures such as the ovaries (5–40%) when the lower half of the body or the cervix is involved.
— Lymph nodes are involved in 10% in stage I disease, 35% in stage II.
— Nodes are involved in increasing number as the myometrial involvement is greater and decrease in the degree of differentiation.

Staging is clinical (FIGO, 1976)

— Clinical staging is less precise than that of cancer of the cervix.
— Staging considers the size of the uterus, palpable evidence of cancer extending beyond the serosal surface of the uterus, spread to the cervix shown by gross lesion or microscopic confirmation by biopsy after fractional curettage.
— Stage 0 — Atypical hyperplasia suspicious of malignancy (still controversial).
— Stage I — Carcinoma confined to the body of the uterus:
  • 1a — uterine cavity ≤ 80 m in length
  • 1b — uterine cavity > 80 m in length
  • Subdivisions
  • Grade 1 — well differentiated
  • Grade 2 — differentiated adenocarcinoma with partially solid areas

- Grade 3 — predominantly solid or entirely undifferentiated carcinoma
— Stage II — Carcinoma has involved the corpus and the cervix (10%). (Simultaneous presence of normal cervical glands and cancer in the same field will give the final diagnosis.)
— Stage III — Carcinoma has spread outside of the uterus but not outside the pelvis (10%).
— Stage IV — Carcinoma has extended outside the true pelvis, or has involved the mucosa of bladder, rectum or both (5%).
— Stage IVa — Spread of growth to adjacent organs.
— Stage IVb — Spread to distant organs.
— Major determinants of spread appear to be poor differentiation, deep penetration of the myometrium and involvement of the cervix.

Prognosis
— Depends on stage, degree of differentiation, depth of myometrial invasion, occult peritoneal involvement, age and general condition of the patient and pelvic node involvement.
— Node involvement lowers the 5-year survival to about 33% even in stage I disease.
— Efficacy of treatment.
— Overall 5-year survival is 60–80%.
— Prognosis is usually good in cancer induced by oestrogen since lesion is early, well-differentiated and rarely penetrates deeply into the myometrium.

Clinical features
— Usual age is 50–70 years.
— Irregular bleeding before menopause.
— Post-menopausal bleeding.
— Watery discharge, may become pink or brown.
— Symptoms related to anaemia due to prolonged bleeding.
— Patient is usually obese, nulliparous or with low parity.
— Tendency to be diabetic and hypertensive.
— Delayed menopause.
— Pain, low-grade fever, bowel or bladder disturbance occur late in the disease.
— There are no early characteristic symptoms.
— Abdominal and pelvic examination are unremarkable except in late cases.
— Speculum examination may reveal discharge of friable tissue or purulent discharge from the cervical os.
— Evidence of cervical or vaginal involvement or the presence of polypoid extension in the cervical canal.
— Uterine enlargement due to tumour growth or evidence of an adnexal mass occur late in the disease.
— Supraclavicular or inguinal node enlargement or the presence

of an abdominal mass are indicators of advanced stage in the disease.

Diagnosis: preclinical cancer

Cytology
- Endocervical and vaginal pool aspirates.
- Cervical scrape improves detection rate to 50–80% of endometrial cancer in post-menopausal women with bleeding.
- Investigation or cytological examination is rarely done in asymptomatic patients.
- Specimen may be obtained from the uterine cavity by the Gravlee-type jet washer or the Isaacs sampler, Barbaro technique of uterine lavage.
- Endometrial brush or other cytosampling technique.

Biopsy of the endometrium
- Curetting is ideal, vabra aspiration, Isaacs or Sherwood samplers may be used.
- If cavity is sampled adequately, it produces few false negative and false positive results.
- Patients at most risk are nulliparous and post-menopausal. It is difficult to obtain samples from obese women using cell samplers.
- If positive results are obtained from asymptomatic patients with early disease a hysterectomy offers an almost 100% cure.

Diagnosis: clinical cancer
- Examination under anaesthesia and fractional curettage should be performed on all patients with irregular and post-menopausal bleeding.
- Uterine size and adnexal pathology should be carefully evaluated.
- Uterine cavity is measured accuraterly using a graduated sound; risk of perforation is high.
- Lesion may be missed if uterine cavity is distorted by fibromyoma.
- Recurrent post-menopausal bleeding with negative curettage indicates a hysterectomy.
- Hysteroscopy and rarely hysterography may help to identify the lesion.
- Ultrasonography will be useful in identifying lesions in the cavity and in the adnexal areas.

Management

Pre-treatment work-up
- Routine history.
- Physical examination.
- Careful pelvic, rectal, recto–vaginal examination.

— Urine analysis.
— Chest X-ray.
— Excretion urography.
— Metastatic — X-ray studies.
— Proctoscopy–sigmoidoscopy if indicated.
— Lymphangiogram.
— Cystoscopy at the time of curettage.
— Barium enema and bone scan if indicated.
— Examination under anaesthesia, and fractional curettage and measurement of uterine cavity.
— Patient is staged accurately.
— Management will depend on the fitness of the patient for surgery, stage of the disease, especially spread to cervix and outside the uterus.
— The two commonly used methods are pre-operative radiation, either external therapy or intravaginal and intracavity, followed by hysterectomy or initial hysterectomy followed by external X-ray therapy and/or intravaginal radiotherapy.

Stage 0

— Depends on the fitness of the patient, her age and desire for future childbearing.
— In selected young patients, repeat curettage in 3 to 4 months after a course of progestational agents or induction of ovulation; in older patients total hysterectomy with conservation of ovaries or removal of ovaries depending on the age of the patient.

Stage Ia G1

— Total hysterectomy and bilateral salpingo-oophorectomy followed by post-operative vaginal radiation.

Stage Ia, G2, G3

— Some prefer external pelvic irradiation pre-operatively followed by total hysterectomy and bilateral salpingo-oophorectomy and post-operative vaginal irradiation.
— Some prefer surgery first, followed by external irradiation and vault radiation.
— Pre-operative radiotherapy may make histological grading of the tumour more difficult, and surgery too is made more difficult.
— If myometrial involvement is one-third or more of its thickness or more than 5 mm, post-operative external irradiation is indicated (if it is not given pre-operatively), followed by vaginal radiation.
— If histological grading is G2 or G3, external radiotherapy should be given post-operatively, followed by vaginal radiation.

Stage Ib

— Pre- or post-operative external irradiation, total hysterectomy and bilateral salpingo-oophorectomy, and post-operative vaginal radiation.

Stage II

— Pre-operative or post-operative external radiotherapy.
— Modified radical hysterectomy (Wertheim's hysterectomy).
— Post-operative vaginal radiation.
— Thirty-seven per cent have lymph node involvement.

Stage III

— If lesion involves only the adnexal structures.
— Pre-operative irradiation.
— Total hysterectomy and bilateral salpingo-oophorectomy.
— Post-operative vaginal irradiation.
— Modified radical hysterectomy may also be done at this stage.

Stage IV

— If spread is limited to the pelvis with bladder and/or rectal involvement.
— External irradiation, intra-uterine and intravaginal radium or caesium.
— Four to six weeks later surgery may be considered — exenteration, anterior or posterior or total, depending on the lesion.
— Distant metastasis:
  • Primary progestational therapy
  • Localised disease not responding to progestational therapy is treated with irradiation
  • Chemotherapy is tried in widespread disease.

Role of radiation therapy

— Adjunctive radiotherapy in a patient with stage Ia G1 disease does little to improve survival.
— Stages beyond Ia G1 disease benefit from radiotherapy — the 5-year survival rate is better.
— It is effective against morbidity and mortality associated with vault recurrence.
— Hence, post-operative vaginal irradiation in all stages is desirable.
— There is controversy regarding the relative effectiveness of pre-operative or post-operative external irradiation.
— The advantage of post-operative external X-ray therapy is that the specimen is available for complete evaluation.
— If the differentiation is poor, extent of myometrial invasion is deeper, spread of disease to the lower uterine segment or upper cervix demands more agressive external X-ray therapy.
— Where no invasion of the myometrium or less than 1 mm with localised disease to the fundus is probable, does not

need X-ray therapy unless the lesion is greater than 2 or 3.
— In the literature there is no evidence to suggest that pre-
  operative external X-ray therapy is more beneficial than post-
  operative external X-ray therapy.
— For localised disease, local radiation using radium, caesium
  or cobalt is adequate; if the tumour is outside the uterus,
  external beam therapy is indicated.

Post-operative irradiation
— Stage Ia G1 should be treated with total hysterectomy and
  bilateral salpingo-oophorectomy followed by vaginal
  irradiation.
— Stage Ia, G2 and G3 are treated with total hysterectomy and
  bilateral salpingo-oophorectomy followed by vaginal
  irradiation and external pelvic irradiation:
  • If myometrial involvement is one-third or more, patient
    will need irradiation despite G1 histological pattern.
— Stage Ib will need vaginal irradiation and external X-ray
  therapy following surgery.
— Stage II disease is ideally treated by a radical hysterectomy
  and pelvic node dissection, if possible followed by external
  X-ray therapy and vaginal irradiation.
— Stage III is treated with total hysterectomy and bilateral
  salpingo-oophorectomy, if possible followed by external X-ray
  therapy and vaginal irradiation.
— Stage IV is treated with surgery followed by radiotherapy to
  vaginal vault, pelvic side wall: progestational agents and
  chemotherapy may be added to the regimen.

Role of surgical treatment
— Total hysterectomy with salpingo-oophorectomy is the
  standard treatment for stage I. This procedure should
  involve, ideally, the upper one-third of the vagina to reduce
  the incidence of vault recurrence.
— Radical hysterectomy and pelvic lymphadenectomy with block
  dissection of parametrial tissue has limited application in the
  treatment of endometrial carcinoma.
— Radical hysterectomy with pelvic lymphadenectomy is
  indicated in young, fit patients with cancer extending to the
  endocervix.
— Patients are often older, obese, diabetic, hypertensive and
  arteriosclerotic and usually not ideal for radical surgery.
— Pelvic exenteration has little place in the management of
  endometrial cancer.

Role of hormonal therapy
— Kelly & Baker (1961) reported the use of 17α-
  hydroxyprogesterone caproate.
— It is recommended in the advanced stage of the disease.

— Drugs used are:
- 17α — hydroxyprogesterone caproate (150–1000 mg weekly i.m.)
- Medroxyprogesterone (400–800 mg weekly i.m.) or tablets daily (100–200 mg).
- Megestrol acetate (20–40 mg tablet).
- Tamoxifen (10–20 mg daily).

— Hormonal effects are mediated by complexes formed by interaction of the steroid and its receptors.
— Tumours that lack receptors are unresponsive to the hormone.
— Progesterone receptor levels are higher in well-differentiated endometrial cancer.
— Progestins lower the levels of oestrogen receptors in normal endometrium and in endometrial carcinoma.
— Anti-oestrogens such as tamoxifen, a non-steroidal drug, would block the proliferative stimulus of oestrogen.
— Tamoxifen would prevent the action of endogenous oestrogen by blocking its interaction with the receptors.

Role of chemotherapy

— In general, there is little room for chemotherapy.
— Patients are often not in ideal condition for chemotherapy.
— May be advocated in poorly differentiated endometrial carcinoma which does not respond to progestins.
— May be given to those who did not respond to surgery, irradiation and progestins.
— Drugs used are:
- 5-fluorouracil
- Cyclophosphamide
- Adriamycin
- Mitomycin
- Cis-platinum

— Drugs may be given singly or in combination.

Recurrent adenocarcinoma and its management

— Primary therapy is with progestational agents.
— Drugs are given in pharmacologic doses.
— Localised lesion may be treated with irradiation.
— Selected patients in good condition may benefit from exenteration operation.
— For distant metastasis, medroxyprogesterone acetate (Depo-Provera), 400 mg intramuscularly per day for 7 days then every 7 to 10 days for a longer period is given.
- 17α — hydroxyprogesterone caproate (Delalutin) 1250 mg is tried.

- Megastrolacetate (Megace) up to 40 mg three times daily.
— Chemotherapy may be tried; probably a combination of drugs is better than single agents.

Management of adenosquamous cancer

— Adenosquamous carcinoma adds a new dimension, not only in diagnosis but in therapy.
— Growth has both malignant-appearing glandular and squamous components.
— In 50% of cases the glandular component is prominent and in 50% the squamous component is prominent.
— Venous involvement is observed in 50%.
— Mean age at detection is 65.5 years.
— Duration of symptoms tends to be short.
— Abdominal and distant spread are common.
— These tumours respond poorly to irradiation.
— Treatment is total hysterectomy and bilateral salpingo-oophorectomy followed by chemotherapy if the disease is advanced.
— Five-year survival is 19–20%.

Summary

— More women are seeking medical examination, and endometrial carcinoma is starting to be identified under age 40 and in a few women in their twenties.
— Misinterpretation of some complex hyperplasias and metaplasias as carcinoma may exaggerate the number.
— Young people with endometrial carcinoma usually have either a chromosomal abnormality or a family history of cancers.
— Oestrogen stimulation after puberty, particularly unopposed by progesterone, and nulliparity are predisposing factors.
— Immunosuppression is associated with endometrial carcinoma in a young woman.
— Patients with polycystic ovarian disease, those who menstruate infrequently and have anovulatory cycles need careful follow-up.
— Less than 3% of endometrial carcinomas develop in woman under the age of 40 years.
— Most tumours are well-differentiated adenocarcinomas.
— Sequential oral contraceptives have been incriminated.
— Twenty per cent of endometrial carcinomas in childbearing age occur in women with Stein–Leventhal syndrome or polycystic ovarian disease.
— Younger patients need careful fractional curettage.

— If lesions are not frankly malignant, repeat the curettage after 4 months and decide further treatment.
— If the condition persists:
  • They need progestational agents
  • Or induction of ovulation
  • Then repeat the curettage.
— If condition is frankly malignant:
  • Will need definitive surgery
— Progesterone:
  • Causes endometrial sloughing
  • Diminishes the number of oestrogen receptors
  • Promotes the intracellular 17-β dehydrogenase which diminishes the endometrial cells' exposure to 17-β oestradiol
— Younger women need accurate diagnosis and careful follow-up.
— There are still problems to be solved regarding the most efficient approach to diagnosis and treatment of carcinoma of the endometrium.
— Increased awareness among the public and physicians has made it possible to pick up the lesion at an earlier stage than previously.
— Early recognition of women at high risk of developing endometrial cancer may reduce the mortality and morbidity associated with the lesion.
— Women on post-menopausal hormone replacement therapy need careful follow-up.
— Treatment is scaled to fit the needs of patient and the extent of disease.
— Five-year survival rates according to clinical stage are:
  • Stage I — 75–80%
  • Stage II — 55–60%
  • Stage III — 35–40%
  • Stage IV — 0–10%

SARCOMA OF THE UTERUS

— These are rare tumours.
— Malignant degeneration in a leiomyoma accounts for half of them.
— May arise from normal myometrial or endometrial stroma.
— Incidence is 1 in 100 000 females above the age of 20 years.
— Accounts for 3% of malignancies of the body of the uterus.
— There are three types: pure sarcoma, mixed sarcoma and mixed müllerian sarcoma.
— Pure sarcomas are composed of only one type of tissue (smooth muscle, connective tissue).

— Mixed sarcoma has two or more components:
  • May be homologus — tumour composed of elements
    normally present in the uterus
  • May be heterologous — tumour composed of elements
    foreign to uterus (cartilage, striated muscle)
— Müllerian mixed tumours have glandular and stromal
  components.
— As a result of the totipotential nature of the mesodermal
  cells, the sarcomatous element can be:
  • Striated muscle
  • Fat
  • Cartilage
  • Bone
  • Other mesenchymal tissue
— Endometrioid sarcoma is a newer name for stromal
  endometriosis, thought to arise in a focus of adenomyosis.
— The leiomyosarcoma is the commonest sarcoma which usually
  originates in smooth muscle cells, from a fibromyoma of the
  uterus.
  • The incidence of malignancy in fibromyoma is in the
    ranges 1 : 100–1 : 800.

Clinical features

— Presents as abnormal bleeding or spotting, or vaginal
  discharge.
— Pain, fever and abdominal mass may occur later.
— Passage of necrotic material vaginally is suspicious of this
  lesion.
— Distant metastases occur soon, most commonly in the lungs,
  liver, lymph nodes and bone.
— This lesion occurs mainly in the age group 45–75.
— Cervical lesion is more common in the reproductive age
  group.
— Vaginal lesion occurs most commonly in chilhood.

Diagnosis

— Cytological examination of material obtained from the uterine
  cavity as in the case of endometrial carcinoma.
— Uterine curettage may be helpful; deeper lesions may be
  missed.
— Rapid enlargement of the uterus in post-menopausal women
  is very suspicious.
— In view of rapid haematogenic spread to distant organs,
  screening of liver, bone and lungs is essential.

Prognosis

— Five-year survival rate differs in the three sub-groups.
— Usual survival ranges are 20–50%.
— Prognosis is poor if tumour has spread beyond the uterus.
— Mitotic rate more than 3 per high-power field, invasion of blood vessel, lymphatics and myometrium carries poor prognosis.
— Tumour arising from previously irradiated area also carries a poor prognosis.

Treatment

— Total hysterectomy and bilateral salpingo-oophorectomy.
— Radiotherapy is relatively ineffective.
— Adjuvant radiotherapy (50–60 Gy/5000–6000 rad) is of some value if tumour is localised to the pelvis.
— Radical chemotherapy may be worth trying as an adjuvant to surgery and/or radiotherapy.
— Leiomyosarcoma is usually resistant to radiotherapy and chemotherapy.

EMBRYONAL RHABDOMYOSARCOMA OF THE VAGINA

— Seen in infancy and childhood.
— It is a mixed mesodermal tumour arising from the cervix or uterine body or vagina.
— Presenting symptoms are offensive, purulent or bloodstained discharge or frank bleeding.
— Seen as a polypoid mass in the upper vagina, hence called sarcoma botryoides.
— Grape-like appearance is due to the marked increase in myxoid ground substance.
— Diagnosis is made by biopsy.
— Extent of the disease is assessed under general anaesthesia.
— Treatment involves exenteration with vaginectomy.
— Pre-operative chemotherapy and irradiation are given to reduce the extent of the surgery.

SUGGESTED READING

Anderson B 1982 Diagnosis and staging of endometrial carcinoma. In: Pitkin R M, Scott J R (eds) Clinical obstetrics and gynaecology. vol 25. p 75–92.
Barber R K H 1982 Management of carcinoma of the endometrium. In: Studd J (ed) Progress in obstetrics and gynaecology, vol 2. Churchill Livingstone, Edinburgh, p 111

Butler E B 1976 The early diagnosis of cancer of the endometrium. In: Langley F A (ed) Clinics in obstetrics and gynaecology. vol 3. Saunders, Philadelphia, p 389

Dewhurst J 1983 Botryoid sarcoma of the cervix and the vagina. In: Studd J (ed) Progress in obstetrics and gynaecology, vol 3. Churchill Livingstone, Edinburgh, p 151

Fox H 1976 The aetiology and pathology of endometrial cancer. In: Langley F A (ed) Clinics in obstetrics and gynaecology, vol 3, Saunders, Philadelphia, p 371

Kistner R W 1982 Treatment of hyperplasia and carcinoma in situ of the endometrium. In: Pitkin R M, Scott J R (eds) Clinical obstetrics and gynaecology, vol 25. p 63

Kolstad P 1982 Advances in the treatment of carcinoma of the cervix and corpus uterus. In: Bonner J (ed) Recent advances in obstetrics and gynaecology, vol 14. p 241

Mackay E V, Beischer N A, Cox L W, Wood C (eds) 1983 Illustrated textbook of gynaecology. Saunders, Philadelphia, p 424

Silverberg S G 1984 New aspects of endometrial carcinoma. In: Fox H (ed) Clinics in obstetrics and gynaecology, vol II p 189

Whitfield C R 1976 Treatment and prognosis of endometrial cancer. In: Langley F A (ed) Clinics in obstetrics and gynaecology, Saunders, Philadelphia, p 407

8. DISEASES OF THE MYOMETRIUM

MYOMA OF THE UTERUS

Introduction

— Common tumour of the uterus is the myoma.
— Twenty per cent of all women over 35 years of age have uterine myoma.
— They frequently have no symptoms.
— Higher incidence in black than in white women; the reasons for this are not known.
— Although the myoma arises from the muscular wall of the uterus, there is always some admixture of fibrous tissue, hence the term 'fibromyoma'.
— Fibromyoma causes problems mainly in childbearing age.
— It is rare before puberty, and usually undergoes atrophy after the menopause.

Incidence

— From autopsy and laparotomy data, 1 in 5 women have the lesion.
— The peak age incidence of symptoms is between 35 and 45 years.
— In Caucasian women the lesions are associated with nulliparity or relative infertility. This is not so in Negro women.

Aetiology

— Growth may be related to oestrogen stimulation, but the evidence is circumstantial.
— Restrictions to childbearing age suggest possible hormonal influence.

Pathology

— Although the initial growth commences in the myometrium (intramural), further extension occurs.
— Inwards to involve the uterine cavity (submucosal, 5%); when pedunculated, forms fibroid polyp.
— Outwards to involve the pelvic cavity (subserosal) when pedunculated moves freely in the pelvis.
— Within the broad ligament (intraligamentous or broad ligament type).
— They usually occur in multiples.
— Subserous pedunculated fibromyoma may get attached to the peritoneum or gut or omentum and may become parasitic myoma, usually rare.
— The location may be cervical or corporeal; the former is less common.
— On section tumour exhibits a trabeculated appearance due to intersection of smooth muscle by interlacing bands of connective tissue.
— There is no definite capsule but the tumour is usually sharply marked off from the surrounding uterine musculature by a pseudocapsule of light areolar tissue.
— Growth is slow and usually ceases after the menopause.

Clinical features

Fibroids can cause polycythaemia probably due to erythropoietin secretion of tumour

Submucous myoma

— Causes the most troublesome symptoms.
— Menorrhagia is common, because of abnormal vessels stretched over the surface and the increased surface area.
— Anaemia is common.
— Infection occurs because of the foreign body type of action, particularly if the myoma becomes submucous, pedunculated and approaches the cervical canal.
— Fibroid polyp produces discharge when infected and irregular bleeding when it is ulcerated.
— Dysmenorrhoea and pelvic pain are other symptoms.
— Large fibromyomatous polyp may present through the cervix and alarming haemorrhage can result.
— Uterine inversion can occur with large fibroid polyp arising from the fundus.
— Pressure symptoms related to urological system may occur.
— Infertility and recurrent abortion are other problems associated with submucous fibromyoma.

Intramural myoma

— May present as an abdominal mass.

— Often produces pressure symptoms, the nature of which
  depends on the site of the tumour in the uterus.
— There is always an associated enlargement of the uterine
  cavity.
— May be associated with menorrhagia and infertility.

Subserous myoma

— Usually asymptomatic.
— May present as an abdominal mass.
— Pedunculated fibroid may undergo torsion and patient may
  present with acute abdominal pain.
— Haemorrhage may occur inside the myoma.
— Haemorrhage may be severe and intraperitoneal if the
  surface vessel ruptures.

Cervical fibromyoma

— It is rare (1–3%).
— Produces early pressure effects, in the region of bladder
  neck, and produces dysuria, frequency and sometimes stress
  incontinence.
— Bleeding, infection, dyspareunia, infertility are other
  symptoms.
— Can cause dystocia in labour.

Complications

— Red degeneration:
  • Typically occurs in the second trimester of pregnancy due
    to ischaemic necrosis
  • Only a large tumour is involved
  • Pain is often severe
  • Conservative treatment is the rule
  • Myomectomy during pregnancy is strongly contra-indicated
    because of the risk of haemorrhage
— Other types of degeneration occur with chronic reduction in
  blood supply:
  • Hyaline degeneration
  • Cystic degeneration
  • Fatty degeneration
  • Myxomatous degeneration
  • Calcification
— Infection and suppuration of submucous fibroid may happen,
  especially following delivery.
— Acute retention, dysuria and repeated urinary tract infection
  may be the presenting symptom when a large fibroid is
  impacted in the pelvis.
— Pressure on the ureter may produce pyelitis hydroureter,
  hydronephrosis.

— Sacromatous changes can occur in the larger fibroid, the incidence being approximately 0.5%.
  • Rapid growth
  • Pain and pyrexia are the warning features
  • Differential diagnosis is benign cellular fibromyoma; mitotic rate, cellular atypia are differentiating features
— Leiomyomatosis is a rare condition in which a benign tumour invades vascular channels, sometimes spreading to inferior venacava or even to the right side of the heart. It is difficult to explain this condition.
— Benign metastasising leiomyomas are benign nodules in relation to peritoneal surfaces and omentum.
— Occasionally a subserous pedunculated fibroid may be associated with ascitis and pleural effusion.
— Pregnancy influences fibromyomas:
  • Rapid growth — red degeneration
— Fibromyoma influences the pregnancy, giving rise to the following problems:
  • Abortion — early pregnancy failure
  • Premature labour
  • Unstable lie
  • Obstructed labour
  • Higher operative delivery
  • Abnormal uterine activity   uterine inertia
  • Post-partum haemorrhage
  • Uterine inversions
  • Puerperal infection
— Rapid enlargement of fibromyoma in pregnancy is due to increased uterine vascularity.
— Tumour often decreases markedly in size after delivery.

Diagnosis

— Symptoms mentioned above, with uterine enlargement.
— Uterus is enlarged, firm, irregular, mobile.
— If the tumour is single, the enlargement is often uniform.
— Tumours do not move separately from the uterus unless they are pedunculated.
— The cervix is often displaced to one side or situated at a higher level.
— When the tumour is larger, difficulty arises in the diagnosis. It should be differentiated from an ovarian cyst, which is closely attached to the uterus.
— If it is an ovarian cyst, uterine cavity is regular and normal; cavity is enlarged and irregular if it is a fibroid.
— If the fibroid has undergone hyaline and myxomatous degeneration, it feels more like a pregnant uterus.

— Carcinoma of the uterine body must be excluded by curettage, especially if bleeding is irregular.
— Infected myoma should be differentiated from inflammatory mass.
— Adenomyoma may simulate the clinical picture of fibromyoma.
— Ultrasonography is useful in diagnosing ovarian cyst, fibromyoma, adenomyoma and inflammatory mass and pregnancy.
— Radiography of abdomen or hip joint may reveal an unsuspected calcified fibroid or pelvic mass.
— Hysterography and curettage may identify submucous fibroid.
— Laparoscopy will also reveal small or asymptomatic fibromyoma.

Treatment

— Anaemia may require correction by iron therapy, or, rarely, by blood transfusion.
— Infection needs treatment.
— The options are conservative management, myomectomy and hysterectomy.

Conservative approach

— This should be adopted when symptoms are absent or minimal.
— When tumours are small (less than 60–80 mm in diameter).
— When they are not of the submucous variety.
— Diagnosis is reasonably certain (ultrasound, laparoscopy).
— In pregnancy; no surgical treatment.
— In post-menopausal women with small fibroids not increasing in size.
— A check-up every three to six months and then yearly is advisable.
— Progestational or antiprostaglandin therapy or Danol may be of value in controlling bleeding if the patient is young or does not want the operation.

Myomectomy

— This should be done if childbearing is essential and the woman wishes to have more children.
— It should be done in those who are infertile.
— In those who refuse to have a hysterectomy but have troublesome symptoms.
— If the size of the uterus is bigger than that of a 12-week pregnancy.
— Complications are related to badly placed incision, poor

repair, accidental damage to the fallopian tubes, peritubal and peri-ovarian adhesions; they reduce fertility.
— Recurrence is common (5–20%).
— Infertile patients need explanation, counselling and to be told the chances of success following surgery.
— Other infertility factors should be excluded.
— Post-operative complications are higher following myomectomy.

Hysterectomy
— It should be done if childbearing is completed or not possible.
— If symptoms are severe.
— If the mass is of a considerable size.
— It causes less systemic upset than a myomectomy.
— Cervical fibroid, broad ligament fibroid cause technical problems at surgery. Ureter and bladder may be injured. This should be identified and rectified immediately.
— Hysterectomy is the definitive treatment.
— Ovaries are usually conserved.

Adenomyosis

This is described in Chapter 10.

Sarcoma of the uterus

This is described in Chapter 7.

SUGGESTED READING

Jones H W Jones S G (eds) 1980 Gynecology, 3rd edn. Williams and Wilkins, Baltimore, p 245
Mackay E V, Beischer N A, Cox L W, Wood C (eds) 1983 Illustrated textbook of gynaecology. Saunders, Philadelphia, p 331

9. DISORDERS OF THE OVARY

INTRODUCTION

— Functional and other non-neoplastic cysts such as endometriomas are common and restricted to childbearing periods.
— Symptoms are related to mechanical effects of the enlarging tumour, special endocrine effects and the presence of complications.
— Malignant tumours are rare in infancy and childhood, more common during the childbearing period, and the incidence increases sharply in the peri- and post-menopausal period.

NON-NEOPLASTIC DISTENSION CYSTS

Follicular and luteal cysts

— These are usually due to excessive pituitary stimulation.
— This in turn produces multiple follicles.
— One follicle unduly sensitive to this stimulus produces a large amount of follicular fluid and fails to rupture.
— A cyst usually measures 50–60 mm in width.
— Overdosage or hypersensitivity to clomiphene or HMG produces bigger follicular cysts.
— A cyst tends to regress spontaneously within a few weeks or, at the latest, 3 months.
— Corpus luteum may become a luteal cyst as a result of excessive haemorrhage into the cavity which remains after ovulation.
— Excessive stimulus from pituitary luteinising hormone or excessive HCG from trophoblastic tissue produce similar lutein cysts.
— These usually regress within a few weeks, or occasionally months (usually three months)

Clinical features
— Usually asymptomatic.
— Pain, usually mild but sometimes severe, is due to rupture of, or haemorrhage into, the cyst.
— May produce urological symptoms such as frequency and dysuria from irritation by the bloodstained fluid.
— Differential diagnoses are ectopic pregnancy, urinary tract infection and appendicitis.

Management
— If ovarian enlargement is detected at pelvic examination and the cyst is 40–60 mm in diameter, no action is necessary if it was considered as functional and non-neoplastic.
— Re-examination in a few weeks' time confirms spontaneous regression if it is a functional cyst.
— If cyst is unchanged, or larger at the end of two months, further investigation such as laparoscopy is necessary.
— At laparoscopy, if the cyst is confirmed, it may be aspirated and the aspirate is sent for cytology.
— Ultrasonography may be useful to assess the follow-up.
— Laparotomy is seldom necessary if the condition is a functional cyst.
— Treatment of any underlying condition.

Theca-lutein cysts

— A corpus luteum becomes cystic and persists in a functional state for longer than the normal period.
— Or the granulosa and theca cells of a follicular cyst become luteinised.
— Or it may be due to stimulation of atretic follicles by abnormally high blood levels of HCG as in trophoblastic disease.
— Ovaries are polycystic and may measure up to 150 mm.
— This condition is usually associated with trophoblastic disease, but also occurs when there is hyperplacentosis, as in:
  • Diabetes mellitus
  • Erythroblastosis fetalis
  • Multiple pregnancy
  • Large fetus
— Condition is similar to the hyperstimulation syndrome when polycystic ovarian enlargement occurs when clomiphene and HMG are given.
— Characteristically, short periods of amenorrhoea are followed by heavier than usual uterine bleeding.
— The endometrium shows a secretory pattern.
— Haemorrhage into the cyst mimics symptoms of ectopic pregnancy.

Management
— Spontaneous regression is usual.
— Very seldom surgical interference is needed; if haemorrhage continues from a ruptured cyst, this is seen at laparoscopy.

Endometriotic cysts

— Involvement of the ovary by endometriosis may occasionally result in considerable enlargement of the cyst, up to 100–120 mm.
— The disease is part of a more general involvement of the pelvic organs by endometriosis.
— Signs and symptoms are characteristic.
— Treatment is described in Chapter 10.

OVARIAN NEOPLASMS

Benign tumours

Cystic teratoma (dermoid cysts).
— It is the commonest benign cystic neoplasm.
— Occurs at all ages, but is more common during the reproductive period and in the first three decades.
— Eighty per cent or so occur in the reproductive age group.
— Elements of all three germ cell layers may be present.
— Those from the ectoderm, such as hair, sebaceous material and teeth are predominant.
— Nervous tissue, often well differentiated, may be seen.
— Occasionally only a single tissue, such as thyroid gland, may be predominant.
— Cysts are rarely larger than 200 mm, smooth-walled, mobile, mostly unilocular, usually have a solid area, the papilla, from which the formed elements arise.
— Bilateral in 10–20% of cases; the contralateral tumour may be small and may be missed.
— Torsion occurs in 5–10%.
— Rupture is uncommon; if it occurs, it produces intense peritoneal reaction due to the irritating nature of the contents of the cyst.
— May cause pressure symptoms or pelvic discomfort.
— Differential diagnosis:
  • Other ovarian and par ovarian cysts
  • Hydrosalpinx
  • Mesenteric cyst
  • Renal cyst

- Pelvic kidney
- Retroperitoneal tumours
- Degenerating fibromyoma
- Full bladder
- Prolapsed caecum
- Loaded colon
— Investigation:
  - Radiography may show teeth and calcification
  - Ultrasonography

Treatment

— Surgical removal.
— Usually cystectomy and reconstruction of the remaining ovary.
— Bisection of the opposite ovary to exclude a similar tumour is essential.

Benign epithelial cysts (cystadenoma)

— There are three types, based on the histology of the lining epithelium and the content:
  - Serous cyst has lining similar to fallopian epithelium
  - Endometrioid cyst has lining similar to endometrium
  - Mucinous cyst has lining similar to cervical epithelium
— Epithelial cysts and tumours are thought to arise from the surface epithelium of the ovary by metaplasia.
— Seen commonly after the age of 20–25 years.
— Usually multilocular; occasionally may be unilocular.
— Mucinous cystadenoma can attain a large size to fill the whole abdomen.
— Signs and symptoms are related to the size and pressure on abdominal contents.
— Pressure symptoms are haemorrhoids, peripheral oedema, varicose veins, dyspnoea, bowel and urinary pressure symptoms.
— Cysts are usually thin-walled, tense, mobile and non-tender.
— Serous cyst adenoma is more common than mucinous cystadenoma, which is more common than endometrioid.
— Mucinous cyst is usually multilocular and contains thick viscid contents.
— Serous cyst is often unilocular or contains few loculi; contents are watery; cysts are nearly always papilliferous and more likely to be bilateral.
— Patients usually present with abdominal mass, or with pressure symptoms or with symptoms of complication such as torsion, haemorrhage or, rarely, rupture.
— Cysts may undergo malignant change.

Treatment

— In the younger age group, if childbearing is required, the

treatment is conservative surgery, cystectomy; other ovary needs to be checked.
— If the woman is near the end of childbearing age, or has completed her family, then salpingo-oophorectomy is performed if the cyst is unilateral; if bilateral, bilateral salpingo-oophorectomy and removal of uterus.

Benign solid tumours
— They are: fibroma and Brenner tumour.
— Fairly rare tumours.
— Fibroma has a firm, whorled, white appearance on cut surface and rarely shows signs of degeneration.
— These tumours are rarely associated with ascitis and hydrothorax (Meig's syndrome).
— Brenner tumour is similar in appearance to fibroma.
— They have greyer or yellowish tint on cut section.
— The diagnosis is usually made on histological examination; Brenner tumour contains islands of clear cuboidal cells called Walthard cell nests.
— Brenner tumour may be seen in association with mucinous cyst adenoma.
— Solid epithelial tumours are derived from ovarian surface epithelium; they take the form of adenoma or papilloma; they are called adenofibroma when there is significant stromal element present and cystadenofibroma when a cystic change is present.

Parovarian cyst
— This originates from a remnant epoophoron or paroophoron of the cranial end of the mesonephric duct, which in the female atrophies during early embryonic life.
— Cyst is situated between the layers of broad ligament.
— It may reach up to 200 m or, rarely, a greater size.
— It is usually unilocular and contains a clear watery fluid.
— Cyst usually displaces the uterus to the opposite side.
— It is usually not mobile and not tender.
— Treatment is surgical removal, and often the fallopian tube is removed with it, since the fallopian tube stretches over and is difficult to save.

Summary

Size
— It is of some help in differentiating between functional cysts and benign tumours.
— Functional cysts are rarely bigger than 60–80 mm.
— A very large tumour filling the whole abdomen is often benign.

— Ultrasonography is useful in identifying the nature of the cyst. If it shows solid areas, it is suspicious of malignancy.

Mobility

— The degree of mobility will not necessarily exclude malignancy.
— Malignant tummours are often fixed and not mobile.
— After hysterectomy, if tumour develops from the ovary it may grow into the broad ligament and is less likely to be mobile.

Bilaterality

— In 15–20% cases, benign tumours are bilateral.
— More commonly cystic teratoma and serous cystadenoma present in both ovaries.
— Benign solid tumours are often unilateral.
— Unilateral solid tumour is often suspicious of malignant tumour, either primary or secondary.

Malignant potential

— Functional tumours almost never become malignant.
— Benign solid tumours and endometriotic cysts almost never undergo malignant change.
— With benign cystic teratoma the risk is 0.5–1%.
— Malignant potential is higher in epithelial cysts, especially serous cyst adenoma.

Diagnosis

— Benign tumours are easily palpable bimanually.
— Pain caused by complications such as haemorrhage, torsion or, rarely, infection makes examination difficult.
— Retroverted uterus ofen poses problems in inexperienced hands.
— There is a distinct tendency for some tumours to occur in specific age groups.
— In infancy and childhood the ratio of benign to malignant tumours is about 3 : 2; the former comprise largely simple cysts and cystic teratomas.
— Functional cysts present after puberty.
— Cystadenomas are more common after the age of 25 years or so.
— The commonest tumours during childbearing years are cystic teratoma, mucinous cystadenoma, luteal cysts and serous cystadenoma.
— The usual ratio of benign to malignant tumours in the reproductive phase is approximately 20:1.
— Endometriotic and functional cysts are uncommon after the menopause.

— Peri- and post-menopausal age groups have a higher incidence of malignant tumours.
— Specialised mesenchymal tumours occurs at any age.
— Presence of ascitis, especially bloodstained, is often suggestive of malignant tumour.
— Diagnosis depends on history, clinical findings and use of investigations.
— Ultrasound may be helpful in differentiating benign and malignant tumours; multiloculation, thick septa, presence of solid areas, complex architecture, fixation and disruption of capsule are highly suspicious of malignancy.
— Differential diagnosis of adnexal masses:
  • Uterine and ligamentous fibromyoma
  • Tubal carcinoma
  • Carcinoma of sigmoid caecum
  • Retroperitoneal tumour
  • Hydro/pyosalpinx
  • Diverticulitis
  • Parovarian cyst
  • Prolapsed caecum
  • Loaded sigmoid colon
  • Pelvic kidney
  • Uterine abnormality
  • Urachal cyst

MALIGNANT TUMOURS OF THE OVARIES

— Ovarian tumours are second in frequency to those of the uterus.
— Ovarian malignancy is responsible for more cancer deaths, because the tumour is often well advanced and widely spread at the time of clinical presentation.
— The malignant potential of ovarian tumours is extremely variable, and this makes treatment and prognosis unpredictable and difficult.

Incidence

— Ovarian cancer is a disease of middle- and upper-class women that occurs primarily in the highly industrialised countries, thus postulating industrial chemicals as a possible cause.
— Incidence is higher in the affluent industrialised countries: Sweden 12 per 100 000, Norway 16 per 100 000, USA white 15 per 100 000, UK 14 per 100 000, Israel 11 per 100 000,

USA black 5 per 100 000, Africa 4 per 100 000, India 3 per
100 000 and Japan 3 per 100 000.
— Japanese women living in the USA have a similar incidence
  to USA women, and this suggests the possible role of
  industrial chemicals in the development of ovarian cancer.
— Asbestos and talc are possible chemical products.
— Ovarian cancer comprises 5% of all female cancers and
  20–25% of genital tract cancers.
— Approximately 1 in 60 (1.4%) of all females will develop it,
  two-thirds of whom will die from their malignancy.
— The incidence rises rapidly after the age of 40 years.
— 20% of ovarian neoplasms are malignant.
— The ratio rises sharply after the age of 40.
— In women over the age of 50 years or more, 50% of tumours
  or more are malignant.

Aetiology

— The ovaries are subject to repetitive hormonal stimulus
  during the reproductive years, and this effect may be a basis
  of some ovarian cancers.
— Suppression of ovarian activity in pregnancy, in the
  puerperium and the use of combined oral contraceptive pills
  is associated with decreased incidence.
— Tumours are more common in the nulliparous and to a lesser
  extent in women bearing children late in life.
— There has been some association with talcum powder and
  asbestos in the past.
— These tumours are more common in industrialised countries.
— Previous history of mumps parotitis is associated with a
  lower incidence of ovarian cancer.
— Higher incidence is noted when there is breast and
  endometrial cancer.
— Ovary follows breast and colon as the commonest site for
  fatal malignant disease in the female.
— The mortality of women in social class I tends to be twice as
  high as that of women in social class V.

Pathology

— In the primitive urogenital ridge, the developing ovary (which
  consists of surface epithelium, germ cells and supporting
  cells) lies in a close relationship to the müllerian,
  mesonephric and adrenal primordia.
— The origin and subtype of malignant tumours are complex.
— There are three groups of cells which give rise to vast
  majority of primary ovarian tumours (Table 9.1):
  • Epithelial tumours

Table 9.1

Cell of origin	Derived tumours	Age group	Frequency	Malignancy
Primary carcinoma Surface epithelium tumours	Serous, mucinous endometrioid Clear cell (mesonephroid) Brenner (transitional cell) Mixed epithelial tumours Mixed mesodermal Undifferentiated carcinoma Unclassified epithelium tumours	Usually after 30 years	Common after 40 years (60–70%)	Variable Often high
Specialised mesenchyme or stromal or sexcord tumours	Granulosa cell Theca cell (thecoma) Fibroma **Sertoli cell tumour** Sertoli-Leydig tumour (androblastoma) Lipid cell tumours Leydig cell tumour Hilus cell tumour Unclassified Gynandroblastoma	Any age usually mature age	Uncommon (5–10%)	Variable Usually low
Germ cell tumours	Dysgerminoma Embryonal carcinoma Endodermal sinus (yolk sac) tumour Choriocarcinoma Gonadoblastoma Teratomas Immature Mature cystic (dermoid) Mature solid Monodermal — stroma ovarii — carcinoid — other	Any age common (15–25 years) Immature Teratoma (6–12 years)	Uncommon (15–20%)	Variable Often high
Non-specialised mesenchyme tumour	Sarcoma	Usually after 40	Rare (<1%)	Often high
Soft-tissue tumours not specific to ovaries Lymphoma/leukaemia Unclassified tumours	—	Usually after 40	Rare	Variable Often high
Secondary carcinoma Colon, stomach, uterus, pancreas, breast, cervix	—	Late reproductive and post-menopausal	Rare (3–5%)	Usually high

- Sexcord — stromal — specialised mesenchymal cell tumours
- Germ cell tumours

— Before puberty, both benign and malignant tumours are found, the former being largely cystic teratomas.
— In the reproductive age, malignant tumours are less than 5%.
— After the age of 40 years the incidence of malignant ovarian tumours increases significantly.
— Malignant tumours derived from the surface epithelium far outnumber the other types in late reproductive age and post-menopausal years:
  - Serous cystadenoma — 50%
  - Endometrioid and mucinous type — 15–20%.
  - Clear cell (mesonephroid) — 5%.
  - Undifferentiated — 10–15%.
— Mucinous cystadenocarcinoma is more common in older patients.

Mesenchymal tumour

— Tumours of the specialised mesenchymal group and germ cell tumours often have complicated mixed histological features.
— The malignant potency of the stromal cell tumour depends on the cell type. Granulosa cell tumours, with or without theca cell component, are the commonest neoplasm, and 15% of these are malignant.
— Thecomas are less common and usually benign.
— Thecomas and granulosa cell tumours produce oestrogen, the effect of which is precocious puberty in the very young and endometrial hyperplasia or adenocarcinoma of the endometrium and post-menopausal bleeding in the older age group.
— The androblastoma (Sertoli-Leydig tumours) cause virilisation following defeminisation; they are the least common and of low-grade malignancy.
— Gynandroblastoma is composed of primitive mesenchymal cells of both female and male derivation:
  - Granulosa and Sertoli and Leydig elements

Germ cell tumour

— Dysgerminoma; tends to occur in young women:
  - In those approximately 20 years old
  - Bilateral in 15%
  - Spreads by lymphatics
  - It is the counterpart of the seminoma in males

- Rare tumour
- Treated by conservative surgery
- It is very radiosensitive

— Gonadoblastoma tends to occur in patients with chromosomal abnormalities or congenital anomalies of the genital tract.
— Teratomas arise from embryonic structures:
  - Benign teratoma consists of mature tissue — dermoid cyst
  - Malignant teratoma consists of immature tissues — teratocarcinoma
— Extra-embryonic germ cell tumours are choriocarcinoma and endodermal sinus tumour:
  - These tumours produce pregnancy-associated plasma proteins
  - Choriocarcinoma — produces HCG and HPL to a lesser extent
  - Yolk sac tumour — produces AFP
  - These can be used as tumour markers in diagnosis and follow-up after treatment
  - Malignant tumours from germ cells had a bad prognosis in the past
  - Chemotherapy using vincristine, actinomycin-D and cyclophosphamide (VAC) are producing better results

Surface epithelial tumours

— These mimic tissues derived from the müllerian or paramesonephric duct.
— Serous cystadenocarcinoma is the malignant counterpart of serous cystadenoma.
— These tumours account for 10% of ovarian neoplasms.
— They are bilateral in about 50% of cases.
— Usually unilocular, with a smooth outer surface.
— The internal papilllae may sprout through the capsule, giving an impression of malignancy.
— The lining cells are cuboidal or columnar, resembling the epithelium of the endosalpinx.
— Mucinous cyst adenocarcinoma is the counterpart of the mucinous cyst adenoma.
— They form 30% to 40% of ovarian neoplasms.
— They are often very large, unilateral or multilocular.
— They are lined by tall columnar mucus-secreting cells.
— They may be found along with Brenner's tumour.
— If the cyst ruptures, the mucus-secreting cells may implant in the peritoneum and produce pseudomyxoma peritonei.
— Endometrioid tumours are often solid tumours.
— They frequently contain elements of serous and mucinous tumours.

— The condition usually carries a good prognosis.
— There is some association with endometrial carcinoma.

Staging of ovarian cancer

Stage I   Growth limited to the ovaries.
    1a   Growth limited to one ovary; no ascitis.
        i. No tumour on the external surface; capsule intact.
        ii. Tumour present on the external surface and/or capsule ruptured.
    Ib   Growth limited to both ovaries; no ascitis.
    Ic   Ia or Ib with ascitis or tumour cells in peritoneal washings.
Stage II   Growth involving one or both ovaries with pelvic extension.
Stage IIa   Involves uterus and/or fallopian tubes.
    IIb   Extension to other pelvic tissues.
    IIc   Same as IIa or IIb with ascitis or tumour cells in peritoneal washings.
Stage III   Growth involves one or both ovaries with:
- Intraperitoneal metastasis outside the pelvis
- Or positive retroperitoneal nodes, or both
- Tumour limited to the true pelvis with histologically proved extension to small bowel or omentum

Stage IV   Growth involving one or both ovaries:
- With distant metastasis
- Pleural fluid containing malignant cells
- Parenchymal liver metastasis

Growth patterns

— Ovarian malignancy is discrete until it reaches 80–100 mm in size.
— Spread is much commoner if the tumour is larger than 100 mm.
— Local spread occurs to tubes, uterus, broad ligament.
— Regional spread occurs to bladder, rectum, sigmoid colon, pelvic side wall and pelvic peritoneum.
— Abdominal spread involves omentum, bowel mesentery, liver and diaphragm.
— Lymphatic spread occurs to the para-aortic nodes and supraclavicular lymph nodes.
— Extra-abdominal spread is rare and very late, and involves lungs and bone.

Clinical features

— Early symptoms of ovarian carcinoma are rarely characteristic except for those tumours producing hormones.

— The peak age incidence is between 40 and 60 years, with the exception of teratomas and mesenchymal tumours which occur at any age.
— They are often found accidentally.
— The disease has often spread beyond the ovary before the diagnosis is made.
— Common complaint is an ache or discomfort in the lower abdomen or pelvis.
— Non-specific symptoms of digestive tract such as epigastric discomfort and feeling of indigestion or dyspepsia are common.
— Pressure symptoms related to bladder and bowel may be present.
— Dyspareunia and dysmenorrhoea.
— Abdominal swelling due to tumour and/or ascitis, often ignored by the patient.
— Thrombo-embolism and leg swelling are bad prognostic signs.
— Weight loss when disease is advanced.
— Menstrual function is not usually affected except by the hormone-producing tumours.
— Symptoms related to secondaries in the liver, lymph nodes and lungs.

Diagnosis

Examination

— If ovary is easily palpable, it needs further investigation.
— Abdominal and combined recto-vaginal examination.
— Site, size, contour, consistency and mobility of lesion should be assessed.
— Restricted mobility and absence of pain are suspicious of malignancy.
— Presence of ascitis.
— Enlargement of abdominal and supraclavicular lymph nodes is an ominous sign.
— Liver enlargement.
— Multiple masses may be felt in the omentum.
— Bilateral ovarian enlargement.
— Ovarian malignancy should be suspected if ovarian lesion is found outside the reproductive age group, solid mass, persistent cystic lesion for more than 3 months and size bigger than 60 –80 mm.

Investigation

— Vaginal cytology may reveal cancer cells in 15–20% of patients.
— Oestrogen levels may be elevated in oestrogen-producing tumours.

— Ultrasound examination may reveal:
  • Presence of multilocular cyst
  • Thick septa
  • Solid areas
  • Attachment to surrounding organs
  • Ascitis
  • Bilateral tumours
  • Liver metastasis
  • Involvement of ureters — hydroureter/pelvis
— Radiography:
  • Chest radiography may reveal hydrothorax and metastasis
  • Assessment of urinary tract and function — intravenous pyelography
  • Bowel by barium study
  • Abdomen may reveal mass, teeth and bone in the mass
  • Lymphangiography is helpful in detecting involved para-aortic nodes
  • Computerised tomography may be of use in the interpretation of abdominal mass
— Laparoscopy may be useful if the mass is small and can also get peritoneal washing for cytology.
— Diagnostic curettage if there is abnormal bleeding.
— Tumour markers:
  • Carcinoembryonic antigen (CEA) is a glycoprotein which is found in the tumour and serum of patients with ovarian malignancy
  • CEA levels were higher in cases of ovarian malignancy and increase with stage of the disease
  • α-Fetoprotein (AFP) is a glycoprotein, found in higher concentrations in teratocarcinoma of the ovary
  • Presence of AFP is found in all ovarian endodermal sinus tumours and in a high percentage of embryonal cell carcinoma of the ovary
  • Carcinoplacental proteins are glycoproteins. Levels are low in epithelial ovarian cancer but a higher level of β-HCG was found in embryonal cell carcinoma and carcinosarcoma of the ovary, and this may be a useful marker in dysgerminoma
  • Human placental lactogen is a polypeptide hormone, found in choriocarcinoma
  • Clinically useful markers in ovarian cancer:
    Choriocarcinoma — HCG
    Dysgerminoma — HCG
    Embryonal cell carcinoma — AFP, HCG
    Endodermal sinus tumour — AFP
    Serous cystadenocarcinoma — OCA, OCAA
    Mucinous cystadenocarcinoma — CEA, OCA, OCAA

(OCAA — ovarian cystadenocarcinoma antigen;
OCA — ovarian cancer antigen)

Differential diagnosis

— Physiological — full blader, loaded colon, pregnancy.
— Congenital — uterine anomaly, pelvic kidney.
— Infective — pyo/hydro salpinx, pelvic abscess, appendicular abscess, diverticulitis, tuberculous peritonitis.
— Neoplastic–fibroid — tumours of colon and rectum, ascitis, retroperitoneal tumour, mesenteric cyst.
— Hormonal — functional cysts of the ovaries.
— Mechanical — hydronephrosis, chronically distended bladder.
— Endometriosis.
— Pregnancy-assocaited — Pregnancy in a uterine horn, chronic ectopic pregnancy, corpus luteum of pregnancy.
— Secondary in the ovaries — from uterine body, stomach, colon, breast.

Management

Prophylaxis

— Careful palpation of ovaries yearly at the annual gynaecological check-up
— Screening using ultrasound may be useful.
— Clamping the pedicle instead of untwisting the pedicle in a twisted ovarian cyst which was suspected to be malignant.

Treatment

— No organ in the body gives rise to as many different histological types of neoplasm as the ovary.
— The vast majority of ovarian cancers (80–90%) are epithelial in origin.
— The stage and histological grading of the malignancy are more prognostic indicators than the type of tumour.

Primary treatment (surgery)

— Adequate pre-operative assessment
— Accurate assessment of stage at laparotomy
— Removal of uterus, tubes, ovaries and omentum
— If ascitis is present, fluid is sent for cytology
— If no ascitis, saline wash of peritoneal cavity for cytology
— Multiple biopsies from mesentery, paracolic gutter, under-surface of diaphragm, and suspicious areas of peritoneum and lymph nodes
— Assessment of liver substance and surface
— For stage I carcinoma of the ovary, total hysterectomy, bilateral salpingo-oophorectomy and omentectomy.

— Simple salpingo-oophorectomy or oophorectomy may be indicated:
  • For younger women with stage Ia disease
  • And favourable histology on frozen section
  • Who wish to preserve their reproductive function
  • And who fully understand the implications
  • Justified if the tumour is a low-grade mucinous cystadenocarcinoma
  • The opposite ovary is biopsided and normal
  • Conservative management is attempted in the younger age group if the tumour is of epithelial origin and low-grade malignancy
  • Once the family is complete, definitive surgery should be considered
— If the disease is advanced, reduction in tumour bulk is advisable which make adjuvant therapy more effective.

Adjuvant therapy
— This includes:
  • External beam irradiation
  • Intraperitoneal instillation of radio isotopes
  • Systemic chemotherapy
  • Immunotherapy
— Adjuvant therapy is not indicated for stage I disease unless:
  • The tumour is poorly differentiated
  • Ascitis was present with positive cytology
  • The cyst was ruptured
— External irradiation
  • All epithelial cancers have the same radiosensitivity, provided the volume of the tumour is the same
  • The whole abdomen and pelvis need irradiation
  • Irradiation to abdomen is limited by the tolerance of the small bowel
  • Therapy is ideal for small tumour nodules and not for bulky extensive residual disease
  • Irradiation of the abdomen is accomplished with mega-voltage units such as the CO^{60} unit or the linear accelerator delivering 30 Gy (3000 rad) to the whole abdomen, with an additional 20 Gy (2000 rad) to the pelvis, a process which takes between 5 and 6 weeks
— The capacity for radiation therapy to eradicate a neoplasm depends chiefly on the volume of the cancer and the oxygenation of the tumour bed.
  • The 5 year survival rate is 57.1% if there was no residual disease
  • 27.5% survival rate if tumour nodule is less than 20 mm
  • 17.2% for nodules between 20 mm and 40 mm
  • 0% for tumour nodules 60 mm or larger

— Complications of radiotherapy may be immediate or delayed:
  • Anorexia, nausea, vomiting, diarrhoea and fatigue
  • Severe gastro-intestinal symptoms may force interruption of treatment
  • Late complications involve the small bowel, include partial or complete obstruction 6 to 18 months following radiation
  • May need resection of bowel and bypass
  • If surgery is delayed, perforation might occur, which is often fatal.
— Radioisotopes:
  • Intraperitoneal instillation of radioisotopes using zinc (Zn^{63}) yttrium (Y^{90}) chromic phosphate ($CrP^{32}O^4$) and gold (Au^{198}) are tried
  • Now only gold and chromic phosphate are used
  • The indication is in stage I cancer which ruptured and spilled malignant cells into the peritoneal cavity
  • Patients with gross residual disease are not suitable for this treatment because the maximum effective tissue penetration of the beta radiation is 3.8 mm
  • Intraperitoneal Au^{198} has been associated with complications and is replaced by chromic phosphate
  • Peritonitis, bowel destruction and fistula formation are related to the gamma emission and to the short half-life of Au^{198} which results in a higher rate of irradiation
  • Radioactive gold has a half-life of 2.7 days with 90% of radiation emitted as beta particles and 10% as gamma radiation
  • Chromic phosphate has a half-life of 14.3 days and emits only beta particles
  • Distant metastasis, large bulk of tumour and parenchymal disease of liver are contra-indication for this therapy
— Chemotherapy:
  • Patients with bulky residual disease following surgery for ovarian cancer will benefit from chemotherapy
  • Single-agent chemotherapy is in general as effective as multiple-agent treatment
  • Alkylating agents such as chlorambucil, melphalan or cyclophosphamide can be used
  • Melphalan is effective in the management of epithelial cancers (1 mg/kg body weight divided over 5 consecutive days every 4 weeks for 12 months). Bone marrow suppression is the major problem, and the drug is usually well tolerated
  • Newer agents such as cis-platinum and JM 8 have been tried, and the results are encouraging
  • The exact method of action of platinum is unknown but some of its effects are similar to the alkylating agents

- Dosage varies from 50 mg to 120 mg/m^2 of body surface area, either singly or in combination given at an intravenous infusion rate of 1 mg a minute
  i. Renal toxicity is the major limiting factor
  ii. Prior to administration of platinum, a rapid infusion of dextrose 5% in water should be given with a mannitol diuresis
  iii. Serum creatinine level should be assayed prior to treatment.
  iv. Dose of platinum should be reduced if the creatinine rises above 1.8 mg
  v. Treatment is given once a month
  vi. Treatment could be given for a long time if bone marrow and kidney functions are normal
  vii. JM8 has lower nephrotoxicity
— Cis-platinum 50 mg/m^2 along with Adriamycin 50 mg/m^2, repeated every 3 to 4 weeks for 10 consecutive courses, are used in some centres
  - Cardiac toxicity is the limiting factor for Adriamycin
  - Cumulative dose should not exceed 450 mg/m^2
  - Bone marrow depression and profound nausea are other complications
  - Combined Cis-platinum and Adriamycin therapy produces clinical cure in 50%
  - Of this 50% of clinical responders, half have no evidence of microscopic disease at second-look laparotomy
  - Success rate depends on the size of the residual tumour
  - A uniform failure rate of treatment has been reported when residual masses approach 100 mm or more
— Hexamethyl melamine was found to be useful in patients who have tumours resistant to alkylating agents, Cis-platinum or Cis-platinum/Adriamycin combinations:
  - Drug is not superior to others
  - It is certainly more toxic
— The 'CHAD' regimen includes the durgs cyclophosphamide, hexamethyl melamine, Adriamycin and Cis-platinum (diamine-dichloroplatinum).
  - This combination is very toxic
  - It needs further evaluation
— Second-look surgery:
  - A second-look operation usually by laparotomy or sometimes by laparoscopy has become routine at many centres
  - If it is a laparotomy, multiple biopsies taken from the pelvic and abdominal peritoneum and peritoneal washing for cytology are also taken
  - Suspicious area is also biopsied

- Attempt at removal of the uterus, tubes, ovaries and omentum is done if they were not removed
- If the second-look procedure is negative, the chemotherapy is stopped and patient is followed up carefully at 3- and 6-monthly intervals, since recurrence is not uncommon
- If there is residual mass, attempt is made to remove it, followed by a change in therapy

— Patients are followed up using clinical examination, ultrasonography, CT scan and chest radiography.
— Immunotherapy has so far not proved to be useful in the management of ovarian cancer.
— Five-year survival rates for primary ovarian carcinoma:

Stage Ia	— 85%
Stage Ib–IIa	— 40%
Stage IIb	— 25%
Stage III	— 15%
Stage IV	— <5%

— Ovarian carcinoma in infancy and childhood.

Ovarian carcinoma in infancy and childhood

— It is rare, accounting for 1–2% of childhood malignancies.
— Common cancers are those of germ cell and specialised mesenchymal origin.
— Lower abdominal pain is the most common complaint.
— Often mistaken for appendicitis.
— Treatment is surgery, either conservative or removal of ovaries depending on the nature, extent of the disease and differentiation.
— Adjuvant therapy may be needed.
— If both ovaries are removed, long-term oestrogen and progestogen therapy will be needed.

Secondary carcinoma (Krukenberg tumour)

— This is uncommon; it comprises approximately 4–5% of ovarian cancers.
— Primary carcinoma is in the genital tract, usually uterine cancer (20%), large bowel, stomach and breast (80%).
— Tumours are bilateral, almost equal in size, nodular and solid.
— Histological examination will show a characteristic signet-ring appearance due to mucus production displacing the nucleus
— Prognosis is poor.
— Treatment is dealing with the primary and the ovarian tumour.
— Few patients survive beyond 6 months.

SUGGESTED READING

Begent R H J 1983 Germ cell tumours. In: Studd J (ed) Progress in obstetrics and gynaecology, vol 3. Churchill Livingstone, Edinburgh, p 174

Benigno B B 1982 Management of advanced ovarian cancer. In: Studd J (ed) Progress in obstetrics and gynaecology, vol 2. Churchill Livingstone, Edinburgh, p 123

Clark D G C, Hilaris B S, Ochoa M 1976 Treatemnt of cancer of the ovary. In: Macnaughton M C, Govan A D T (eds) Clinics in obstetrics and gynaecology, vol 3. Saunders, Philadelphia, p 159

Coppleson M (ed) 1981 Gynaecological oncology: fundamental principles and clinical practice, vol 2. Churchill Livingstone, Edinburgh

Dembo A J 1983 Radiation therapy in the management of ovarian cancer. In: Disaia P J (ed) Clinics in obstetrics and gynaecology, vol 10. Saunders, Philadelphia, p 261

Disaia P J (ed) 1983 Clinics in obstetrics and gynaecology, vol 10. Saunders, Philadelphia

Govan A D T 1976 Ovarian tumours: clinical and pathological features. In: Macnaughton M C, Govan A D T (eds) Clinics in obstetrics and gynaecology, vol 3. Saunders, Philadelphia, p 89

Piver M S 1983 Importance of proper staging in ovarian carcinoma. In: Disaia P J (ed) Clinics in obstetrics and gynaecology, vol 10. Saunders, Philadelphia, p 223

Rosenheim A 1983 Radio isotopes in the treatment of ovarian cancer. In: Disaia P J (ed) Clinics in obstetrics and gynaecology, vol 10. Saunders, Philadelphia, p 279

Smith L H, Oi R H 1984 Detection of malignant ovarian neoplasms. A review of the literature. In: Detection of the patient at risk: clinical, radiological and cytological detection. Obstetrical and gynaecological survey, vol 39, p 313

Smith L H, Oi R H 1984 Detection of malignant ovarian neoplasms. A review of the literature, II. Laboratory detection. p 329

Smith L H, Oi R H 1984 Detection of malignant ovarian neoplasms. A review of the literature, III. Immunological detection and ovarian cancer — associated antigens. p 346

Van Nagel Jr J R 1983 Tumour markers in ovarian cancer. In: Disaia P J (ed) Clinics in obstetrics and gynaecology, vol 10. Saunders, Philadelphia, p 197

Wiltshaw 1981 The management of Stage I carcinoma of the ovary. In: Studd J (ed) Progress in obstetrics and gynaecology, vol 1. Churchill Livingstone, Edinburgh, p 229

Young R H, Scully R E 1984 Ovarian sexcord — stromal tumours: recent advances and current status. In: Fox H (ed) Clinics in obstetrics and gynaecology, vol II. Saunders, Philadelphia, p 93

10. ENDOMETRIOSIS AND ADENOMYOSIS

ENDOMETRIOSIS

Introduction

— Endometriosis is the presence of endometrium in aberrant sites.
— It was probably first recognised in 1860 by Von Rokitansky.
— It is a problem during menstrual life.
— More common in those with uninterrupted menstruation for periods exceeding 5 years.
— The cause is not fully understood.
— Viable endometrial cells can be found in the majority of women in the pelvis during menstruation.
— Why implantation takes place in some is unclear.

Definition

— Endometriosis is defined as the proliferation and functioning of endometrial tissue outside the uterine cavity.

Aetiology

— Main mechanism of spread is direct to the myometrium (adenomyosis).
— Reflux of menstrual fluid through the fallopian tubes — this leads to implantation on the ovaries, uterosacral ligament, pouch of Douglas, tubes and other pelvic structures.
— Retrograde menstruation is probably the main cause. Reflux bleeding is often found at laparoscopy or at laparotomy at the time of menstruation.
— Viable endometrial cells are present in the peritoneal fluid in more than 50% of women during menstruation.
  • During laparoscopy, a flow of blood from the fimbriated end of the tube has been noted in some menstruating women

- Endometriosis is most commonly found in dependent portions of the pelvis
- Endometrial fragments from the menstrual flow can grow both in tissue culture and following injection beneath the abdominal wall
- When the cervix of monkeys was transposed so that menstruation occurred into the peritoneal cavity, endometriosis developed

— Recent theory is that in ovulating women there is a high sex steroid hormone content in the peritoneal fluid of the pelvis and this inhibits implantation and/or growth of endometrial tissue.

— Regurgitation of endometrial fragments through the fallopian tubes at the time of menstruation is a common occurrence.

— High levels of ovarian steroids, oestradiol and progesterone, in the peritoneal fluid inactivate the endometrium and prevent rooting and developing.

— If hormone contents are low, as in luteinisation of an unruptured follicle (LUF syndrome), the endometrial tissue survives.

— Endometrium is a potent source of prostaglandin F_2 alpha.

— Prostaglandin affects ovum transport and ovarian function, and also induces luteolysis or post-implantation abortion.

— In endometriosis the peritoneal fluid contains a higher level of PGF_2 alpha which alters tubal motility, ovum release and steroidogenesis.

— Endometriosis in more distant sites can be explained by lymphatic or bloodstream spread.

— The other main theory is that müllerian epithelium may be displaced during fetal development or arise *de novo* by metaplasia.

— Recent thoughts are directed towards the possibility of genetic and familial influence and auto-immune pathogenesis.

— Direct implantation of endometrial tissue may happen at the time of uterine surgery.

— at time of surgery — caesarean or episiotomy following delivery

Pathology

— The cardinal histological features of endometriosis are:
- Ectopic endometrial glands and stroma
- Evidence of fresh haemorrhage (red cells and haemosiderin pigment) or old (haemosiderin-laden macrophages)
- Abundance of inflammatory cells and fibrous connective tissue indicating an intense reaction
- It is the endometrial stroma and not epithelium or glands that is responsible for the haemorrhage

— Clinical appearance varies with the location and duration of activity of the lesion.
— Commonest site is the ovary, and in the majority of women both ovaries are involved, though not to the same extent.
— The tendency is for cystic structures to form, varying from tiny bluish or dark brown blisters to large chocolate cysts, sometimes attaining large size (200 mm).
— There is considerable fibrosis and puckering of the ovarian surface in the region of the cyst.
— Adhesion to neighbouring structures occurs because of intermittent rupture, usually during or just after a period.
— Contents of the endometrial cyst produce local peritonitis and fibrosis.
— Early lesions on the pelvic peritoneum appear as multiple 'blueberry' spots or 'powder-burn' lesions.
— As time and disease advance, scar tissue involves all pelvic organs, the uterus becomes fixed and retroverted and the pouch of Douglas gets obliterated.
— Disease spreads into rectovaginal septum, posterior vaginal fornix, cervix, wall of rectum, sigmoid colon, bladder, ureter, small bowel, round and uterosacral ligament.
— In 5–35% of cases the bowel is involved, in 10–20% the lower urinary tract is involved.

Incidence

— 25–50% of infertile women have endometriosis.
— Not uncommon in the teenage group.
— Not confined to nulliparous women.
— Condition does exist before menarche and in black women.

Clinical features

— Median age is 25–30.
— Under the age of 20 years it is uncommon; if it occurs, it is possibly due to obstructive malformation of the lower genital tract (acute anteflexion and retroflexion).

Infertility

— Endometriosis is often diagnosed when a woman is examined and investigated for infertility (by laparoscopy).
— 30–40% of women with endometriosis will be infertile.
— 15–30% of infertile women will have endometriotic lesions.
— Infertility is probably due to the effect of endometriosis on tubal motility and function.
— Ovulation may be inhibited, dyspareunia reduces the frequency of intercourse.
— Abortion is significantly more common.

Pelvic pain

— Dysmenorrhoea and dyspareunia are the main symptoms; the pain also affects work and sexual function.

— Dysmenorrhoea is secondary in type; the pain is due to swelling or bleeding of ectopic endometrium and tends to be unilateral.

— As disease advances, the pain is bilateral, constant and worse before the period and persists for days after the onset of bleeding.

— Pain gets worse with age.

— In some women there is no pain.

— In many women there is pain but no palpable mass in the pelvis.

— Dyspareunia is deep and internal; it may be localised to one part of the pelvis — worse premenstrually and pain persists for some hours after intercourse.

Urological symptoms

— Frequency, dysuria are common and, rarely, haematuria at the time of menses.

— Obstruction of the pelvic part of the ureter due to disease or due to adhesion may produce hydronephrosis and infection.

Bowel symptoms

— As a result of direct involvement of the sigmoid colon and rectum or indirectly from pressure of adjacent lesions in the ovary or other pelvic structures.

— Pain during defecation, melena, premenstrual and menstrual diarrhoea and constipation are some of the symptoms.

Menstrual symptoms

— Menorrhagia occurs more often in adenomyosis.

— Irregular bleeding can occur with cervical and vaginal lesions.

— Amenorrhoea is rare, but occurs when ovarian function is totally destroyed.

Less common symptoms

— Abdominal mass, bowel obstruction, peritonitis from rupture of the cyst, ectopic pregnancy, nodule in the abdominal scar, acute appendicitis due to involvement of the wall of the appendix.

— There is no correlation between symptoms and the extent of the disease; site and functional activity are probably important.

— 10–15% of cases are asymptomatic.

Signs

— These vary according to the stage of the disease.

— Endometriosis is staged depending on the extent of the disease.

— Acosta et al (1973) staged the disease into mild, moderate and severe degrees:
- Mild — Scattered fresh lesions
  - No scarring or retraction
  - No adhesions around tube and ovary
- Moderate — Involves ovaries with some scarring and retraction or contains small endometriomas
  - Minimal peri-ovarian or peritubal adhesions
  - Small endometriotic lesions present in the anterior and posterior peritoneal pouch, with some scarring and retraction
- Severe — Involves ovaries
  - Size of endometriomas is > 20 mm
  - Adhesions around tubes and ovaries with almost total absence of mobility
  - Thickening of uterosacral ligaments
  - Involvement of bowel and urinary tract

— Kistner (1977) classified endometriosis into four stages:

— Stage 1 (mild) (30–40%):
- Lesions are small, 5 mm or less
- Confined to the surface of the pelvic peritoneum, including the ovaries
- No scarring, adhesions or fixity
- Localised tenderness may be present
- Pelvis often feels normal

— Stage 2(a) (moderate) (40–50%):
- Scarring and retraction appear
- Mild adhesions around the ovaries and/or tubes
- Ovarian endometrial cyst measures 5 mm or less
- It is subdivided into .1, 2, 3, depending on the area of the endometrial lesion

— Stage 2(b):
- Lesions are larger
- Palpable nodules
- Ovarian cysts larger than 5 mm
- Moderate adhesions around the ovaries and tubes
- Fimbriae of the tubes are free

— Stage 3 (severe) (15–25%):
- Major part of pelvis is affected
- Uterus is fixed and retroverted
- Ovarian lesions are extensive and fixed
- Tubes are blocked by direct involvement or by adhesions

— Stage 4 (extensive) (10–15%):
- Involvement of bowel and bladder
- Uterus is fixed, third-degree retroversion
- Pouch of Douglas is obliterated

— Proper staging of the disease gives a clear picture of

prognosis and allows better comparison of treatment method and results.

Diagnosis

— Often suspected after a careful history is taken.
— Presence of cyclic symptoms referable to the lower abdomen.
— Careful inspection and bimanual examination will reveal nodularity or swelling — tenderness and fixity.
— Rectovaginal examination may be helpful.
— Deviation of cervix, fixed mass, fixed retroverted uterus are other features.
— Examination under anaesthesia and laparoscopy confirm the diagnosis.
— For histological diagnosis both glandular and stromal tissue must be present.
— Ultrasonic examination will show one or more cysts separate from the uterus, but the outline of cyst wall is irregular and often not smooth.
— Laparoscopy confirms the diagnosis made on a clinical basis.

Differential diagnosis

— Pelvic inflammatory disease.
— Fibromyoma.
— Ectopic pregnancy.
— Appendicitis.
— Diverticulitis.
— Neoplasia of ovary, uterus, bowel, bladder.
— Psychosomatic pain.

Treatment

— This depends on:
  • Severity and presence of symptoms
  • Extent of the disease
  • Age of the patient
  • Need for reproductive function
  • Patient aptitude
  • Tolerance of medical treatment
  • Whether previous conservative surgery has been undertaken
  • Severe side-effects of medical treatment
— The aim is to reverse or eliminate the disease process.
— Relieve symptoms and facilitate childbearing if this is desired.
— In stage 1, disease can be treated by drug therapy or conservative surgery, and the chance of recurrence is small (about 10%).

— Stage 2 requires conservative surgery and drug therapy; the recurrence rate is 50%.
— Stages 3 and 4 need radical surgery, removal of endometriotic lesion, ovaries and uterus. Pre-operative drug therapy may reduce the extent and the risk of surgery, which is often difficult.
— In general, drug therapy and/or conservative surgery are used in cases of infertility.
— In older women who do not wish to bear children, or in whom symptoms are severe and the disease is extensive, more radical surgery is indicated.
— Basis of treatment is the inhibition of endometrial growth, and this can be achieved by physiological means (pregnancy), pharmacological techniques (inhibition of hormone production or blocking hormone receptors in the endometrium) or surgery (removal of the ovaries and thus prevention of hormone stimulus of the endometrial tissue).

Prophylaxis

— For family planning, oral contraceptive pills are better. They reduce endometrial growth in the uterus, hence reflux and regurgitation problems are minimised.
— Insufflation of the tube or dye test or hysterosalpingogram should be avoided at or near the time of menstruation or after curettage.
— Cervical stenosis or spasm cause reflux or regurgitation.
— Operations on the genital tract should be scheduled in the post-menstrual phase.
— Caesarean section, hysterectomy, uterine repair may cause implantation, and care must be taken to avoid this.
— Explanation, reassurance and counselling of the patient are an essential part of the treatment.

Drug treatment

— The aim is to cause atrophy of the ectopic endometrium, with mimmum side-effects, by the anti-oestrogenic effects of progestogens, the avoidance of endometrial shedding by giving hormones continously or by blocking of receptors in the ovary or ectopic endometrium.
— Oral contraceptive pills given continously or intermittently may cure the problem. But the side effects are high, including the risk of thrombo-embolism.
— Progestogen (norethisterone 10–20 mg daily) or dydrogesterone (Duphaston 10–30 mg daily) have fewer risks than oestrogen and progesterone compounds, but may cause depression. Treatment is given for a period of nine months. Antidepressant drugs will help.
— Oral Provera (medroxyprogesterone acetate) (30 mg/day) and injectable Depo-Provera have also been used.

— Recently, a long-acting gonadotropin-releasing hormone (GnRH) agonist has been used to create a pseudomenopause for the treatment of endometriosis. *Inhibits gonadotrophin secretion*
— Danocrine (200–800 mg — Danol, Danazol), is the most effective drug, but is very expensive. It is a synthetic derivative of ethinyl testosterone.
- Side-effects are due to mild androgenic effect (acne, oily skin and facial hair, hirsutism, deepening of voice)
- Anabolic effect (overweight problem)
- Hypo-oestrogenic effect (vaginal and breast atrophy)
- Central nervous system symptoms (depression, anxiety, fatigue)
- Gastro-intestinal symptoms
- Muscle spasms and cramp
- Depression is less common with this drug
- This drug inhibits the midcycle surge of FSH, LH, inhibits ovulation and ovarian steroid production
- Success rate of removal of endometriosis (60–90%)
- Pregnancy rate is approximately 70%
- Long-term hormonal therapy without surgery is useful in patients with symptoms but with little in the way of palpable masses
- Diagnosis should be established by laparoscopy before treatment is initiated
- Laparoscopy is used at the end of the medical treatment (6–9 months) to assess response to medical therapy and treatment is prolonged if there are residual lesions
- Medical treatment is given if disease recurs following conservative surgery.

Surgery (conservative/radical)

— Conservative surgery involves diathermy using a bipolar technique at laparoscopy or at laparotomy.
— Excision of small lesion and peritonisation.
— Release of peritubo-ovarian adhesions using a microsurgical technique.
— Tubal reconstructive surgery when endometriosis involved the wall of the tube.
— Dilatation of the cervix.
— Ventrosuspension.
— Pre-sacral neurectomy for pain.
— To avoid adhesions, meticulous dissection using a microsurgical technique, good haemostasis, peritonisation, use of a post-operative steroid, intraperitoneal dextran may prevent or reduce adhesions.
— Radical surgery (hysterectomy and bilateral salpingo-oophorectomy) is indicated for stage 3 disease — surgery could be difficult and may need repair of bladder, ureter and

bowel due to injury at the time of surgery — pre-operative drug therapy is helpful.
— If oophorectomy is performed, small-dosage oestrogen replacement therapy is indicated along with progestins if menopausal symptoms are severe.

Radiation

— Radiotherapy is indicated for a patient with severe symptoms or who is unsuitable for surgery and did not respond to drug therapy — rarely used.

Prognosis

— The more extensive the lesion, the more likely it is to recur.
— Once it recurs, the chance of a cure is further reduced.
— Hence regular follow-up examination is ideal for 5 years. Laparoscopy is done to check response to medical treatment at the end of the course.

Pregnancy rate

— Varies in the range 0–85%.
— Depends on the extent of damage to the ovary and tube.
— A rate of 75% conceive in mild cases. 50% conceive in moderate cases and 35% in severe cases.
— There is disturbed ovulation, disturbed corpus luteum function; risks of abortion and ectopic pregnancy are higher.
— Pregnancy does not cure the disease; patient reverts back to anovulation and may need induction of ovulation to prevent recurrence.

ADENOMYOSIS

Definition

— Adenomyosis, also known as endometriosis interna, is a relatively common condition in which areas of endometrium, both glands and stroma, are found in the myometrium.

Incidence

— 20–40% of parous women in their forties and fifties have adenomyosis in the hysterectomy specimens.
— Incidence is higher in patients with uterine body cancer, fibromyoma and uterine polyp.

Pathology

— The distinctive microscopic characteristic is the presence of islands of typical endometrial tissue scattered throughout the muscle layer; endometrial glands are surrounded by typical endometrial stromal cells.
— Occasionally the endometrium is of the functioning type.
— More frequently the endometrium is of the immature, non-functioning type.
— There is considerable generalised myometrial hypertrophy.
— The enlargement of the uterus produced by adenomyosis is often symmetrical and rarely greater than 2 or 3 times the normal size.
— Occasionally one or more discrete adenomyomas may grow to moderate size and project into the uterine cavity.
— There is no capsulation as seen in fibromyoma.
— Cut section of the myometrium shows small dark spaces.
— Occasionally there is spread to the myometrium by endometrial stroma without glands; in rare cases invasion of lymphatic channels can be seen.
— Adenocarcinomas developing in these aberrant islands are rare.

Clinical features

— There are many points of similarity between endometriosis and adenomyosis.
— Adenomyosis affects 40-year-old parous women, but endometriosis is a disease of younger, infertile women.
— Menorrhagia and dysmenorrhea are the two most frequent symptoms.
— Increasingly severe dysmenorrhoea in the 4th and 5th decade, colicky in nature, is a characteristic feature.
— Pelvic discomfort and dyspareunia are other symptoms.
— Occasionally bleeding may be irregular.

Diagnosis

— Definite diagnosis is made at surgery and following pathological examination.
— Condition should be suspected if women at 40 or after develop dysmenorrhoea, menorrhagia and dyspareunia.
— Uterus is usually symmetrically enlarged 2 or 3 times the normal uterine size and mobile unless endometriosis co-exists.
— 13% of patients with adenomyosis have endometriosis, and then symptoms related to that condition are present.
— Fibromyoma, endometrial hyperplasia or polyp may co-exist.

Treatment

— Usually diagnostic curettage will have been done as the initial step.
— A trial of menstrual suppression therapy with a progestin or danazol may be tried in the younger patient if curettage in ineffective.
— Hysterectomy with conservation of ovaries is the conventional treatment.
— An expectant approach may be considered if patient is approaching the menopause.

STROMAL ENDOMETRIOSIS

Introduction

— It is a rare condition.
— Acts more like a neoplasm.
— Histologically solid masses of cells resembling endometrial stroma are found in the myometrial wall.
— Other features of neoplasm are uncommon, mitoses are few, pleomorphism is slight.
— Histologically it is divided into 3 grades.
— Grade I shows a histological picture identical with ordinary adenomyosis except it is made up entirely of stromal elements — clinically it is benign.
— Grade II shows endometrial stroma invading the musculature but may also show endolymphatic and intravascular invasion; it is locally invasive in the pelvis; distant metastasis does not occur.
— Hysterectomy may cure it; death may occur from local extension.
— Grade III shows malignant features histologically and clinically.
— It is called endometrial sarcoma.
— Hysterectomy and bilateral salpingo-oophorectomy is the treatment if lesion is beyond the uterus.
— If the lesion is confined to the uterus, a hysterectomy is done.
— Progesterone therapy may be useful in some patients.

Clinical features

— The peak incidence is in the 35–50 age group.
— The condition does not regress on removal of the ovaries.

— Metastasis does occur, but rarely; behaves like a low-grade sarcoma.
— Clinically, patients present with menorrhagia or post-menopausal bleeding and pelvic pain.
— Urological symptoms may be present if the ureters are obstructed by metastasis in the pelvis.
— Diagnosed at surgery and subsequent histological examination.
— Prognosis is usually good.
— Differential diagnosis is from haemangiopericytoma characterised by a concentric arrangement of pericytes around the capillaries

SUGGESTED READING

Barnes A B Wenneberg C N, Barnes B 1983 Ectopic pregnancy. Incidence and review of determinant factors. Obstetrical and gynecological survey, vol 38. p 345

Brosens I, Koninckx P, Boeckx W 1981 Endometriosis. In: Hull M G R (ed) Clinics in obstetrics and gynaecology, vol 8. Saunders, Philadelphia, p 63

Jones H W, Rock J A 1980 Other factors associated with infertility. Endometriosis externa, fibromyomata uteri. In: Pepperell R J, Hudson B, Wood C (eds) The infertile couple. Churchill Livingstone, Edinburgh, p 145

Schneider G T 1983 Endometriosis — an up-date. In: Studd J (ed) Progress in obstetrics and gynaecoloty, vol 3. Churchill Livingstone, Edinburgh, p 246

Speroff L Glass R H, Kase N G (eds) 1984 Clinical gynecologic endocrinology and infertility, 3rd edn, Williams & Wilkins, Baltimore, p 493

Vorys N, Boutselis J G Neri A S 1980 Endometriosis. In: Gold J J, Josimovich J B Gynecologic endocrinology, 3rd edn. Harper & Row, New York, p 414

11. DISPLACEMENT OF THE UROGENITAL TRACT

INTRODUCTION

— In genital prolapse there is, as a result of weakness or attenuation of supporting tissues, an abnormal descent of one or more of the pelvic viscera.
— The chief supporting structures are:
  • The radiating paracervical ligaments.
  • These attach to the adjacent pelvic wall and the various condensations of the pubo-urethral and pubocervical fascial complex.
  • Part of this complex forms the supporting septum which separates the vagina from the urethra and bladder anteriorly.
  • A similar condensation separates the vagina from the rectum posteriorly.
— In general, pelvic organs are supported by the pelvic diaphragm (levator ani muscles).
— Pelvic diaphragm contracts reflexly in response to sudden increases in intra-abdominal pressure.
— Impairment of the pelvic support is due to:
  • Trauma associated with childbirth
  • Progressive weakening associated with age
  • Oestrogen lack after the menopause
  • Conditions which cause a rise in intra-abdominal pressure
— Because of the intimate relationship of the lower birth canal to the bladder neck, disorders of the control of micturation are often associated with uterovaginal prolapse.

AETIOLOGY

— The three main organs of the pelvis are the bladder and the upper urethra anteriorly, the uterus and vagina centrally, and the sigmoid and the upper rectum posteriorly.

— They pass through the central hiatus of the pelvic diaphragm formed by the two levator ani muscles.

— They are attached to the margins of the levatores ani muscles by fascial condensations.

— The viscera rest on the upper surface of this diaphragm.

— Coughing, laughing and sneezing raise intra-abdominal pressure, which causes a reflex contraction of levatores ani muscles, which in turn strengthens the supports and narrows the hiatus.

— The hiatus gets drawn forwards towards the symphysis pubis by the puborectalis part of the levator ani muscles.

— It also serves to close the hiatus and prevent herniation of the pelvic and abdominal viscera.

— Damage to the levator ani muscles usually occurs during childbirth. The damage consists of overstretching and/or tearing of the margins of the hiatus by the fetus as it passes through the pelvic diaphragm during the second stage of labour.

— This type of injury allows a 'drop-down' type of prolapse.

— A similar mechanism is responsible for the overstretching and/or tearing of the fascial septa of the vagina on the front and back walls.

— This allows protrusion into the vagina of the bladder and urethra anteriorly (cystocele, urethrocele) and the rectum posteriorly (rectocele).

— The major uterine supports run anteriorly (pubocervical ligament), laterally (transverse cervical or cardinal ligaments) and posteriorly (uterosacral ligaments).

— Whereas distension injury during childbirth is often inevitable, particularly if the baby is large, traction injury to the above ligaments is largely avoidable.

— Commonly seen in patients:
  • Who push down prematurely in labour.
  • Or extraction on the baby before full dilatation of the cervix.
  • Or in those in whom a credé or Dublin-type manoeuvre has been used to express the placenta.

— Vault prolapse is rare. It occurs after vaginal or abdominal hysterectomy (1 in 250 operations approximately):
  • When the supporting structures have not been fixed adequately to the vault.
  • The integrity of the repair has been undermined by haematoma or infection.
  • Congenitally deep pouch of Douglas has not been dealt with adequately.

— Some women suffer from a congenital weakness of connective tissues throughout the body.

- Vault prolapse is not uncommon in this group.
- Often these women have not borne children.
— Ageing leads to a slow weakening of both pelvic floor musculature and a loss of elasticity and strength of the fascial condensations.
— Loss of oestrogenic support after a spontaneous or surgical menopause may be a further factor.
— Chronic elevation of intra-abdominal pressure may act as a precipitating factor, due to:
  - Chronic cough
  - Constipation
  - Heavy lifting
  - Large intra-abdominal tumours
  - Ascitis
  - Pregnancy
  - Obesity

DEFINITION

— The downward displacement of the uterus and/or vagina towards or through the vaginal introitus.
— The bladder, urethra, rectum and bowel may be secondarily involved.
— Prolapse has three degrees of severity:
  - First degree: decent of the cervix to the introitus.
  - Second degree: decent of the cervix, but not the whole uterus, through the introitus.
  - Third degree: procedentia, descent of the cervix and the whole uterus through the introitus.

INCIDENCE

— This differs widely, largely because of differences in childbirth practices, parity, pelvic anatomy and cultural habits.

CLINICAL FEATURES

— Even extensive relaxation of the outlet may be entirely symptom-free.
— Pressure and heaviness in the vaginal region especially after prolonged standing.

— Awareness of a lump protruding from the vagina, which is worse on standing or straining and disappears on lying down, or when pressure is applied to it.
— Pain is often absent, but backache is a common complaint.
— Difficulty in emptying the lower bowel, relieved by pressing on the rectocele from the vagina.
— Dyspareunia and loss of libido.
— Disturbances of micturition:
  • Chronic cystitis with frequency and dysuria associated with residual urine in the prolapsed bladder
  • Replacement of cystocele to effect complete voiding helps
  • Urgency and stress incontinence due to instability of the detrusor muscle and to bladder neck damage
  • In rare cases, acute retention of urine can occur.
— Discharge, often bloodstained, occurs when the cervix prolapses outside the introitus due to stasis, chafes against clothing or inner thighs and becomes ulcerated and/or infected.
— Ureteric obstruction occurs in gross long-standing prolapse, leading to hydronephrosis and eventual uraemia.

DIAGNOSIS

— Lump presenting in the vagina.
— Patient is asked to strain down in dorsal position to assess the degree of prolapse.
— Examination in the Sims' position shows more precisely the anatomical disturbance.
— Sims' speculum is used posteriorly to assess the degree of descent of the bladder (cystocele) and the descent of the uterus on straining down.
— Sims' speculum is applied anteriorly to visualise posterior vaginal wall descent (enterocele, rectocele), upper third (enterocele), lower two-thirds (rectocele).
— Cysts in the anterior or lateral vaginal wall may be confusing if not palpated.
— Urethral diverticula may also be mistaken for urethrocele.
— With long-standing third-degree prolapse with decubitus ulceration, the possibility of cervical cancer should be ruled out.

MANAGEMENT

Investigation

— If a Papanicolaou smear has not been done in the previous 12 months, this should be done.
— Microscopy and culture of urine.
— In long-standing third-degree prolapse, an assessment of urological system is advisable.
— Since patients are often elderly, cardiovascular and respiratory function should be assessed if there are clinical indications.
— Patient should be advised to lose weight if she is overweight.
— Reduce or stop cigarette smoking.
— Improve diet if patient has problems of constipation.
— Post-menopausal atrophic changes in the vagina should be treated with a course of low-dose oral oestrogen or topical application.
— Prophylactic antibacterial therapy is useful for major procedures because of the potential pathogenicity of the vaginal flora.
— If there is decubitus ulceration of the cervix, the patient should be admitted for a rest and replacement of the uterus inside the vagina and packing of the vagina until the ulcer heals.

Prophylaxis

— Avoidance of perineal overstretching during labour and adequate repair thereafter.
— Adequate post-natal pelvic floor exercises.
— Appropriate use of hormone replacement therapy in some post-menopausal women.
— Adequate treatment of chronic chest problems.
— Avoidance of obesity or loss of weight.
— Appropriate treatment will depend on:
  • Severity of the symptoms
  • Asymptomatic first-degree prolapse does not require treatment
  • Patient's age, parity and her desire for further pregnancies
  • Patient's sexual activity
  • Presence of aggravating features such as obesity, smoking, constipation and chronic cough
  • Presence of urological symptoms
  • Severity of uterovaginal prolapse
  • Other gynaecological problems such as menorrhagia

Conservative management

— Pelvic-floor exercises will improve the tone of the levators ani muscles in the young parous women.

— Ring or shelf pessary may be used either for a short- or long-term basis.

— Conservative management is indicated:
- When women are old, frail and medically unfit for surgery
- When women refuse to have surgery
- During pregnancy or immediately after delivery
- When a woman is waiting to come in for surgery

— A modern portex pessary seldom causes the same amount of infection and vaginal ulceration seen with the rubber watch-spring type.

— The patient should be seen at intervals of 3 to 4 months for assessment.

— Anti-bacterial and/or oestrogen vaginal cream may be given for intermittent use.

Surgical treatment

— Whatever surgical approach is considered, it is important to remember that prolapse is not a life-threatening condition, but surgery has its morbidity and occasional mortality.

— Where there has been distension injury to the vaginal fascia (cystocele, rectocele) the operation of colporrhaphy (anterior and/or posterior) is appropriate.

— Anterior repair is less effective in improving stress incontinence.

— Posterior repair is often avoided in the younger woman unless there are major relaxation problems.

— Posterior colporrhaphy is usually combined with perineorrhaphy, which involves approximation of the lower and inner part of the puborectalis muscle and repair of the structures of the perineal body.

— Traction injury or other weakness of uterine supports is usually dealt with by vaginal hysterectomy, together with shortening and plication of cardinal and uterosacral ligaments.

— If preservation of uterus is desired for childbearing, Manchester (Fothergill) repair is appropriate.

— Manchester repair involves dilatation of the cervix, anterior repair, amputation of the vaginal portion of the cervix and its repair, shortening of the paracervical ligament, with or without posterior colpoperineorrhaphy.

— Caesarean section is necessary in any subsequent pregnancy.

— Vaginal hysterectomy is the ideal operation for uterovaginal

F

prolapse in the presence of benign uterine pathology, as long as the uterus is not enlarged to a size greater than the equivalent of a 12-week pregnancy.
  - It is the operation of choice if an enterocele is present — uterosacral ligaments are used to obliterate the hernial sac
  - For-third degree prolapse
— The main disadvantages are the development of an enterocele and/or vault prolapse following vaginal hysterectomy.
— Their correction can pose considerable surgical problems, particularly if sexual function is to be preserved.

Post-operative care

Catheter
— Urinary retention is common after repair procedures:
  - Due to trauma to urethra and bladder neck during dissection
  - Causes oedema and dysfunction
  - Pressure of a pack in the vagina
  - Reflex bladder inhibition from sutures in the vagina and perineum
— An indwelling catheter is often used for the above reasons for 2–5 days (Foley catheter via the urethra or suprapubic catheter).
— Initially continous closed drainage followed by intermittent emptying will allow the earlier return of normal bladder function.
— With a suprapubic catheter it is easy to assess the residual urine after voiding.
— A residual urine volume of less than 100 ml is satisfactory.
— Urinary antiseptic is used if a catheter is used.
— If an indwelling catheter is not used, it is important to monitor urinary output and suprapubic discomfort and fullness.

Vaginal pack
— A pack soaked in antiseptic emulsion or solution is often used for 24 hours.
— The pack aids in haemostasis and in prevention of haematoma formation, and has an antibacterial effect.
— The pack also prevents adhesions of adjacent suture lines on the anterior and posterior vaginal wall.

Complications
— These are related to vaginal repair surgery:
  - Lower urinary tract infection
  - Wound infection
  - Urinary retention

- Haemorrhage
- Thrombo-embolic disease
- Late complications are dyspareunia and recurrence

Colpocleisis *(Le Fort operation)*

— This operation is indicated:
  - In massive procedentia
  - Failure of other operative procedures
  - Involves closing the vagina
  - It is easily and quickly performed
  - Should be performed as a last resort
  - Usually successful procedure
  - Has minimum complications
  - Vault prolapse may need abdominal and vaginal approach

RETROVERSION OF THE UTERUS

Definition

— The axis of the uterus lies posterior to the axis of the vagina.
— The terms 'version' and 'flexion' as applied to the uterus should be differentiated.
— Flexion applies to the axis of the uterine body in relation to that of the cervix.
— The uterus may adopt any position from anteversion and anteflexion (the normal state) through the erect or intermediate position, to retroversion and retroflexion.

Incidence

— In 10–25% of women the uterus is in a retroverted position.
— This figure increases in the reproductive age period as a result of acquired pathology.
— Mobile retroversion of the uterus is a variant of normal, occurring in over 25% of women.
— Retroversion is divided into three degrees:
  - First degree: the fundus is vertical or pointing towards the sacral promontory.
  - Second degree: the fundus is in the hollow of the sacrum but not below the level of the cervix.
  - Third degree: the fundus of the uterus is below the level of the cervix.

Aetiology

— Congenital: the condition persists into adult life as a result of developmental deficiencies.
— Acquired: retrodisplacement of a previously normally placed uterus:
  • Puerperal
  • Adnexal disease, inflammatory disease or endometriosis
  • Neoplasms — large myoma in the anterior wall of the uterus
  • Trauma — debatable
— Position of anteversion is usually maintained by the anterior pull of the round ligament on the upper part of the uterus.
— It is also maintained by the upward pull of the uterosacral ligaments on the back of the cervix.

Clinical features

— Simple, uncomplicated retrodisplacement of the uterus is often entirely symptom-free.
— Only a few problems appear to be significantly related to the mobile retroversion of the uterus:
  • Dyspareunia due to trauma to the prolapsed ovaries
  • Infertility due to the displacement of the cervix is debatable
  • Dysmenorrhoea and backache may be noted
  • In rare cases incarcerations which occurs late in the first trimester of pregnancy cause acute retention of urine.
— The situation is different with fixed retroversion; symptoms depend on the primary disorder, such as inflammatory disease and endometriosis.

Diagnosis

— The first clue is given by the upward- and forward-pointing cervix on speculum examination.
— On bimanual examination the body of the uterus is difficult to palpate.
— Combined retrovaginal examination will confirm the uterine position.
— Pain may be experienced as with coitus when the sensitive ovaries are being compressed.
— Mobility of the uterus needs to be assessed digitally or using uterine sound.
— If endometriosis or other pathology is present in the pouch of Douglas and the uterosacral ligaments, considerable tenderness may be present on examination.
— Differential diagnosis includes other pelvic masses behind the

uterus such as ovarian tumours, fibro-myoma, loaded rectum and lesions in the sigmoid colon.

Management

— If the primary mobile retroversion is associated with symptoms, a Hodge pessary test is usually applied.
— A Hodge pessary works by putting tension on the posterior fornix.
— When the pessary is in position, the patient and her partner should be unaware of its presence.
— It is left in situ for 2 to 3 months, provided the uterus is kept anteverted.
— If retroversion and symptoms recur after removal of the Hodge pessary, a type of suspension procedure is usually carried out.
— Most procedures depend on shortening the round ligament.
— Simple plication of the round ligament is usually less effective as compared with Gwillim's ventrosuspension operation.
— Laparotomy or laparoscopy may be used to shorten the round ligament.
— Too much shortening may cause pain during pregnancy.
— Treatment of secondary retroversion due to pelvic pathology needs dealing with the primary pathology and shortening of the round ligament to keep the uterus anteverted.

SUGGESTED READING

Dewhurst C J (ed) 1981 Integrated obstetrics and gynaecology for post-graduates, 3rd edn. Blackwell, Oxford

Feroze R M 1978 Vaginal hysterectomy and repair. Clinics in obstetrics and gynaecology, vol 5. p 54 Saunders, London.

Jones H W, Jones G S (eds) 1980 Gynecology, 3rd edn. Williams & Wilkins, Baltimore, p 208

Mackay E V, Beischer N A, Cox L W Wood C (eds) 1983 Illustrated textbook of gynaecology. Saunders, London, p 293

12. DISORDERS OF THE LOWER URINARY TRACT

INTRODUCTION

— Disorders of the lower urinary tract are of considerable importance because of their frequency and the social disability they cause.
— In many gynaecological disorders such as prolapse, endometriosis and benign and malignant disease, the lower urinary tract may be involved.
— Diseases of the lower ureter, bladder and urethra may cause symptoms which may be diagnosed as gynaecological disorders.
— The incidence of incontinence in women over the age of 70 years is 15–20%.
— The incontinence in the older woman is usually due to loss of central nervous control along with atrophy and damage to the sphincter mechanism.

ANATOMY OF THE LOWER URINARY TRACT

— The ureters enter the pelvis, passing over the bifurcation of the common iliac artery.
— At the level of the cervix the ureter turns medially just below the uterine artery to enter the base of the bladder.
— The bladder occupies the space between the symphysis pubis anteriorly and the uterus posteriorly.
— The bladder rests on the pelvic diaphragm.
— The urethra passes through the levator hiatus in front of the vagina and traverses the urogenital diaphragm.
— The bladder neck region is attached to the posterior aspect of the pubic rami by condensations of the pubocervical fascia and is supported posteriorly by attachment to the lower part of the uterus and the upper part of the vagina.
— The trigone of the bladder is the triangular area at the base

of the bladder bounded by the internal urethral meatus and the openings of the ureters.
— Extension of the detrusor muscle fibres around the proximal urethra form the so-called internal or intrinsic sphincter of the bladder.
— Internal sphincter maintains continence at rest.
— During micturation the fibres are drawn up in a similar manner to that which occurs during labour with the lower uterine segment, the muscle fibre no longer acting as a sphincter.
— No doubt there is some argument about the existence of an internal sphincter of the bladder.
— Being composed of smooth muscle fibres, the sphincter is involuntary.
— An external sphincter does exist and consists of voluntary muscle within the urogenital diaphragm.
— The sympathetic nervous system (T11 to L3) inhibits the detrusor muscle, while the parasympathetic system (sacral 2, 3, 4) activates it.
— Sensory fibres subserve pain and proprioception.
— Parasympathetic fibres largely convey information on filling.
— Both divisions relay information from the trigone.

PHYSIOLOGY

Factors maintaining continence

— Urethral pressure.
— Posterior urethrovesical angle.
— Bladder tone.

Urethral pressure

— Urethral pressure is maintained by the thick folded uroepithelium, intrinsic smooth muscle, elastic fibres and extrinsic striated muscle.
— The intra-urethral pressure at rest is approximately 950 m of water, and this is well above the bladder pressure both at rest and during normal rises of pressure.
— The urethral diameter is very small; even a low wall tension will resist a high intraluminal pressure.
— The levator ani muscles, unlike the above muscles, are fast responders and are utilised largely for resisting sudden rises of intra-abdominal pressure and stopping the stream after it has commenced.
— Unless the proximal urethra (bladder-neck area) is above the level of the pelvic diaphragm, intra-abdominal pressure will

act only on the bladder and then create a marked pressure differential between this organ and the urethra.

— Urinary continence is dependent upon maintenance of a pressure differential between bladder and urethra.

— The pressure in the urethra exceeding that in the bladder (urethral closure pressure) maintains the continence.

Posterior urethrovesical angle

— This is an indication of the integrity of the pubovesical and pubourethral ligaments which support the bladder neck anteriorly.

Normal bladder tone

— If the bladder is over-filled pressed upon, it has a high resting tone.

— Or is also irritable (dyssynergia).

— The normal closing pressure in the urethra may be overcome and incontinence will result.

Response to bladder filling

— If a patient's bladder is filled with sterile water, or normal saline at a rate of approximately 60 ml per minute, there is little increase in intravesical pressure.

— The intravesical pressure normally remains below 100 mm to 200 mm fof water because of the phenomenon of adaptation.

— After 175 ml to 250 ml has run in, the patient will experience a feeling of fullness and a first desire to void.

— Desire gradually subsides and with further filling to 350–500 ml there is again a normal desire to micturate.

— Second desire is voluntarily inhibited until a convenient time and place is available.

— Stimulus to void is probably related largely to activation of gravity receptors at the base of the bladder in addition to stretch receptors in the bladder wall.

— The limit of tolerance lies in the range 500–800 ml and decreases slowly after the age of 40–50 years.

Normal emptying

— In the infant, micturation is activated by a purely spinal reflex, which later develops into a conscious process with integration of smooth and striated muscle action.

— In normal micturition there is a contraction of the detrusor muscle which induces an opening of the bladder neck, and together with this there is a relaxation of the pelvic floor and external sphincter.

— Usually there is little or no hesitance at the commencement of voiding.

— The mean flow rate is 15–20 ml per second.
— At the end of voiding the external sphincter and bulbocavernous muscle contract, forcing urine in the urethra and then out or back into the bladder.
— If there is bladder neck obstruction, normal milking back is prevented and when the voluntary muscles relax there may be terminal dribbling.

URINARY INCONTINENCE

— There are a number of types of incontinence, and some are of importance to the gynaecologist.
— Diagnosis and assessment depend on careful history, then on the investigations:
  • Frequency of micturation by day and by night
  • Volumes of urine passed
  • Urgency and urge incontinence
  • Difficulty in starting stream
  • Dribbling at the end of micturition
  • Incontinence, urge, stress, continuous
  • Amount of urine lost
  • Bed wetting at night
  • Feeling of incomplete emptying
  • Pain on micturition, beginning, during and at end
  • Blood in the urine
  • Aggravation by intercourse
  • Relation to the menstrual cycle
  • Relation to medication
  • Presence of discharge from urethra
  • The time of onset of the current problems
  • Severity, duration, frequency of occurrence
  • Precipitating factors
— Incontinence may be due to:
  • Congenital abnormality
  • Genito-urinary fistulae
  • Overflow incontinence
  • Stress incontinence
  • Detrusor instability

Congenital abnormality
— Ectopic ureter opening into the vagina.
— Ectopia vesicae.
— Both require surgical treatment.

Genito-urinary fistulae
— A genital fistula is an abnormal communication between some part of the genital canal and the urinary tract.

— Genito-urinary fistulae are divided into four groups:
  • Ureterovaginal fistulae which usually follow hysterectomy (radical surgery)
  • High vesicovaginal fistulae which can follow lower segment caesarian section, uterine rupture, hysterectomy or radiotherapy for carcinoma of the cervix
  • Mid-vaginal vesicovaginal fistulae may be caused by pressure necrosis after prolonged obstructed labour or colporrhaphy
  • Peri-urethral fistulae and urethral fistulae mostly due to pressure necrosis or trauma by rotational forceps

Aetiology

— The commonest cause of genital fistulae in past years was obstetrical trauma, direct injury or pressure necrosis.
— Occurs mainly in the developing countries.
— There is considerable reduction in the incidence of obstetrical fistulae, due to improvement in obstetrical management.
— Surgical trauma, usually abdominal hysterectomy, vaginal repair or urological procedures on the bladder neck are responsible for urogenital fistulae in the developed countries.
— Other causes are the destruction of tissue by malignant tumours, ulceration due to foreign bodies, especially vaginal pessaries, radiotherapy.
— In rare cases infection, cervical cerclage during pregnancy and road traffic accidents may cause fistulae.
— Ureterovaginal fistulae are complications resulting from radical (Wertheim) hysterectomy, when the ureters are displaced by tumours or when they are involved in pelvic inflammatory disease and endometriosis.

Symptoms

— Continuous leakage of urine from the vagina.
— May be only a slight dribble in some women, and they may pass some urine via the urethra.
— In some women there is flow of urine from the vagina and no urine is voided via the urethra.
— Irritation of the vagina, vulva and perineum is produced by the constant leakage.

Diagnosis

— It is easy to make the diagnosis.
— Exact location and nature of the fistula are not always easy to determine.

— Simple atony of the sphincter following difficult delivery and surgery may produce intermittent leakage and usually occurs after sneezing and coughing; this should be differentiated from true incontinence.
— Fistulae can be usually visualised in the knee–chest position, especially if they are small.
— Larger fistulae can easily be palpated.
— Very small fistulae may be identified by filling the bladder with methylene — blue-coloured sterile water, and observing the escape of the bluish fluid.
— Cystoscopic examination gives valuable information.
— Occasionally intravenous or retrograde pyelogram or both may be necessary.

Treatment

— Small fistulae, unless produced by malignant disease, occasionally close spontaneously.
— This is often facilitated by:
  • Postural treatment
  • Limitation of fluid
  • Urinary antiseptics
  • Indwelling catheter with continuous suction drainage
— If a spontaneous cure does not occur, surgery is indicated but should be deferred to allow maximum tissue healing.
  • Approximate intervals will depend on the cause
  • With a fistula following surgery, one should wait for 10 to 12 weeks.
  • In cases of fistula following obstructed labour, the interval needs to be 3 to 6 months.
  • Fistula following radiation may need a year or more to provide adequate healing following surgery.

Pre-operative assessment

— Assessment of general health.
— Urine and sensitivity.
— Intravenous pyelogram and urethrogram.
— Cystoscopic examination.
— Assessment under anaesthesia.
— If fistula is associated with radiotherapy for neoplasm, a biopsy of the edge should be taken to exclude tumour activity.

Operative closure

— The approach may be vaginal or transvesical.
— Ideally the patient should be referred to centres or surgeons or gynaecologists with special expertise.
— Most urethrovaginal and vesicovaginal fistulae can be repaired vaginally by gentle dissection and repair in layers.

— The bladder wall closure should be meticulous and watertight.
— Over 70% of fistulae can be closed at the first attempt, which should be the best attempt for success.
— Following operation, continuous closed bladder drainage is necessary for 10 days.
— Some physicians use cortisone to minimise fibrosis and prophylactic antibiotics to prevent infection.
— An abdominal approach is necessary if the fistula involves ureters.

Overflow incontinence

— In this condition the bladder becomes filled to capacity and intermittent dribbling occurs as further urine flows into the bladder from the ureters.
— In the female the main cause is disturbance of the nerves supplying the bladder, so that there is loss of sensation of fullness (afferent supply) or loss of motor nerves to the bladder muscle (efferent supply).
— Trauma to the spinal cord, nervous disorders such as multiple sclerosis, or surgery (radical hysterectomy), extreme old age, debility, can cause this condition.
— Urethritis and painful vulvitis, trauma to the vulva, can cause reflex inhibition of micturition.
— Diagnosis is confirmed by catheterisation which reveals a large volume of urine.
— A retroverted incarcerated pregnant uterus may produce retention with overflow, usually between 10 and 14 weeks.
— Impacted fibromyoma, ovarian tumour and hysteria cause retention with overflow.
— Urethral stenosis as an isolated condition may affect the elderly patient.
— Malignant disease involving the lower urinary or genital tracts may occasionally be the cause of overflow incontinence.

Treatment
— Catheterisation as soon as possible.
— Suitable drug to control infection.
— If there is diminished detrusor function, drugs such as bethanechol (10–30 mg) or Carbachol (1–4 mg) may be given.
— Treatment of the primary cause.

Stress incontinence
Definition
— It is a leakage of urine through the urethra after a sudden increase in intra-abdominal pressure, thereby increasing

intravesical pressure, without a compensating increase in intra-urethral pressure.
— In this condition there is a weakness of the bladder neck and/or urethra which is not able to withstand sudden increases in intravesical pressure.
— Such increases are usually secondary to rises in intra-abdominal pressure but may be the result of detrusor instability.
— The condition is usually graded mild, moderate and severe, according to the degree of pressure rise necessary to cause the patient to lose urine involuntarily.
— In mild stress incontinence the loss of urine occurs during vigorous sporting activity, coughing or sneezing.
— In severe cases, loss occurs with a mild cough or sudden change in posture.

Aetiology
— There are two basic causes: overstretching and/or damage to the muscle fibres at the bladder neck, overstretching and/or damage to its supporting ligaments.
— The above conditions allow the bladder neck to descend through the hiatus of the pelvic diaphragm.
— Continence in the female is achieved because the urethrovesical junction and proximal urethra are above the pelvic floor muscles and therefore intra-abdominal structures.
— Any rise in intra-abdominal pressure is transmitted equally to the bladder and proximal urethra, which preserves the pressure gradient and maintains the positive urethral pressure.
— In genuine stress incontinence most of the urethra is below the pelvic floor.
— Hence increased intra-abdominal pressure will increase the intravesical pressure, and not urethral, and a small amount of urine will be lost.
— Funnelling of the bladder neck on exertion or straining without detrusor activity, a short functional length of the urethra, loss of posterior urethrovesical angle are associated features in stress incontinence.

Clinical features
— Patient is usually parous and is often over 40 years of age.
— Childbirth, pelvic surgery and post-menopausal hormonal changes may adversely affect the condition.
— Congenital lesions such as a short urethra, relaxed bladder neck syndrome and female epispadias may cause stress incontinence.
— It is common for patients to experience stress incontinence for the first time in pregnancy, with improvement after delivery.

— The amount of urine escaping is usually small because of the immediate voluntary contraction of the external sphincter; also intravesical pressure increases only for a few seconds.
— It is common for patients to experience stress incontinence even with little urine in the bladder.

Investigation
— History.
— Examination.
— Specific tests.
— Urodynamic tests.
— Past history:
  • Medical and surgical history, STD, polio, surgery to spine or genito-urinary tract, cerebral, spinal and pelvic trauma.
  • Gynaecological surgery
  • Rapid or very slow labour, large infants
  • Enuresis, urinary infection, haematuria
  • Family history of diabetes, enuresis
  • Social history — drug abuse, excessive intake of alcohol and/or smoking
— Present complaint:
  • Duration of the symptoms
  • If symptoms are continuous or intermittent
  • If incontinent, type, amount of loss, degree of social inconvenience
  • Presence of urgency incontinence
  • Voiding difficulties, initiation, stream termination
  • Frequency — diurnal and nocturnal
  • Urinary infection
— In stress incontinence, micturition is normal, urine loss is small and the patient can interrupt the flow.
— Examination to demonstrate incontinence, uterovaginal prolapse, any other pathology and post-menopausal atrophic changes in the vagina.
— Specific tests:
  • Urine microscopy and culture
  • Cystoscopy
  • Intravenous pyelogram to exclude congenital abnormalities, calculi and other lesions
  • Bonney's test, in which the bladder neck is supported well up behind the symphysis pubis by the index and middle fingers placed in the lateral vaginal fornices. Prevents passage of urine on coughing. Test, if positive, indicates that surgical elevation of the bladder neck area will cure the symptoms
— Urodynamic tests:
  • Uroflowmetry will differentiate abnormal from normal voiding

- Cystometry tests the filling function of the bladder (bladder capacity)
- Intravesical and abdominal pressure (rectal) are measured simultaneously
- By subtracting the rectal from the intravesical pressure, intrinsic bladder pressure can be determined
- Cystometry should ideally be done in the supine and erect position, since instability may not be detected in the supine position in some women.

— Micturition cystourethrography is useful in assessing the anatomical relationship of the urethra, urethrovesical junction and bladder base, pictures being taken at rest, during coughing or bearing down and at the beginning, middle and end of micturition.

— Videocystourethrography (VCU) combines measurement of bladder pressure, urine flow and volume. It is especially helpful for the assessment of detrusor instability and neurological disturbances.

- VCU is indicated when urge and stress incontinence symptoms present
- Stress incontinence with frequency and nocturia
- Perpetual wetness
- Failed surgery for stress incontinence
- Adult enuresis
- Abnormal neurological signs

— Urethral pressure profile.

— Use of Urilos nappy test.

Treatment

— The major decision to be made is whether the symptoms are sufficient to warrant surgery, if so what component, if any, of dyssynergia is present that will persist after bladder neck repair.

— The need for surgery should be decided by the patient after she has been informed of the risks of surgery and the prospects of cure.

Physiotherapy

— Perineal exercises are useful prophylaxis after childbirth and in patients with milder problems.

Drug therapy

— Hormone therapy in post-menopausal women is usually useful.

Mechanical devices

— Vaginal ring pessary and Hodge pessary are found to be useful in some patients.

— Inflatable devices which exert pressure within the vagina to elevate the bladder neck have been tried.

— Electrical devices have been used with certain amount of benefit in those awaiting and unfit for surgery.
— A large-sized vaginal tampon may prove useful for a short period.
— An implantable artificial sphincter can be inserted, an inflatable cuff being used to occlude the bladder neck.

Surgery

— Restores the position of the proximal urethra as an intra-abdominal structure.
— Increases the urethral closure pressure.
— Increases the functional urethral length.
— Increases the support to bladder neck and therefore its competence.
— The type of surgery usually depends on whether there is a significant degree of cysto-urethrocele and/or uterine prolapse.
— Anterior colporrhaphy is the conventional surgery for stress incontinence and anterior vaginal wall prolapse. It cures stress incontinence in 50–60%.
— Primary suprapubic procedures are reported to have success rates of 80–90%.
  • Urethropexy by the Marshall-Marchetti and Krantz technique involves suturing the para-urethral and paravesical tissues to cartilage of the symphysis pubis or periosteum of the pelvic ramus and back of the pubic bone
  • Colposuspension by the Burch technique involves suturing the paravaginal fascia to the ileopectineal ligament on the same side
  • Urethrovesical slings using either muscular or fascial strips or Mersilene gauze are also useful, and this requires a combined vaginal and abdominal approach

Causes of failure

— Poor evaluation of pathology.
— Larger dyssynergia component (instability).
— Persistence of precipitating factors such as smoking, constipation, overweight, chronic cough.
— Wrong operation and poor technique.

Urinary diversion procedure

— Used as a final resort in patients in whom all other methods have failed.
— Construction of an ileal bladder is the method of choice.

Detrusor instability

— Stress incontinence and urge incontinence may coexist.
— Bladder instability is characterised by urge incontinence.

Incidence

— Sphincter disturbance — 40%
— Combined sphincter disturbance and bladder instability — 20%
— Bladder instability (motor type) — 20%
— Bladder instability (sensory type) — 10%
— Other (reflex, overflow, extra-urethral) — 10%

Definition

— Bladder or detrusor instability (dyssynergia) means faulty co-ordination of muscles usually acting in harmony.

Pathophysiology

— Disturbance is in the detrusor muscle of the bladder wall which does not accommodate correctly to normal filling pressure and contracts spasmodically and often without warning.
— The gradient between vesical and urethral pressure will determine whether incontinence will result.
— Urgency of micturation is a strong sensation of the desire to void.
— This may precede an uncontrolled detrusor contraction and the leakage of a large amount of urine (urge incontinence).
— Urgency usually results from either a sensory disturbance, irritation of the otherwise normal bladder wall by inflammation, calculus, neoplasia or funnelling of the bladder neck which allows urine to come into contact with the proximal urethra, thus exciting detrusor reflex activity.
— It may also result from motor disturbance, often indicating bladder instability.
— If the patient has a strong external sphincter, she may be able to control micturition temporarily.
— Unduly rapid filling of the bladder for, e.g. diuretics, excess alcohol intake, may stimulate detrusor activity.
— Same effect occurs when there is an acute rise in intra-abdominal pressure.

Aetiology

— The cause of the primary instability of the detrusor remains unknown.
— Upper motor neuron lesion such as multiple sclerosis.
— Inflammation tends to exacerbate the condition.
— Oestrogen deficiency in post-menopausal women.
— Bladder outflow obstruction, rare in women.

Clinical features

— Urgency of micturition.
— Urge incontinence.
— Frequency during day and night.
— Enuresis.

Investigation

— Urine examination using microscope for protein, sugar and culture.
— Serum urea and electrolytes.
— Full blood count.
— Cystoscopy, excretion urography.
— Flow-rate estimation, ml/second (normal is above 15–20 ml/s, but this depends on age).
— Neurological assessment is necessary.
— Cystometry using sterile water or saline will measure bladder capacity, bladder tone response to filling.
— Video cystourethrography.
— In patients with bladder instability, the capacity of the bladder may be less than normal.
— Filling pressure is more than 20 mm or more.
— Bladder responds to a rapid increase in pressure (e.g. bearing down, especially if standing or during rapid filling) by detrusor contraction and opening of the vesical neck.

Management

Psychological aspects

— There may be a significant psychogenic component to the disorder.
— Emotional stress, psychosomatic symptoms should be treated.
— Patient education as to the nature of the disorder is helpful and is important.

Bladder drill or training

— Patient is admitted to assess the extent of her problem.
— She is instructed to pass urine by the clock during the day.
— The interval starts at 30 minutes and gradually increases.
— When good progress is made, she is sent home to continue with the bladder drill.
— Bladder drill is very effective and does not involve expensive equipment or surgery.

Drug therapy

— Drugs with anticholinergic activity may be beneficial.
— Anticholinergic drugs:
  • Emepromium promide (Cetiprin)
  • Flavoxate (Urispas)
  • Dicyclomine (Merbentyl)
  • Propantheline (Pro-banthine)
— Antidepressant agents:
  • Imipramine (Tofranil)
  • Amitriptyline (Tryptizol)
  • Diazepam (Valium)
— Betamimetic agents:
  • Orciprenaline sulphate (Alupent)

— Hormones:
  - Oestrogen replacement therapy (orally or vaginally)

Surgery

— Prolonged bladder distension.
— Bladder neck operations.
— Urinary diversion.

VOIDING DIFFICULTIES

The urethral syndrome

— Recurrent episodes of frequency and dysuria not associated with any significant abnormality in the urinary tract.
— There may or may not be associated infection.

Aetiology

— It is usually due to a combination of proliferation of organisms in the introitus and the failure of the urethral defence mechanisms to prevent the bacteria invading the lower urinary tract.
— Significant bacteriuria ($> 10^5$ organisms/ml) is present in 50% of the cases.
— Infective causes:
  - Lack of personal hygiene
  - Conditions which promote vulvovaginitis
  - Commonest infective agents are normal bowel flora
  - Other common organisms are *T. vaginalis*, *N. gonnorrhoeae* and *Chlamydia trachomatis*
— Gynaecological causes:
  - Possible cervical ectropion is an association
  - Method of contraception
  - Post-menopausal oestrogen deficiency
— Chemical or allergic reactions:
  - Soaps
  - Douches
  - Deodorants
  - Contraceptive foam, pessaries, cream
  - Anti-oxidants in condoms
  - Nylon underclothes
— Sexual causes:
  - Frequent and clumsy sexual activity
  - Masturbation with a foreign body
  - Associated with first intercourse (honeymoon cystitis)
— Psychological causes:
  - Anxiety
  - Neuroticism
  - It is difficult to be certain what produces what

— Bladder problems:
- Bladder outlet obstruction is rare in women
- Detrusor instability is not uncommon
- Bladder tumour

— Multiple sclerosis may present with similar symptoms.

Investigation

— History.

— Haematuria needs full investigation.

— Cystoscopy, urethroscopy and excretion urography.

— Full gynaecological examination.

— Microscopy and culture of urine.

— Urine is tested for protein and glucose.

— Occasionally urodynamic investigation.

Treatment

— Improve perineal and introital hygiene.

— Antiseptic douching and bathing should be avoided.

— Increase in fluid intake.

— Potassium citrate may help.

— Avoid nylon underclothes.

— Appropriate treatment of vulvovaginitis and persistent vaginal discharge.

— Short course of hormone replacement therapy in post-menopausal women with atrophic changes.

— Urethrotomy may be helpful in some.

— If there is bladder neck obstruction, it can be treated by endoscopic incision of the bladder neck.

— Psychotherapy may also be helpful in some.

Neurogenic bladder disorders

— Damage to the nerve supply may interfere with the control of micturition by blocking motor pathways of inhibition or contractility or abolishing sensory appreciation of bladder filling, causing precipitous micturition without warning to the patient.

— A hypotonic bladder is produced by a lower motor neuron lesion — surgical trauma to the parasympathetic motor nerves S 2-3-4 at the time of radical Wertheim hysterectomy.

— Hypertonic bladder results from an upper motor neuron lesion.

— In multiple sclerosis there initially be a hypertonic detrusor which later becomes hypotonic, with progressively rising outflow resistance from a spastic pelvic floor.

— Impaired control may follow stroke, cord lesions or mental clouding associated with arteriosclerosis, metabolic toxins, drugs.

— The incidence rises to 15% in females over the age of 65.
— Neurological examination is essential.

URETHRAL DISORDERS

Urethritis

— Inflammatory disorders of the urethra are fairly common.
— Sexually transmitted disease (STD) forms a major part of these; gonococcus and Chlamydia trachomatis.
— Trichomonas, moniliasis and certain viruses also produce problems.
— Disease is limited to the distal half to two-thirds of the urethra and is often part of vulvovaginitis.
— Infection involves the mucosa and para-urethral glands.
— Honeymoon cystitis is probably related to frequent and/or vigorous coitus.
— A urethral meatus tethered to the anterior part of the hymen is a common cause of honeymoon cystitis.
  • Adequate coital lubrication
  • Altered coital position
  • Hormone replacement therapy in the post-menopausal women
  • Frequent daytime voiding and increased fluid intake
  • Avoiding excess moisture
  • Avoiding and excluding allergic and chemical reaction to contraceptives, deodorants and detergents should prevent episodes of honeymoon cystitis and urethritis

Symptoms
— Dysuria.
— Frequency.

Diagnosis
— Reddened urethral orifice.
— Purulent exudate from the meatus.
— Milking of the urethra will show the discharge for culture and microscopy.
— Urethroscopy.

Treatment
— Appropriate antibiotics.
— Urinary antiseptic.
— Oestrogen if there is atrophic change.

Urethral caruncle

— It is a common condition.
— Occurs many years after the menopause.
— There is vaginal atrophy.
— It results in the exposure of the urethral mucosa which becomes swollen due to chronic infection and pouts like a red cherry posteriorly from the external meatus.
— The patient may present with bleeding, usually post-coital, dyspareunia and pain.
— Treatment is by electrocoagulation diathermy after biopsy and curettage to exclude endometrial carcinoma if there is a history of bleeding.
— Oestrogen cream could be applied.

Urethral prolapse

— Prolapse of the urethral mucosa is uncommon.
— Occurs in the very young and in the very old.
— Cause is straining, and lack of oestrogen.
— Treatment is excision with suturing of the urethral mucosa to the circumference of the external urethral meatus.

Urethral diverticulum

— It is present in 2–4% of adult females.
— Rarely diagnosed.
— Symptoms are relatively non-specific.
— Symptoms may be:
  • Frequency of micturition
  • Dysuria, especially after intercourse
  • Dribbling
  • Urgency
  • Incontinence
  • Urethral or pelvic pain
  • Dyspareunia
  • Haematuria
  • Vaginal discharge
  • Vaginal lump

Diagnosis

— Palpation anteriorly in the vagina confirms the swelling.
— When pressed, few drops of urine may be seen from the meatus.
— It is not easy to diagnose the condition using urethroscopy.
— Micturating cystourethrogram often demonstrates the lesion.
— Differential diagnoses are:
  • Abscess of Skene's gland

- Urethral tumour
- Cystocele
— Treatment is surgical excision or marsupialisation.

Urethral stenosis

— Urethral narrowing usually occurs at the bladder neck or at the meatus.
— May be congenital or the result of neoplasm, diverticulum, infection or injury.
— Patient gives history of recurrent cystitis and poor urinary stream.
— Diagnosis is suggested by a low urinary flow (<15 ml/second).
— Urethroscope shows blanched meatal mucosa on passage of a 28F or smaller scope and bleeding on its withdrawal.
— There will be trabeculation of the walls of the bladder.

Treatment
— This depends on the cause:
- Frequent dilatation of urethra
- May need to repeat at 3-monthly intervals
- Occasionally a plastic operation may be necessary
- Urethrotomy
- Treatment of causes such as cyst or tumour

SUGGESTED READING

Bates C P, Taylor M C 1984 Clinical investigation of bladder function. In: Symonds, E. M, Zuspan F B (eds) Clinical and diagnostic procedures in obstetrics and gynaecology. Part B, Gynaecology, Dekker, New York, p 57
Beck R P 1979 Urinary stress incontinence reviewed. In: Stallworthy J, Bourne G (eds) Recent advances in obstetrics and gynaecology, vol 13. Churchill Livingstone, Edinburgh, p 211
Beck R P 1984 An overview of urinary stress incontinence. In: Symonds E M, Zuspan F P (eds) Clinical and diagnostic procedures in obstetrics and gynaecology. Part B, Gynaecology. Dekker.
Fantl J A 1984 Urinary incontinence due to detrusor instability. In: Mattingly R F (ed) Clinical obstetrics and gynaecology, vol 27. Harper & Row, New York, p 474
Jordan J A, Stanton S L (eds) 1981 The incontinent women. Scientific Meeting of the RCOG.
Marchant D J 1984 Clinical evaluation of urinary incontinence and abnormal anatomy and pathopysiology. In: Mattingly R F (ed) Clinical obstetrics and gynaecology, vol 27. Harper & Row, New York, p 434
Mattingly R F, Davis L E 1984 Primary treatment of anatomic stress urinary incontinence. In: Mattingly, R F (ed) Clinical obstetrics and gynaecology, vol 27. Harper & Row, New York, p 445
Smith P B 1979 The management of the urethral syndrome. British Journal of Hospital Medicine 22:578
Stanton S L (ed) 1978 Gynaecological urology. In: Clinics in obstetrics and gynaecology, vol 5. Saunders, Philadelphia
Stanton S L, Tanagho E (eds) 1980 Surgery of female incontinence. Springer, Berlin
Stanton S L (ed) 1984 Clinical gynecologic urology. Mosby, New York

13. INFECTION OF THE GENITAL TRACT

LOWER GENITAL TRACT INFECTION

Introduction

— Infections of the cervix, vagina and vulva are common gynaecological lesions.
— Often the urethra is infected.
— Majority of infections need specific therapy.
— Post-pubertal infections are often associated with sexual activity.

Factors maintaining the health of the lower genital tract

— Vagina is usually empty and is full of organisms that live in harmony with the host.
— When the natural defences of the body (local and/or general) are depressed, the resident flora may produce problems.
— Vaginal pH, epithelial status and introital closure help to maintain the integrity of the lower genital tract.

Vaginal pH

— Vaginal acidity is protective against infections.
  • It depends mainly on oestrogen
  • Oestrogen acts on vaginal epithelium
  • This in turn produces glycogen
  • Lactobacilli produce lactic acid
  • This in turn reduces the pH of the vagina to 3.5–4.5
  • Low pH prevents the growth of other bacteria
— Vaginal acidity is reduced when there is lack of oestrogen at:
  • Pre-puberty
  • Postpartum period
  • Post-menopausal status
— Vaginal acidity is reduced when there is excessive mucus production from the cervix.
— Vaginal pH is reduced by seminal fluid, menstrual blood, douching and progestin therapy.

Epithelial status

- The thickness and thus the resistance of the epithelium depends on oestrogen level.
- A fall in hormone level makes the epithelium thinner, fragile and susceptible to infection.
- Sexual activity will produce trauma to vaginal epithelium if the vagina is dry and this facilitates infection.
- Vaginal pessaries can produce trauma.
- Forgotten tampons will damage the epithelium and produce infection.

Introital closure

- Vagina is usually kept closed by the surrounding muscles.
- This closure effect may be damaged by childbirth.
- Lack of closure allows the perineal micro-organisms to gain access into the vagina.
- Ascending infection from the perineal and perianal region may be associated with poor hygiene and toilet technique.
- Scarring from previous infection may produce obstruction and recurrent infection.
- Cervical ectropion and chronic cervicitis may produce excessive mucus, which raises the vaginal pH.
- Immunoglobulin in the cervical mucus, especially IgA and with specific immune cells, macrophages and polymorphs keep the vaginal flora under control.

Underclothes and cosmetics

- Tight-fitting nylon clothes produce heat and moisture and promote infection.
- Cosmetics and chemicals upset the vaginal flora and vaginal pH.

Sexual activity

- If coital activity is rough and excessive, it may introduce organisms from the perineum and perianal regions to the vagina.
- Trauma.
- Certain coital techniques.
- Sexually transmitted diseases may be introduced.

VAGINAL DISCHARGE

- Needs action if it wets the underclothes or if protection is necessary.
- Common in the reproductive period.
- It is a common complaint.
- May be associated with:
  - Backache

- Pruritus
- Irritation
- Urinary tract symptoms
- Post-coital bleeding

Aetiology

Physiological
— Main contribution is from the cervix, especially at mid-cycle.
— At the time of coitus.
— In pregnancy the columnar epithelium expands on to the ectocervix as a result of oestrogenic stimulus.
— The discharge is usually clear, though it may be mucoid or white.
— Quantity varies right through the menstrual cycle.
— During oestrogen-containing medication such as the oral contraceptive combined pill, there is excess discharge.
— Intra-uterine devices also cause discharge.

Pathological
— Infections of the vulva, vagina and cervix most commonly cause discharge.
— Sometimes infection of the endometrium and endosalpinx may also produce discharge.
— Benign and malignant lesions of the genital tract may also produce discharge.

Investigation

History
— Nature of discharge (mucoid, serous, purulent).
— Colour (white, yellowish, green).
— Bloodstained or not.
— Duration (continuous or intermittent).
— Quantity (needing protection).
— Relation to menstrual cycle.
— Relation to sexual activity and technique.
— Pregnancy.
— Drug therapy.
— Previous episodes and treatment.
— Medical condition.
— Associated symptoms.
— Hygiene practices.

Examination
— General examination.
— Examination of vulva, vagina and cervix under good light.
— Bimanual examination.

— Swabs from the urethra, Bartholin's gland orifice, cervix and rectum for microbiology.
— Poor correlation between symptoms and abnormalities detected suggests investigation to exclude psychosomatic problems.

Non-sexually transmitted infections causing vaginal discharge

Staphylococcal infection
— Not common.
— Classical tampon toxic shock syndrome.
— Associated with fever, vomiting and diarrhoea, aches, pains, skin erythema, hypotension, may lead to death.
— Check for kidney, liver, muscle and blood involvement.
— Treatment is to correct shock, hypotension; following hospitalisation appropriate antibiotics, Methicillin or Flucloxacillin.

Sexually-transmitted infection

Aetiology
— Gonorrhoea.
— Syphilis.
— Chancroid.
— Lymphogranuloma venereum.
— Granuloma inguinale.
— *Trichomonas* infection.
— Herpes simplex.
— Papilloma virus.
— Chlamydia.
— *Mycoplasma*.
— Gardeneralla vaginalis.
— Sometimes fungal infection.
— Less commonly Group B streptococci, cytomegalic virus, actinomycosis, hepatitis B virus, *Schistosoma*.
— Gonorrhoea continues to be a problem.
— Syphilis is largely controlled.
— Increase in STD is due to:
  ● Greater sexual freedom
  ● Reduction in the use of barrier methods
  ● Drug use
  ● Greater freedom in travelling and mobility
  ● Changes in sexual behaviour

[Handwritten annotation:]
Principles of STDs
1) commonly multiple
2) often (asymptomatic
3) low infectivity
4) Infect anyone!

Fungal infections

— Organism is *Candida albicans*.
— Grows well at a low pH (5–6.5).
— Common in pregnancy, in the reproductive period.
— Common in obese women.
— Common in diabetes.
— Common following oral contraceptive combined pill use.
— Common following use of antibiotics.
— Immunosuppressive therapy causes this infection.

Clinical features

— The infection may be totally asymptomatic.
— There is minimum discharge externally.
— It produces intense pruritus and soreness.
— May spread to labia, upper thigh and intergluteal folds.
— May cause dyspareunia in severe infection.
— May be associated with urological symptoms.
— Examination reveals brick-red areas underneath the curd-like precipitate in the vagina and vulval area.
— When discharge is examined characteristic hyphae and spores are seen.

Treatment

— Specific antifungal creams or pessaries may be useful (nystatin, miconazole, Econazole).
— Resistant infection may respond to 1% gentian violet paint.
— In recurrent infections oral medication using nystatin or Ketoconazole may be helpful for patient and partner.
— Reduction of weight and treatment of diabetes are helpful.
— Effective prompt treatment of fungal infection when the patient is on antibiotics and immunosuppressive therapy.

Trichomonas vaginalis

— This flagellated protozoon is thought to originate in the bowel.
— It is usually a problem after the onset of sexual activity.
— It is found in the male and may reinfect his partner.
— Incidence varies: 1% or less among healthy asymptomatic women, 20–30% in women attending a venereal disease clinic.
— Can co-exist with gonococcal infection.

Clinical features

— Discharge is profuse, thin, frothy and yellow-green in colour.
— There is often a characteristic odour.
— The cervix and vagina appear diffusely reddened and show a punctate appearance.
— Vagina is tender.

— Causes dyspareunia.
— Diagnosed using culture from a charcoal swab placed in stuart medium, also using saline preparation and viewing it under a microscope.

Treatment

— Metronidazole 600–1000 mg/day for 7 days.
— Tinidazole 2 g daily for 7 days.
— Side-effects are nausea and alcohol intolerance.
— Sexual partner should be treated.

Herpes simplex

— Herpes simplex infection is a major problem.
— It is short-lasting but may recur frequently.
— Associated with severe discomfort and inability to work; it also has a tendency to spread.
— Physical and emotional distress of this disease is significantly higher than with most other STDs.
— Virus has a high infectivity; 80% of susceptible women will become infected following contact with infected male.
— Virus lies dormant in the body between attacks.
— Incidence of genital herpes infection is 5–10 times more common than primary syphilis.
— Immunity develops after 1 or 2 attacks.
— Baby is at greater risk at birth if the mother has active infection.

Clinical features

— Produces acute inflammation.
— Caused by herpes simplex virus 2 (HSV2).
— If oral genital sex practice is prevalent, then HSV1 is also isolated.
— The incubation period is usually 3–7 days, but may be up to several weeks.
— Labial and peri-anal skin may be involved.
— Initially an indurated tender papule develops.
— Then vesicles develop and break down into a shallow ulcer which is extremely painful.
— There is associated erythema, discharge and swelling.
— Inguinal nodes are often involved.
— Symptoms are burning, itchiness, hyperaesthesia, watery discharge and severe dyspareunia.
— If peri-urethral area is involved, then patient suffers from dysuria, retention of urine.
— General symptoms are malaise, headache, neuralgia.
— Can affect the rectum, and patient develops related acute proctitis.

— Many attacks are often subclinical and usually involve the vagina and cervix.
— The reason for activation and deactivation of HSV2 is not clear.
— Acute phase usually lasts for 3–5 days, during which time there is free viral shedding and the disease is most infective.
— Healing occurs by day 8 or 10.

Diagnosis

— History.
— Presence of crops of vesicles or shallow small ulcers.
— Stained smear shows mutlinucleate cells with chromatin condensed against nuclear membrane; eosinophilic inclusion bodies are also present within the cell.
— Viral isolation can be made from the vesicular fluid or material scraped from the ulcer.
— HSV1 is identified in 10–14% or more of patients with acute genital herpes. Seldom seen in recurrent attacks or in those who use corticosteroids and cancer therapy.
— Blood antibody level will differentiate the primary and secondary infection.
— Swabs are taken into transport medium and held at 4°C or below prior to despatching to virology laboratory.
— Differential diagnosis includes other STDs, Behçet's syndrome and other ulcerative lesions.

Treatment

Prophylaxis

— When there is a possible history of herpes infection in the male partner, he needs investigation and treatment.
— Use of barrier methods for contraception may provide a certain amount of protection.
— Physical and emotional stress often precipitates attacks, hence attention should be paid to this and treatment started immediately.

Definitive therapy

— Ice pack may relieve the discomfort.
— Soothing local creams, but not cortisone-based, and analgesics to relieve pain.
— Idoxuridine is a topical antiviral, used every 5 minutes for 30 minutes and the interval gradually increased.
— Better results are achieved when the concentration of idoxuridine is 20% or more dissolved in dimethyl sulphoxide.
— Application of idoxuridine is only for 3 days because of skin maceration.
— Acyclovir 3% ointment is a newer drug.
— Silver nitrate solution, 10% application on the ulcer promotes healing.

— Saline sitz bath is soothing.
— Providone-iodine (Betadine) is useful to control secondary infection.
— Laser therapy may also be useful.
— Indwelling catheter may be necessary in acute phase with retention of urine.
— Systemically acting drugs will be of value for the relief of symptoms, reduction of viral shedding and extent of spread in the nervous system.
— Patient is counselled and advised to use barrier methods for contraception.
— A new compound zinc preparation (Zinvit) may reduce the frequency of attacks.

Papilloma virus (Condylomata acuminata)

— The genital wart virus is one of the papilloma virus.
— Identified as an intranuclear particle.
— Incubation period ranges from weeks to months.
— Highly infective once the lesion develops.
— It is sexually transmitted, and 50% or more will be affected.

Clinical features

— The initial lesion is usually single and soon spreads.
— This lesion is pink or white in colour, softer, friable than the common skin wart.
— The growth is excessive in the moist areas.
— Ulceration and secondary infection cause a thicker purulent discharge, and sometimes bleeding occurs.
— It grows rapidly and gets bigger in pregnancy.
— The site of lesion is usually the external genitalia but it may involve the vagina and cervix.

Diagnosis

— Characteric appearance.
— A flat type may look like condylomata lata.
— Histology shows a thick papillary squamous epithelium with thickening and elongation of rete peg's, acanthosis, parakeratosis together with fine dermal projections which are oedematous and infiltrated with chronic inflammatory cells.
— Should be differentiated from neoplasia, benign papilloma, verrucous carcinoma, giant condylomata and vulval carcinoma.
— Colposcopic examination of the cervix has shown that the incidence of lesion is 0.5–1%.

Treatment

— Small lesions may be treated with 20–25% podophyllin.
— May need repeat application.

— Solution is applied to the lesions only.
— Not suitable in pregnancy or if the lesion is too large and friable.
— Electrocautery and laser therapy under general anaesthesia.
— Surgical excision.
— Contacts need tracing.
— Advice regarding hygiene.

Chlamydia

— *Chlamydia trachomatis* has been incriminated in the majority of non-gonococcal urethritis in the male.
— Significant number of women may develop chronic cervicitis and salpingitis.
— The disease is usually isolated from sexually promiscuous population.
— Often found in the partners of the affected people.
— The incidence in the venerology clinic is 20–60%.
— In the family planning clinic it is only 2–6%.
— Produces conjunctivitis in babies born to affected mothers.
— Less commonly babies may develop trachoma, neonatal pneumonia and enteritis.

Clinical features

— Often produces mild symptoms in the female.
— Vaginal discharge may develop.
— Discharge may be watery or purulent.
— Can produce cervicitis and salpingitis.
— Cervix may look red, inflamed; there may be micro-abscess and loss of epithelium in severe infection.
— Produces chronic pelvic inflammatory disease and sterility.
— Reiter's syndrome may occur.
— Perihepatitis develops as in gonococcal infection.

Diagnosis

— The organism is a small, gram- negative intracellular bacterium; it is often missed on routine study of the discharge.
— Duration of symptoms is often prolonged but is less severe than gonococcal infection.
— Micro-immunofluorescence.
— Isolation in tissue culture.
— Fluorescent antibody.
— Giemsa and complement fixation are less efficient in isolating or diagnosing the condition.

Treatment

— Tetracycline is the drug of choice.

Mycoplasma

— There are many similarities between infections produced by the *Mycoplasma* group and by *Chlamydia*.
— It produces urethritis and prostatitis in the male.
— It produces cervicitis and salpingitis in the female.
— There are three species: *M. hominis*, *M. fermentans* and *Ureaplasma urealyticum*.
— These organisms have no cell wall, but contain both DNA and RNA.
— Approximately one-third of babies are colonised with *Mycoplasma* from the mothers' genital tract.
— The organisms mostly disappear until sexual activity starts.
— These organisms produce vaginitis and cervicitis and are implicated as a cause of early abortion.
— May produce salpingitis and puerperal infection.

Treatment

— Tetracycline 500 mg. 6 hourly, 7–14 days.
— This will cure co-existing gonorrhoea.
— Cotrimoxazole is also effective.
— Partner needs investigation and treatment.

Gardeneralla vaginalis

— The role of this organism in vaginal infection is not clear.
— It is a facultative anaerobe.
— It is a small gram-negative rod.

Clinical features

— Discharge is greyish-white and malodorous.
— Sometimes it is frothy.
— Symptoms are pruritus, frequency, dysuria, dyspareunia and post-coital bleeding.
— Infection is related to a rise in pH in the vagina.

Treatment

— Use Tinidazole or Metronidazole.

Gonorrhoea   Gram Negative intracellular diplococci

— This is a highly contagious disease.
— Affects both mucosal and glandular structures.
— Involvement of rectum and mouth will depend on the coital practice.
— Affects the eyes of neonates if mother has active infection in the birth canal at delivery.
— Incubation period is usually 3–7 days but may vary considerably.

Gonorrhoea does NOT cross the placenta

G

Incidence

— Varies considerably.
— Average rate is 1:250.
— In certain communities it is much higher.
— Factors contributing to its high prevalence:
  • Rapid incubation period
  • High degree of infectivity
  • Low immunity
  • Presence of asymptomatic carriers
  • Increased rate of casual sexual relationships
  • Efficiency of health care system, such as health education, special clinics, contact tracing
  • Type of contraception
— Incidence is higher in venerology clinics (25–30%) and lower in correctional institutions (5–10%) and in general clinics (0.5–5%).

Clinical features   *80% asymptomatic*

— Endocervicitis results in a purulent vaginal discharge.
— The colour varies: it may be white, creamy, yellow, green, brown and sometimes bloodstained.
— May be offensive and bubbly.
— Presence of other pathogens such as trichomonads and mixed bacteria may produce variable symptoms.
— Urethritis is not uncommon and causes dysuria.
— Bartholin's gland may be affected and may produce acute bartholinitis or even abscess.
— Ascending infection produces acute salpingitis and oophoritis.
— Pelvic peritonitis and perihepatitis may develop.
— Secondary infection due to aerobic and anaerobic organisms often supervenes.
— Often permanent damage occurs unless prompt diagnosis and adequate treatment are given.
— Common sequelae include:
  • Recurrent episodes of infection
  • Dyspareunia
  • Dysmenorrhoea
  • Sterility
  • Menorrhagia
  • Chronic pelvic pain
— It is important to exclude oral and rectal lesions if patients coital habits suggests the possibility.
— Vulvovaginal infection in the pre-pubertal period is uncommon (0.5%).
— Generalised infection is uncommon (1–2%).
— Joint involvement and skin lesions are manifestations of general disease.

Diagnosis

— History of exposure to a male who has the infection or develops it soon after the exposure.
— History of the patient's symptoms and their relationship to the sexual contact.
— History of previous infection and treatment.
— When baby develops ophthalmia neonatorum, the most likely cause is the infection in the mother.
— Swabs from the endocervix, orifice of Bartholin's gland, urethral meatus, rectum and oropharynx, depending on the patient's coital practice.
— Bimanual examination may reveal bilateral tenderness in the pelvis.
— Blood should be taken for serological studies to exclude syphilis and should be repeated 8–12 weeks later.
— Charcoal swab taken from all suspected orifices and sent in Stuart transport medium for culture and sensitivity.
— Fluorescent staining methods may show gonococci in direct smear.
— Sexual partner needs adequate investigation and treatment.

Treatment

— Acute uncomplicated cases — aqueous procaine penicillin G 4.8 million units.
— Oral probenecid 1 g is given half an hour before the administration of penicillin to delay renal excretion.
— Ampicillin 3.5 g or amoxycillin 3 g are effective as a single dose.
— Lactamase-resistant cephalosporin derivatives will cure more than 95% of patients.
— If patient is sensitive to penicillin, or the organism is resistant to this drug, tetracycline 1 g followed by 500 mg 6-hourly for 5 days, or doxycycline twice daily is useful.
— Trimethoprim/sulphamethoxazole 1 tablet or capsule twice daily for 5 days.
— Streptomycin 2 g i.m., but this drug has no effect on *Treponema pallidum, Chlamydia trachomatis* or *Ureaplasma urealyticum.*
— Penicillin G is effective against pharyngeal infection.
— In pregnancy, penicillin or erythromycin is used.
— When the infection involves the upper genital tract (20%) or is generalised, therapy should be continued for 2 to 3 days after the symptoms subside.
— In severe infection 10–20 million units of penicillin per day initially intravenously, then ampicillin 0.5 g 6-hourly for 5–6 days.
— Tetracycline and metronidazole may be added to the regimen

of treatment if the symptoms suggest any other type of infection already described.
— Two negative cultures after completion of treatment are considered as evidence of cure.
— Failure rate is high when the rectum is involved.
— If infection recurs, it may be due to a resistant strain or reinfection.
— For resistant strains, use a beta lactamase-resistant drug such as spectinomycin 2 g i.m. or cefoxitin 2 g i.m. together with probenecid.
— In cases of reinfection, prompt and meticulous contact tracing and education are necessary.

Prophylaxis
— Barrier methods protect against infection.
— Gonorrhoea is asymptomatic in 50–80% of females; if a man developes gonorrhoea after contact, then the asymptomatic woman should be traced.
— Women who have sexual contact with a man who is known to have the infection should be treated.
— If the male partner is suspected of having gonococcal infection, then the woman needs investigation for confirmation prior to treatment.
— Adequate and appropriate antibiotic regime including probenecid.
— Routine bacteriological examination as part of the follow-up programme.
— Systematic contact tracing and treatment.
— Testing of patients with resistant disease for penicillinase-producing organisms.
— 50% of females and 5% of males remain asymptomatic and spread the disease.

Granuloma inguinale

Clinical features
— If starts as a painless nodule.
— It breaks down into an ulcer which soon extends into the vulva and peri-anal region.
— Spread occurs to inguinal nodes by subcutaneous infiltration.
— Clinical features are discharge, dyspareunia swelling and ulceration.

— Causative organism is *Donovania granulomatis* related to the *Klebsiella* group.
— Intracellular Donovan bodies are found on microscopic examination of the exudate or from crushed tissue smear.

- The differential diagnosis are lymphogranuloma venereum, condylomata lata, condylomata acuminata, carcinoma and conditions causing lymphadenitis and lymphoedema.
- Secondary infection is common.
- The disease is more prevalent in the tropics and subtropics.
- Heat, humidity, poor hygiene are predisposing factors.
- This condition is moderately contagious and auto-innoculable.

Treatment
- Tetracycline 1–2 g daily for 2–3 weeks.
- In pregnancy erythromycin 1–2 g daily for 2–3 weeks.
- Social and hygiene measures are important.

Lymphogranuloma venereum

Clinical features
- Initial lesion is a small papule or vesicle which appears 1–2 weeks after contact.
- It then breaks down in 1–2 weeks to produce a relatively painless ulcer.
- Two to three weeks later inguinal lymphadenitis develops.
- Often multiple nodes are involved, matted together and adhering to the skin.
- Later the matted lymphadenitis produces an abscess and breaks down into multiple sinuses.
- Proctocolitis and pelvic lymphadenitis may develop in some women.
- If rectum and intestines are involved, the woman may develop stricture and later obstruction.
- In some women, a peri-anal and rectovaginal fistula may develop.
- Once the lymphatic blockage occurs, elephantiasis of the vulva will develop.
- This disease is caused by a member of the *Chlamydia* group.
- It responds to the usual antibiotics.
- Extensive damage to the lymphatic system may not be cured.

Diagnosis
- Serological tests are of most value (micro-immunofluorescence technique).
- A complement fixation test is used to assess the effect of treatment.

Treatment
- Tetracycline.
- Erythromycin.
- Sulphisoxazole is an alternative.
- Abscess may need drainage.

Chancroid

— The causative organism is *Haemophilus ducreyi*, a Gram-negative organism.
— It produces soft chancre which is painful.
— It involves lymph nodes in the inguinal region and produces a painful swelling.
— Regional lymphadenitis develops in 1–2 weeks.
— Suppuration and abscess formation is common.
— Aspiration of pus allows laboratory confirmation.
— Sulfisoxazole is effective if given for 10–14 days.
— Amoxicillin 500 mg three times a day, together with calvulanic acid 125 mg three times daily for 7 days is an alternative.

Syphilis

— This used to be the dominant venereal disease.
— Its incidence has fallen dramatically.
— Reliable serological testing in all pregnant women has helped to control the disease.
— There is no acquired resistance of this organism to penicillin.
— The long incubation period allows contact tracing.

Incidence

— In the developed Western world the incidence is 1 : 1000 to 1 : 5000.
— Higher incidence is reported in the developing world.
— More common in poorer urban communities and in homosexuals.

Clinical features

Primary syphilis

— Incubation period is in the range 10–80 days.
— Then one papule appears, usually painless, which is the primary lesion.
— Mucosa of the lower genital tract is vulnerable to this infection.
— Rarely seen in the mouth or the anorectal region, depending on the coital habits.
— After 7 days or so, papule becomes a solitary non-tender indurated ulcer — the chancre.
— Usually the chancre heals in 2–6 weeks.
— There may be enlargement of one or two discrete lymph nodes
— If no treatment, the next stage develops.

Secondary syphilis

— Develops in 6 weeks' to 6 months' time.

— Skin rash, including palms and soles, develops.
— Painless shallow mucosal ulcerations will develop gradually.
— Condylomata lata are flat wart-like growths on the skin of the external genitalia and peri-anal region.
— Then myalgia, headache and lymphadenopathy may develop.

Teritary syphilis

— Formation of gummas, which are painless tumours.
— This usually takes years.
— Gummas may develop in the cardiovascular system, neurological system and in the liver.

Diagnosis

— Dark-field examination and direct fluorescence microscopy of material from the suspicious lesions.
— The spirochaete, *Treponema pallidum*, is a slender organism about 7–14 microns in length.
— Each has 10–15 regular spirals and is tapered at each end.
— Dark-field examination of material from mucosal ulcer may be diagnostic.
— Condylomata lata are the most infective of the syphilitic lesions.
— Serous exudate teems with the organism.
— In secondary and tertiary stages, serological tests are more useful and reliable.
— In very late syphilis, serological reactivity may be lost.
— In pregnancy the reverse occurs, false positive tests being more common.
— VDRL (venereal disease research laboratory) and RPR (rapid plasma reagin) detect antibodies not specific to the *Treponema*.
  Confirmation by FTA (fluorescent treponemal antibody absorption test) or TPI (treponema immobilisation test) is essential.
— Reagin and treponemal serological tests cross-react with the treponema responsible for yaws (*Treponema pertenue*).
— Yaws are common in South-East Asia and Pacific areas.
— Low unchanging titre (1:8) in a patient who has either lived in or emigrated from a yaws-endemic area is strongly suggestive of this disease.

Treatment

— For primary and secondary syphilis:
  • Benzathine penicillin G 2–4 million units in 2 divided doses i.m. and repeated 1 week later
  • Course is coupled with probenecid 500 mg three times daily
  • Tetracycline or erythromycin 500 mg orally 4 times daily for 2 weeks

- Serological tests should be done at 1, 3, 6 and 12 months to see the disease is cured
- VDRL reverts to negative within 2 years if treatment has been adequate
- Tests using treponemal antigens are likely to remain positive despite adequate treatment.

— Later stages of the disease:

- Need referral to special clinics; hepatic, cardiovascular, neurological lesions will need treatment
- Neurosyphilis should be excluded by lumbar puncture and study of spinal fluid
- A longer course of penicillin is needed for neurosyphilis
- Aqueous procaine penicillin G 2–4 million units every other day for 10 injections along with probenecid

Atrophic vaginitis

— It is associated with low oestrogen level.
— Renders the vagina more susceptible to infection.
— Pessaries may aggravate the condition.
— Infection may be due to commensal organisms, common aerobic and anaerobic infections.
— The discharge is usually non-offensive, yellow in colour, slight to moderate in amount.
— Pruritus is not a common complaint.
— Examination reveals a diffuse reddened vagina with haemorrhagic areas instead of a pale vagina.
— Treatment is either topical oestrogen cream and appropriate medication if there is infection.
— Oral small-dosage hormone replacement therapy for a short time may also be useful to build the epithelium.

Other conditions

— Benign or malignant lesions.
— Frequent douching, lubricants, deodorants.
— Foreign body such as pessary, tampons, IUCD.
— Oxyuris infestation.
— Fistulae.
— Poor toilet hygiene.
— In rare cases endometriosis of the cervix and vagina.

Treatment

— Deal with the primary precipitating factor.

CERVICITIS

Introduction

— Inflammation of the cervix is usually associated with a similar process in the vagina.
— Cervix is often involved in acute gonococcal infection which affects columnar rather than squamous epithelium.
— Cervix may be involved in *Chlamydia*, herpes simplex and papilloma virus infection.
— Infection becomes chronic because of obstruction to gland openings by fibrosis or overgrowth of metaplastic squamous epithelium.
— Lacerations following delivery and abortion can get infected.

Clinical features

— Vaginal discharge.
— Nature of discharge depends on infecting organisms.
— Pruritus may be present.
— Patient may complain of pelvic discomfort and dyspareunia.
— Purulent exudate may be seen at the external os of the cervix or coming out of the endocervical canal.
— Cervix may appear red and inflamed.
— In erosion of the cervix, the columnar epithelium may be more susceptible to attack by the vaginal organism and produce secondary cervicitis.
— Actual ulceration is pathological; it may be due to malignancy, syphilis and, rarely tuberculosis.
— In the tropics cervix may be affected by schistosomiasis.

Treatment

— Nature of organism should be identified by culture and sensitivity tests.
— Cervical smear should be done.
— If cervix looks frankly infected, parenteral antibiotics should be given.
— Surface infection will respond to local applications of cream or suppositories.
— In chronic conditions electrocautery or cryotherapy may be used.
— Cryotherapy is better, heals faster; secondary haemorrhage and stenosis are rare.
— Cryoprobe may be used.
— Patient should be advised to refrain from sexual activity for 2–3 weeks following therapy.

— Following cryotherapy there may be vaginal spotting or watery discharge for 2–4 weeks.
— Laser therapy is useful but it is expensive.

BARTHOLINITIS

Introduction

— Bartholin's glands are prone to infection, being placed at the vaginal introitus.
— Gonococcus, streptococci, staphylococci, coliform and anaerobes are the common organisms.
— Initial infection produces fibrosis and narrowing of the distal part of the duct.
— This gives rise to cyst formation of the duct, stasis of secretion which gets infected chronically.

Clinical features

Acute bartholinitis

— Marked tenderness and pain in the introital area.
— If infection is gonococcal, the urethra is also often involved and the patient may have urological symptoms.
— Often presents as an abscess.
— Usually presents as red inflamed tender swelling at the posterior aspect of the labia majora.
— Often there is fever and general malaise.
— Sometimes a large inflamed infected sebaceous cyst may cause confusion.
— It is important to exclude gonococcal infection.

Chronic bartholinitis

— Presents usually as a small tender lump.
— Causes symptoms when infection recurs.

Treatment

— In the acute phase, the patient needs admission to hospital.
— Antibiotics should be given (Cotrimoxazole or penicillin and metronidazole).
— Liberal use of analgesics for pain.
— If abscess forms, it should be marsupialised under anaesthesia.
— Saline bath post-operatively helps healing.
— Single incision and drainage are often not satisfactory; recurrence is common.

— Progressive enlargement and persistence of symptoms are suspicious of underlying neoplasm.
— In rare cases surgical excision of the duct and gland may be necessary.

VULVOVAGINITIS IN CHILDHOOD

Introduction

— Commonest gynaecological complaint.
— Reasons for this are:
  - Poor hygiene
  - Anus and vaginal introitus are very close
  - Lack of oestrogen
  - Vaginal epithelium is thinner and fragile
  - Lactobacilli are few or absent
  - Vaginal pH is high

Clinical features

— Vulvitis is usually a primary lesion in children; the spread to the vagina is secondary.
— Symptoms are itching, burning, discharge, stain on the underclothes and dysuria.
— Other sites of infection should be looked for: skin, throat and ear.
— If symptoms mainly occur at night, pinworm infestation should be considered.
— Diabetes, and antibiotic therapy may predispose to *Candida* infection.

Diagnosis

— General examination.
— Inspection of the vulva and introitus.
— Transparent tape swab from the peri-anal region and repeat for 2–3 days.
— Swab if possible for culture.
— Rectal examination to check for foreign bodies in the vagina.
— Visualisation of the vagina under anaesthesia may be necessary.

Treatment

— Hygiene regarding cleaning and bathing.
— Faecal smearing due to poor cleaning after bowel action should be corrected.

— May be advisable to clean the vulva after micturition.
— Calamine lotion or weak hydrocor tisone cream may relieve symptoms.
— Application of dienoestrol cream at night for a few days will improve epithelial resistance.
— Loose-fitting cotton panties are desirable.
— Pinworm infestation will respond to piperazine syrup or tablets.
— Other family members should be checked and treated for pinworms.
— For fungal and *Trichomonas* infection, local or oral therapy is given.
— If a foreign body is present (1–2%), it should be removed under general anaesthesia.
— Specific infection such as gonococcal needs specific therapy, and the family needs to be checked and treated.
— Physiological discharge may be excessive 1 or years before menarche; it only needs reassurance.

INFECTION OF THE UPPER GENITAL TRACT

Definition

— Clinically, pelvic inflammatory disease (PID) is defined as an acute febrile illness in a woman with pelvic pain and signs of genital infection.

Epidemiology

— 70% of all women with salpingitis are aged under 25 years.
— 30% have their first infection before the age of 30.
— 75% are nulliparous.
— The age-related risk of developing PID in sexually active young women is:
  • Aged 15 years — 1 in 8
  • Aged 16 years — 1 in 10
  • Aged 24 years — 1 in 80
  • Usually related to promiscuity.
— Approximately 250 million women a year will develop gonococcal infection in the world.
— In England and Wales the incidence of PID has recently increased significantly.
  • The incidence of gonococcal infection has increased in women more than in men
  • The increase is mainly in the age group of 16–24 years

— Pelvic inflammatory disease is one of the major gynaecological complaints in African countries.
— The reasons for increased incidence of PID are:
  • Increase in world population
  • Greater increase in the urban population
  • Liberalised attitudes to sex
  • The considerable reduction in the age at first sexual activity
  • Increased travelling and casual sexual encounters

Bacteriology

— *Neisseria gonorrhoeae.*
— *Chlamydia trachomatis.*
— Anaerobic organisms:
  • Bacteroides — *B. fragiles*
  • Peptococcus
  • Peptostreptococcus
— *Mycoplasma hominis* and *Ureaplasma urealyticum.*
— Other organisms:
  • Coliforms
  • *H. influenzae*
  • Streptococci
— PID can be classified as primary and secondary.
— Primary PID is due to:
  • Sexually transmitted diseases caused by *N. gonorrhoeae, C. trachomatis, M. hominis* and *U. urealyticum* (70% of all cases)
  • Ascent of endogenous vaginal and peri-anal flora (usually anaerobic organisms)
  • Following surgery and investigations such as D and C, HSG, tubal insufflation, termination of pregnancy, insertion of IUD (15% of all cases)
— Spread from inflamed and infected appendix.
  • Associated with diseases such as schistosomiasis and filariasis (accounts for 1% of all cases)

Pathogenesis

— Majority of infections of the upper genital tract are sexually transmitted.
— Condition is rare in women who are not sexually active.
— The incidence of post-abortal and post-partum pelvic inflammatory disease (PID) has shown a relative decrease.
— Peritonitis and septicaemia may occur which may be fatal.
— Damage may occur to the tubal epithelium with subsequent sterility and higher incidence of ectopic gestation.

— Prophylactic antibiotics in selected obstetrical and gynaecological operations have reduced pelvic infection.
— Laparoscopic examination has made possible early diagnosis and prompt treatment.

Clinical features

— Chronic pelvic pain is the main feature in 20% of this group. 60–70% will be infertile and/or have dyspareunia.
— Heavy prolonged periods.
— In 15–20% infertility is the problem.
— Incidence of ectopic pregnancy increases by 7 to 10 times.
— With each episode of PID the risk of sterility and ectopic gestation increases.

Diagnosis

— Classical clinical features of acute PID:
  • Acute pelvic pain
  • Pyrexia 38–39°C
  • Tender adnexae with unilateral or bilateral adnexal mass
  • Raised ESR and white cell count
  • Clinical diagnosis is accurate in only 50–60%
— Differential diagnoses are:
  • Acute appendicitis
  • Inflammatory condition of other organs
  • Endometriosis
  • Ectopic pregnancy
  • Corpus luteum haemorrhage
  • Ovarian cyst
  • Symptoms may be present in 20% of women without pelvic pathology
— Laparoscopy is the most reliable method of diagnosis:
  • Laparoscopy may show erythema of fallopian tube, oedema and swelling of tube and seropurulent exudate on the surface of the tube
  • If PID, is mild the tubes are mobile and patent
  • If PID is moderate, tubes look florid and less mobile
  • If severe, tube-ovarian abscess or mass may be seen
  • Inflammation is usually bilateral
  • Swabs could be taken from the pouch of Douglas or from the tubes
  • Peritoneal fluid can be taken for culture
— In some countries culdocentesis is done to obtain fluid for culture.
— Other diagnostic measures include:
  • Posterior fornix swab, not usually helpful

- Cervical and urethral swabs may be helpful
- Microscopy of vaginal wet preparation for leucocytes may be useful
- C-reactive proteins in plasma are elevated in acute problems

Management of acute PID

— Initial choice is usually empirical.
— If the culture and sensitivity of organisms are not compatible with initial treatment, or there is no improvement in signs and symptoms within 48 hours, the drugs need to be reviewed.
   - The penicillins — Ampicillin, Mezlocillin, Azlocillin, Mecillinam and its oral analogue, Pivmecillinam
   - Cephalosporins — Cefoxitin
   - Metronidazole
— Surgery is indicated:
   - If there is a tubo-ovarian abscess — drain it.
   - Large pyosalpinx — drain it.
   - If large bilateral tubo-ovarian masses or abscesses are not responding to antibiotic therapy.

Gonococcal infection

— Spread to upper genital tract occurs in 10–15%.
— Spreads via mucosal surfaces.
— Women on oral contraceptive pills have a significantly reduced incidence of upward spread of gonorrhoea; this may be due to resistance to passage through the less receptive cervical mucus.
— Damage caused by the gonococcal organism often paves the way for other pathogens, both aerobic and anaerobic.
— Laparoscopic examination may reveal swollen and reddened fallopian tubes with purulent exudate from the fimbrial ends.
— Fimbrial ends often become closed, and peritoneal adhesions often follow.
— Blockage of fimbrial ends causes pyosalpinx, which later becomes hydrosalpinx.
— Ovary may be involved and may be involved in tubo-ovarian mass or abscess.

Clinical features   *Gonorrhoea — doesn't affect peritoneum so much*
— History of sexual contact.
— Symptoms of lower genital tract infection.
— Lower abdominal pain, malaise and fever.
— Nausea and vomiting may occur later.
— In rare cases, symptoms are referable to generalised spread

of the disease, pain in the peripheral joints, lesions in heart, skin, liver and meninges.
— Fitz-Hugh and Curtis syndrome is seen in about 10%, caused by gonococcal and chlamydial infection. The syndrome involves:
  - Perihepatitis
  - Nausea and vomiting
  - Pain in the right upper quadrant
  - Positive Murphy's sign
  - Pain in the shoulder tip
  - Friction rub on examination
— Later perihepatic violin string adhesions develop and cause persistent right upper abdominal pain.
— In the acute phase with gonococcal infection the patient appears flushed, and movement is often painful.
— Moderate pyrexia and tachycardia are common.
— Lower abdomen is very tender (often bilateral).
— If peritonitis develops, there is guarding and release tenderness.
— Pelvic examination may reveal evidence of urethritis and cervicitis.
— Cervical excitation pain is bilateral.
— Adnexal mass may be felt.

Diagnosis

— The infection is confirmed by isolation of the gonococcus from the lower genital tract, urethra, cervix and anus.
— Laparoscopy and swab and peritoneal fluid for examination and culture.
— Differential diagnoses are:
  - Other type of tubo-ovarian infection, aerobic and/or anaerobic
  - Appendicitis
  - Haemorrhage from corpus luteum and follicle or other cyst
  - Ectopic pregnancy
  - Torsion of the tube, ovary
  - Urinary calculus
  - Endometriosis

Treatment

— Aqueous penicillin G, in severe cases intravenous regimen, the dose ranging 10–20 million U/day.
— Ampicillin 0.5 g. 4 times daily for 10 days (i.v./i.m./oral).
— Tetracycline 0.25–0.5 g. 4 times daily for 10 days (i.m./i.v./oral).
— Newer cephalosporins (Cephotaxime, Cephuroxime) are very effective.
— Bed rest, intravenous fluid and analgesia are necessary.

— Blood culture if there is any suspicion of blood spread.
— The condition usually improves rapidly.
— Adequate rest and therapy are essential.
— If improvement is not adequate consider *Chlamydia*, and anaerobic infection should be suspected.
— Follow-up and initial serology is mandatory to exclude syphilis.

Non-gonococcal infections

— Usual organisms
  • *Chlamydia*
  • *Mycoplasma*
  • Entericc pathogens
  • Aerobic organisms
  • Anaerobic organisms
— The above organisms often take over after other bacteria have caused damage to tubes and ovaries.

Clinical features

— Symptoms and signs are similar to those described under gonococcal infection.
— Usually the infection in the lower genital tract is less obvious or absent.
— Infection may be precipitated from:
  • A specific sexual episode
  • Organisms already in the birth canal
  • Pathogenicity has been altered by menstruation
  • Presence of IUD
  • Instrumentation

Diagnosis

— History
— Examination.
— Swabs from the cervix, urethra, vagina, anus for microscopy and culture.
— Laparoscopic examination and swabs and aspirate from the tube and the pouch of Douglas for microscopy and culture.
— A variety of organisms are involved.

Treatment

— The penicillins. The ampicillins are not useful because they are not stable to beta-lactamases, therefore have no activity against beta-lactamase producing *E.coli*. These are ineffective against *Pseudomonas aeruginosa* and Bacteroides fragilis.
— The introduction of the beta-lactamase inhibitor, clavulanic acid, may help to overcome many of these problems.
— Cephalosporins and cephalexin are active against coliforms, *Klebsiella*, *Proteus mirabilis*, gonococci.

— Cefuroxime is stable to the actions of many beta-lactamases and is highly active against *N.gonorrhoea* and *H.influenzae*. It is given parenterally.
— Cefoxitin is also stable against beta-lactamases and highly effective against gram-negative organisms and *B.fragilis*; it is given by injection.
— Aminoglycosides — gentamicin is still a useful parenteral antibiotic, effective against most Gram-negative bacteria.
— Metronidazole is invaluable in the treatment of infections due to *Bacteriodes*, *Clostridia* and many anaerobic streptococci. It is well absorbed, given orally and rectally.
— Hence the choice of drugs in the management of non-gonococcal infection should include a cephelosporin and metronidazole
— If IUD is in situ, it is removed 2–4 hours after the commencement of chemotherapy.
— If it is unilateral, actinomycotic infection is a possibility; this needs a prolonged course of penicillin.
— For chlamydial infection, tetracycline or erythromycin is ineffective.
— *Mycoplasma* infection responds to tetracycline or erythromycin.

Post-abortal infections

— Risk of infection with spontaneous and legally induced abortion is low.
— It is much higher in illegally induced abortion, which is very rare.
— There is a tendency for infection to spread to the parametrium to produce cellutitis and the patient may develop septicaemia.

Clinical features

— History of interference, abortion, termination.
— Symptoms depend on the type of organism and severity of infection.
— Pyrexia may be mild to moderate, malaise and tachycardia may be present.
— Associated bloodstained, serous or purulent vaginal or cervical discharge may be present.
— Discharge may be foul-smelling.
— Marked pelvic and lower abdominal tenderness may be present.
— Patient can develop shock from:
  - Bacteraemia with gram-negative organisms (*E.coli*)
  - One of the enteric organisms, a gram-positive organism (streptococcus), the clostridial group (*C.welchii*)

- Endotoxaemia
- Patient may develop intravascular coagulation.
- There may eventually be coagulation failure.

Diagnosis

— History.
— Examination.
— Speculum examination — this may reveal products of conception.
— Swabs from the vagina, cervix and from the peritoneal cavity if laparoscope was used.
— High leucocyte count — greater than 15 000/cmm.
— High temperature, tachycardia and rigor are associated with septicaemia.
— Septic shock or other evidence of endo- or exotoxaemia occurs in 1–5% of illegal abortions.
— Blood culture for aerobic and anaerobic organisms.

Treatment

— Antimicrobial therapy should cover both aerobic and anaerobic organisms.
— If there are retained products of conception, these need removal 12 hours after antibiotic therapy unless there is heavy bleeding.

Pelvic abscess

— Pelvic absecess is the end result of acute infection.
— Needs drainage if not responding to medical treatment.
— Approximately 0.2–2% of gynaecological admissions are associated with pelvic abscess.
— Incidence depends on the incidence of STD, control of infection, practice of illegal abortion.

Clinical features

— History of one or more episodes of PID or pelvic surgery.
— Pelvic pain, pyrexia, malaise, anorexia.
— Pain on micturition or defecation.
— Mucus diarrhoea.
— Dyspareunia.
— Pelvis is tender on examination.
— Boggy hot soft mass in the pouch of Douglas or in the fornices.

Treatment

— If the diagnosis is in doubt, laparoscopy or laparotomy may be necessary.
— Wide-spectrum antibiotics and metronidazole are given.
— Colpotomy to drain the pus may be necessary.
— In rare cases laparotomy and drainage may be needed.

CHRONIC PELVIC INFLAMMATORY DISEASE

— It occurs as a consequence of acute pelvic inflammatory disease.
— Tuberculosis.
— Rarely actinomycosis.
— Chronic PID is due to inadequate treatment of acute PID.
— Loss of surface epithelium prevents complete resolution.

Non-granulomatous infection

— The chronicity is usually related to inadequate treatment.
— The patient may have presented too late or was wrongly diagnosed and is receiving inadequate medication.
— Loss of epithelium, intramural and extramural adhesions and reduced vascularity render the tubes and ovaries susceptible to further bacterial attack.

Clinical features

— History of previous episodes of PID.
— Secondary dysmenorrhoea and dyspareunia.
— Intermittent purulent vaginal discharge.
— On examination, tender adnexal masses may be felt.
— Uterus is retroverted and fixed.
— Laparoscopy may reveal multiple adhesions with tubal distortion.
— Treatment is conservative or radical surgery if medical treatment fails.

Tuberculosis

Incidence

— This varies greatly according to socio-economic and public health conditions.
— Usually parallels the incidence of pulmonary and abdominal tuberculosis.
— Primary sites of infection are usually the lungs or abdomen.
— Spread is usually haematogenous, which occurs in adolescence.
— Rarely see in active form.
— Causes ill-health and sterility.
— The incidence is reducing with improved public health, standard of living and effective drug therapy.

Pathogenesis

— Fallopian tubes are initially infected.
— Endometrium is involved secondarily.
— Tubes may look normal externally in the early stages.
— As disease progresses, pyosalpinx may develop or the patient

may develop salpingitis, isthmica nodosa and, rarely, hydrosalpinx.
— Associated with miliary tuberculous peritonitis, numerous tubercles may be seen on the surface of the tubes and pelvic cavity.
— Fallopian tubes look thickened, dilated and surrounded by dense adhesions.
— Ovaries are involved in one-third of patients, sometimes with formation of chronic tubo-ovarian abscess.
— Uterine lesion is usually confined to the endometrium.
— In rare cases the cervix and the vagina are also involved.

Clinical features

— The disease is rarely symptomatic unless the lesion is advanced.
— Symptoms are similar to chronic PID produced by other organisms.
— Symptoms are:
  • Sterility
  • Lower abdominal pain
  • Asthenia
  • Menstrual problems
  • Vaginal discharge
  • Symptoms related to infection in other sites (lung, abdomen, kidney and bone)
— Pelvic findings are similar to those of chronic PID.
— Uterus may be retroverted and fixed, and there may be adnexal masses.

Diagnosis

— Condition is suspected if the disease is prevalent in the place.
— Positive personal and family history of tuberculosis.
— Careful general physical and pelvic examination.
— Loss of weight, mild pyrexia, anaemia, tachycardia; absence of response to treatment should raise suspicion.
— Chest radiography.
— Mantoux test.
— Late premenstrual endometrial curettage for histology and bacteriology.
— Menstrual blood culture.
— Laparoscopic examination.
— Suspicious HSG appearance performed on an infertile patient.
— Search for primary or other foci should be made (lungs and kidneys).
— Differential diagnosis:
  • Sarcoidosis — bacteriology is negative
  • Actinomycosis
  • Schistosomiasis

Treatment
- — Adequate and prolonged drug therapy is essential.
- — Effective drugs are:
  - Ethambutol (25 mg/kg/day for the first 3 months)
  - Isoniazid (300–400 mg/day for 9–12 months)
  - Rifampicin (450–600 mg/day for 9–12 months)
- — The last two drugs are bactericidal.
- — Streptomycin 750–1000 mg/day for the first 3 months is an alternative to ethambutol.
- — Combination of the above three drugs will make the patient non-infective in 2–4 weeks.
- — Failure to treatment is due to:
  - Inadequate regimen
  - Poor patient compliance
  - Drug toxicity
  - Bacterial resistance
- — Indications for surgery:
  - Failure to respond to drug therapy
  - Persistence of symptoms
  - Presence of pelvic abscess in the pouch of Douglas
  - Presence of tubo-ovarian abscess
  - Grossly damaged fallopian tubes
  - Ascitis

Prognosis
- — With modern chemotherapy, a cure is usual.
- — Anatomical distortion may persist.
- — Sterility is usually permanent.
- — If tubes are not damaged, pregnancy is possible.
- — There is a higher incidence of abortion and ectopic gestation.

SUGGESTED READING

Baker D A 1983 Herpes genitalis. In: Charles D (ed) Clinics in obstetrics and gynaecology, vol 10. Saunders, Philadelphia, p 3

Brown I 1982 The management of pelvic abscess. In: Studd J (ed) Progress in obstetrics and gynaecology, Vol 2. Churchill Livingstone, Edinburgh, p 274

Butler E G, Stanbridge C M 1985 Condylomatous lesions of the lower female genital tract. In: Fox H (ed) Clinics in obstetrics and gynaecology, vol, 11. Saunders, Philadelphia, p 171

Jones H W, Jones G S (eds) 1980 Gynecology. Williams and Wilkins, Baltimore, p 268

Mackay W V, Beischer N A, Cox L W, Wood C (eds) 1983 Illustrated textbook of gynaecology. Saunders, Philadelphia, p 255 and 282

Monday P E 1983 Chlamydial infections in women. In: Studd J (ed) Progress in obstetrics and gynaecology, Vol 3. Churchill Livingstone, Edinburgh, p 231

14. ECTOPIC PREGNANCY

In ectopic pregnancy there is an implantation of the fertilised ovum in a site outside the uterine cavity. The spectrum of clinical presentation is quite varied. It ranges from a slight discomfort to severe shock. The condition may lead to death from acute haemorrhage.

DEFINITION

— The term ectopic pregnancy is applied to pregnancy following implantation of the fertilized ovum on any tissue other than the mucous membrane lining the uterine cavity.

INCIDENCE

— Ectopic pregnancy occurs approximately 1 in 100 clinically recognised pregnancies (range 1 in 50–250).

— The rate depends on the prevalence of pelvic inflammatory disease and the use of IUD in the particular community.
— The most common site for the ectopic pregnancy is the fallopian tube.

AETIOLOGY

Factors affecting the passage of the fertilised ovum into the uterine cavity:
— The ovum is normally fertilised in the outer one-third of the fallopian tube and takes 4–5 days to reach the uterine cavity.
— In 25–30% of cases the damage to the tube is the result of a previous inflammatory disease (PID).
  • Reduced ciliary activity and muscle peristalsis will delay the transportation of the fertilised ovum

- PID delays the sperm migration towards the end of the tube
— PID is caused by:
  - Sexually transmitted diseases (gonorrhoea)
  - Post-abortal and post-partum infection
  - Post-gynaecological operative infection
  - Pelvic tuberculosis
  - Following appendicitis
  - Use of IUD
  - *Chlamydia* infection
— PID produces damage to muscle, cilia, and produces a blind gutter due to adhesions.
— Endometriosis in the wall of the tube and in the pelvis affect the condition of the tube and mucous membrane.
— Congenital abnormality of the tube such as hypoplasia, tortuosity, diverticula, accessory ostia are other causes.
— Tumours, cysts, pelvic endometriosis, previous surgery in the pelvis, in the tube, uterine fibromyoma may affect the functions of the fallopian tube.
— However, in 50% of cases the tube appears histologically normal.
— Progesterone-containing IUD and progesterone-only pill are associated with higher incidence of ectopic pregnancy.

FACTORS INHERENT IN THE EMBRYO

— Embryonic maldevelopment and gross chromosomal defects are a common finding.
— Fertilisation of the contralateral ovum with external migration of the conceptus.
— Delayed ovulation and/or premature menstruation which causes reflux of the ovum that is either passing down the tube or even has already entered the uterine cavity.
— In about 4–5% of patients the corpus luteum is on the side opposite to that of the ectopic pregnancy.

PATHOLOGY

— 95% of ectopic pregnancies occur in the fallopian tube.
— Majority are in the fimbrial end (10–20%), ampullary portion (40–50%) and isthmus (15–25).
— Interstitial or cornual implantations are uncommon (5–10%).
— Abdominal, ovarian and cervical implantations are rare (3–5%).

— Most abdominal implantations are secondary to ruptured tubal gestation.
— Co-existence of intra-uterine and extra-uterine ectopic pregnancies is unusual.
— Bilateral tubal gestation is rare, though reported in the literature.
— The outcome depends on the site of implantation.
— In the ampullary portion of the tube, the usual sequence is either tubal abortion or tubal rupture, usually into the peritoneal cavity.
— In the narrow middle part of the tube, early rupture (6–8 weeks) is inevitable into either the peritoneal cavity or, rarely, into the broad ligament.
— In the interstitial portion of the tube, a longer gestation is usual — rupture occurs during 10–16 weeks gestation, with a heavy haemorrhage that may be life-threatening.
— A missed or incomplete abortion may occur in any part of the tube.
— Once the fertilised egg has implanted into the tubal mucosa, early nidation changes are similar to intra-uterine pregnancy.
— The erosive action of the trophoblast causes penetration of the tubal muscle wall and gradually produces the rupture of the fallopian tube.
— The trophoblast invades blood vessels and causes bleeding into the lumen or into the wall or the peritoneal cavity.
— The embryo usually dies, although very few survive and reach full term.
— Bleeding into the lumen of the tube cause haematosalpinx.
— Microscopically, the presence of chorionic villi is the diagnostic feature.

OUTCOMES OF TUBAL PREGNANCY

Tubal rupture

— This causes intratubal bleeding and slow bleeding from the fimbrial end.
— Perifimbrial haematoma.
— Intraperitoneal haemorrhage — acute and slow leakage.
— Broad ligament haematoma.
— Pelvic haematoma in the pouch of Douglas.

Tubal abortion

— Actual separation of the whole products of conception from the tubal wall with mild bleeding from the fimbrial end.

— May cause perifimbrial haematoma.
— Dead embryo may be passed into the peritoneal cavity.
— This condition is often not recognised.
— Usually causes minor bleeding which in general ceases spontaneously.

Secondary abdominal pregnancy

— It is very rare to have a primary abdominal pregnancy.
— Usually it is secondary to tubal rupture, and the fetus becomes extruded and attached to the peritoneal surface and gut.
— The placenta is probably attached partially to the tube and later grows out and becomes attached to the peritoneum and gut.

Broad ligament or intraligamentary pregnancy

— When tubal rupture occurs away from the mesenteric border into the leaves of the mesosalpinx, the embryo escapes and becomes attached.
— Sometimes the pregnancy may advance to a late stage.

Spontaneous regression

— Many embryos may pass unrecognised.
— Embryos succumb at a very early phase with regression of the placenta and pregnancy symptoms.
— Symptoms are too mild for the woman to seek medical attention.

Mummification of the fetus

— This may occur in an unrecognised ruptured tubal pregnancy.
— Extensive calcification may convert the fetus into a so-called lithopedion
— Fetal bones may be passed vaginally, rectally or through the abdominal sinustract.

Endometrial change

— Uterine mucosa responds by a decidual reaction to the hormonal stimuli set in motion by the implanted fertilised ovum.
— If the conceptus is alive, the decidual reaction is maintained.
— Death of conceptus provides a breakdown of decidua which may be passed as fragments or as a whole-decidual cast.

— When curettage is done, the decidual reaction is present only in 30%. This is because the decidual lining might already have been passed.
— Finding of decidual reaction to progestational hormones without villi may also occur.
— In 1954 Arias–Stella described certain changes in the endometrial glands in response to the presence of trophoblast:
  • Cellular enlargement
  • Significant hyperchromatosis
  • Pleomorphism and mitotic activity
  • Nucleus is exfoliated into the gland lumen
  • Generalised tendency to appear neoplastic
— The incidence of Aria–Stella reaction occurs in ectopic or other pregnancy in 5–75% of cases.

SPECIAL SITES

Ovarian pregnancy

— Gestation sac occupies the site of the ovary.
— Sac is attached to the uterus by the ovarian ligament.
— Tube looked healthy.
— Ovarian tissue is demonstrated in the wall of the sac.
— Rupture occurs relatively early.
— Differential diagnosis from other type of haemorrhagic ovarian cyst (follicular, luteal, endometriotic).
— Association of ovarian ectopic pregnancy and IUD.
— Ovary could be conserved at surgery.
— Tubal rupture and extruded conceptus may sometimes get attached to the ovary.

Cervical pregnancy

— It is uncommon, but very dangerous.
— Causes expansion of cervix.
— Rupture of the sac and abortion occurs.
— Severe haemorrhage may occur due to the proximity to branches of the uterine artery.

Cornual (interstitial) pregnancy

— It is rare and is located in that part of the tube which traverses the uterine wall.
— Late rupture is more likely (12–18 weeks).

— Risk of major haemorrhage is high.
— Condition is rarely diagnosed before rupture.

Abdominal (peritoneal) pregnancy

— Both primary and secondary abdominal pregnancies are rare.
— Usually it is secondary to tubal rupture.
— The fetus may develop fully and survive, but the woman usually presents as an acute abdominal emergency in mid-trimester.
— If the woman presents early, ultrasonic scan will show a different appearance of fetus, higher up and outside the uterus.
— There is often a history of an episode of abdominal pain and slight vaginal bleeding early in pregnancy which is often treated as threatened miscarriage.
— Maternal serum AFP may be elevated.
— Ultrasound scan shows oligohydramnios, no clear uterine outline around the sac, and the uterus usually appears as a separate mass.
— Fetal prognosis is poor (11% salvage is reported).
— When laparotomy is carried out, the fetus is usually removed, the cord is tied and the placenta is left inside the abdomen.

Combined intra- and extra-uterine pregnancy

— There are few cases reported.
— Diagnosis is difficult.
— Ultrasound examination may be helpful.
— Bilateral tubal pregnancy alone or with intra-uterine pregnancy also are reported but rare.

Post-hysterectomy ectopic pregnancy

— Fimbria may protrude through the vaginal vault.
— It is a rare condition.
— Sometimes conception might have occurred just before surgery.
— Often the condition is self-limited and may not need operative intervention.

Embryo and fetus

— Often no embryo is seen.
— When present it is often malformed.
— Fetal death is common.

CLINICAL FEATURES

History

— Patient is usually in her mid-twenties.
— Use of IUD and mini-pill for contraception.
— History of previous ectopic pregnancy (10%). Recurrence is 5–10 times more common after it has occurred in the past.
— Previous history of PID (10–35%), pelvic surgery, tubal surgery. Sterilisation (3–4%) and appendectomy.
— Infertility investigation and treatment.

Symptoms

— Amenorrhoea (65–80%).
— Lower abdominal pain (95+%), initially unilateral then spreads.
— Vaginal bleeding (65–85%).
— Classical presentation occurs in approximately 80%.
— In 10–15% there is no bleeding.
— Bleeding is often darker, slight and persistent.
— Pregnancy symptoms occur in 50%.
— Clinical features may be very variable.
— Pain is usually unilateral then spreads — cramping in nature, due to tubal distension and blood in the peritoneal cavity.
— Pelvic haematocele causes rectal and bladder symptoms.
— Occasionally patients may present with acute severe pain due to rupture and heavy haemorrhage.
— Patient may be in shock.
— She frequently complains of shoulder-tip pain due to irritation of diaphragm.
— Average duration of amenorrhoea is 7 weeks.
— Five to ten per cent will give history of fainting.
— Nausea, vomiting, diarrhoea are other symptoms.

Examination

— Picture will vary depending on the amount of blood loss.
— Temperature is often normal or slightly elevated.
— Twenty per cent will be clinically shocked.
— Lower abdominal tenderness, guarding or rebound tenderness may be present.
— Often there is some reflex bowel distension due to blood in the peritoneal cavity.
— In rare cases a bruise-type discoloration around the umbilicus (Cullen's sign) may be seen in extraligamentary rupture.
— Severe pain on moving the cervix when the pelvic examination is done is suggestive of ectopic gestation.

— In 30% a mass may be felt.
— Softening and bluish coloration of the cervix is present in 20–25%.
— Careful examination may reveal uterine enlargement, usually never more than of 6–8 weeks' duration.
— A firm clinical diagnosis is possible in about 50% of patients.

Special investigation

— Beta-HCG in the urine or in blood.
— Ultrasound examination.
— Culdocentesis.
— Laparoscopy.

Differential diagnosis

— Pregnancy complication (threatened, incomplete, missed abortion).
— PID.
— Subacute appendicitis.
— Complications of ovarian cyst.
— Dysfunctional uterine bleeding.
— Endometriosis.
— Urinary tract problem.
— Pregnancy with ovarian cyst complications.

MANAGEMENT

Confirmation of diagnosis

— Pregnancy test:
  • Will be positive in less than 50%
  • Beta-HCG assay will be positive if viable trophoblast is present
— Ultrasonic examination:
  • Not very reliable unless the sac is intact and
  • amenorrhoea is 6–8 weeks
  • Shows slightly enlarged uterus without gestation sac
  • Blood in the pouch of Douglas shows transonic area
  • Uterine fibroid and ovarian cyst are easily identified
— Culdocentesis:
  • Blood removed from the pouch of Douglas via needling through the posterior fornix
  • High incidence of false positive and negative results
  • If blood is drawn (old), then this suggests intraperitoneal bleeding has occurred

— Laparoscopy:
  - Usual procedure for the doubtful case
  - Usually patient is prepared for laparotomy
  - Examination under anaesthesia and curettage alone are never done unless laparoscopy is normal and ultrasound excludes intra-uterine pregnancy.

Treatment

— This is undertaken immediately for all patients in whom blood loss is obvious.
— In those the diagnosis is strongly suspected on the basis of clinical or laboratory findings, ultrasound examination and/or laparoscopy.
— It is essential that the patient in severe pain and/or shock should have her condition explained and be reassured.
— Her wishes regarding future childbearing must be discussed.
— Technique varies depending on the nature of the pathology.
— Milking the products or securing fimbrial haemostasis is all that is needed in some patients.
— Partial or total salpingectomy is the usual procedure.
— A more conservative salpingectomy operation has been done in special circumstances.
— Removal of blood and blood clot is essential to prevent adhesions.
— Blood loss should be replaced.
— For Rh-negative women, anti (D) gammaglobulin is given, provided there is no antibody.
— As soon as haemostasis is achieved, contralateral tube and ovary should be checked; if they are grossly damaged, conservative surgery is done on the affected side.
— Hysterectomy may be needed to secure haemostasis in 1–2% of ectopic pregnancies, especially in interstitial pregnancy.
— In cornual pregnancy, wedge resection may be necessary and repair of the remaining uterus.
— In cervical pregnancy, cavity is curetted and packed firmly; if bleeding continues ligation of the uterine artery may be necessary — internal iliac artery ligation in patients needing childbearing function or hysterectomy may be needed if bleeding is severe.
— In abdominal pregnancy, the fetus is removed and placenta is left inside after the cord has been ligated.

Prognosis

— Approximately 5% of maternal deaths are due to ectopic gestation. 1:1000, ectopics will die.

— Chance of future successful pregnancy depends on a number of factors, mainly the normality of the remaining tubes and presence of other infertility factors.

— Approximately 40–60% of patients will become pregnant after surgery.

— 10–20% of these pregnancies will be another ectopic pregnancy.

— In the past conservative surgery was practised in 5–10%, now it is in 30–40%.

SUGGESTED READING

Adler M W 1980 Trends for gonorrhoea and pelvic inflammatory disease in England and Wales and for gonorrhoea in a defined population. American Journal of Obstetrics and Gynecology 138:901

Beral V 1975 An epidemiological study of recent trends in ectopic pregnancy. British Journal of Obstetrics and Gynaecology 82:775

Bonnar J 1974 Progesterone-only contraception and tubal pregnancies. British Medical Journal 1:287

Brenner P F, Roy, Mishell D R 1980 Ectopic pregnancy. A study of 300 consecutive surgical treated cases. Journal of the American Medical Association 243:673

Fox H Buckley C H 1984 Current concepts of endometriosis. In: Clinics in obstetrics and gynaecology, vol 11. Saunders Philadelphia, p 279

Kadar N 1983 Ectopic pregnancy. In: Studd J (ed) Progress in obstetrics and gynaecology, vol 3. p 305

Rannevik G, Starup J, Doberyl A (eds) 1983 Current concepts on endometriosis. In: Proceedings of the Symposium of the Scandinavian Association of Obstetricians and Gynecologists. Acta Obstetrica et Gynecologica Scandinavica Suppl 123:7

15. DISORDERS OF MENSTRUATION AND ASSOCIATED PROBLEMS

INTRODUCTION

— Between the menarche and menopause, women have a great deal of ill-health attributable to the reproductive system.
— Menstruation is a cyclic phenomenon involving partial shedding of the endometrium with associated loss of blood.
— It occurs usually every 21 to 35 days during the reproductive years.
— Cycle length outside the above range occurs in 1–2% of women.
— Irregular menstrual periods are much more common at the extremes of reproductive failure.
— Menstrual bleeding lasts for 4 to 5 days, although the normal range is 1–7 days.
— Blood loss is normally less than 80 ml, the average being 30–40 ml. Losses in excess of 80 ml are classed as menorrhagia.

MENSTRUAL PROCESS

— The withdrawal of ovarian hormones' support coupled with accumulation of other hormones or enzymes within the endometrium leads to a spasm of the spiral arterioles.
— This leads to ischaemia and finally rupture of the spiral arterioles.
— Vascular lakes form in the endometrium separating the bulk of the endometrial layer, which is shed as small fragments admixed with blood from the open vessels.
— Experimental evidences suggests that prostaglandins are implicated in the endometrial shedding and myometrial contraction which accompany menstruation.
— Both PGE_2 and PGF_2-alpha in the endometrium and menstrual fluid show a marked increase immediately preceding and during menstruation.

H

- Calcium stabilisation is related in part to the ratio of prostaglandin to progesterone.
- This ratio is upset as prostaglandins increase and progesterone falls late in the cylce and membrane stability is lost, with resultant menstruation.
- Endometrial repair is largely independent of oestrogen and is relatively rapid.
- It begins between the second and third cycle days and is complete by the fifth day.
- Uterine contractility is strongest during menstruation and weakest at mid-cycle.
- In the luteal phase the contractions tend to be of lower frequency but higher amplitude.
- Recent studies suggest that antiduretic hormone has a role in the uterine contractility during the menstrual cycle.
- The regular menstrual cycle does not usually begin suddenly at the menarche or stop suddenly at the menopause.
- What initiates the menstrual cycle is not easy to explain.
- In childhood, gonadotropic and ovarian activities are low.
- At puberty, gonadotropin secretion increases, causing ovarian follicular development and oestrogen secretion.
- The first menstrual flow follows an endometrial build-up in response to oestrogen from the ripening follicles.
- The peak of oestrogen secretion is often insufficient to trigger the mid-cycle surge of GnRH and thus LH, so ovulation does not occur.
- Oestrogen secretion builds up the endometrium, and eventually inhibitory feedback of oestrogen to hypothalamus results in withdrawal of FSH.
- The follicle undergoes regression, oestrogen level falls and the endometrium breaks down and is shed.
- Ovulation occurs with increasing follicular oestrogen levels which produce GnRH surge and LH surge.
- Ovulation occurs less frequently after the age of 40 years, although the cycle remains regular.
- With increasing age, ovulatory cycles become fewer, cycles become irregular and the flow becomes less and eventually stops around 50 years.

ABNORMAL MENSTRUATION

Excessive uterine bleeding (menorrhagia)

- This is reported to occur in 5–10% of women. It may be either prolonged or heavy, or both.
- It is abnormal if the cycle is less than 21 days and the

duration of loss more than 7 days, or the volume of loss is such that menstrual pads of adequate absorbency cannot cope with the flow.

— Excessive loss is usually estimated to be that in excess of 80 ml per cycle.

— In the management of abnormal uterine bleeding there are two aims: one is to arrest the immediate bleeding if it is so excessive as to threaten health; and the other is the prevention of future similar occurrences; determining the cause of bleeding is crucial to prevent recurrence.

Aetiology

— The first problem in evaluating abnormal bleeding is to establish that the bleeding is uterine in origin.

— Once the bleeding has been determined to be uterine in origin, the differentiation between an organic or anatomical cause and a dysfunction of the neuro-endocrine system should be made.

— Abnormal bleeding may be associated with an ovulatory or anovulatory cycle.

— Abnormal bleeding associated with an ovulatory cycle is ordinarily organic in aetiology.

— Anovulatory uterine bleeding is primarily a disease of menarcheal and perimenopausal patients.

— Women with a moderate to heavy alcohol consumption tend to menstruate for fewer days.

— Alcohol affects uterine contractility and oestrogen metabolism and may be a direct cause of a shortened cycle.

— Cigarette smokers are five times more likely to have abnormal bleeding.

— It may be associated with abnormal prostaglandin metabolism.

— There is an increased incidence of psychological disturbance, chiefly anxiety and depression.

— Psychological factors may alter endocrine function by acting on the hypothalamic–pituitary–ovarian axis.

— Ovarian steroid hormones may affect in a number of ways the amount of blood lost:
  • The endometrium may be stimulated excessively by high prolonged or unopposed oestrogen production
  • The local uterine haemostatic mechanisms may be affected
  • Uterine contractility may be affected
  • The production of prostaglandins may be increased, which might affect vascular and uterine smooth muscle
  • The excessive prostacyclin in the endometrium enhances vasodilatation

— Abnormal bleeding may occur with many common endocrinopathies: ovarian disease such as polycystic ovarian disease, functional ovarian tumours, endometriosis and pelvic inflammation affecting the ovary.

— Abnormal function of the pituitary, thyroid or adrenal glands, diabetes mellitus, use of hormone contraceptives or oestrogen therapy produce abnormal bleeding.

— Marked weight change will also affect menstrual function.

— Bleeding disorders (deficiences of Factors 5, 7, 10; platelet disorders; Von Willebrand's syndrome), hypothyroidism, chronic hepatic disease and congestive cardiac failure may cause excessive menstrual loss.

— Excess loss may be associated with surface ulceration related to fibromyoma, or submucus fibromyoma, polyp, carcinoma, a foreign body such as IUD, inflammation — endometrial hyperplasia, adenomyosis and uterine abnormality.

— Complications of pregnancy such as abortion and ectopic pregnancy may cause abnormal bleeding.

Diagnosis

— Determine the degree of abnormality, the duration, the time of maximal loss, whether clots are passed and blood runs away.

— Associated symptoms such as pain, lethargy, dyspareunia should be ascertained.

— Complications of pregnancy, and endocrine, psychological and haematological causes are elicited

— General and pelvic examination will clarify aspects of the history and pinpoint pelvic pathology.

Investigations

— Haemoglobin and full blood examination are required to establish the presence and type of anaemia.

— Haematological investigation includes bleeding and clotting time, capillary fragility, platelet count and estimation of relevant clotting factors.

— Investigation of thyroid, adrenal, ovarian or pituitary function may be needed. Plasma LH, FSH, oestrogen, progesterone, androstenedione and testosterone assays may be useful.

— Diagnostic curettage is often necessary to exclude uterine pathology, especially in women of 35 years of age or over — it is rarely indicated in the younger age group.

— When the cause is not apparent and the condition is persistent, laparoscopy and possibly hysteroscopy may be useful in revealing unsuspected diseases such as intra-uterine

— polyp or small ovarian tumour, endometriosis or pelvic inflammatory disease.
— Often a cause is not found to account for the symptoms.

Pathology

— The endometrium may show a secretory phase which may be complete or mixed with a proliferative phase.
— It may show only a proliferative phase.
— It may show cystic glandular hyperplasia, usually occurs towards the end of the reproductive phase.
— It may show adenomatous hyperplasia which may or may not be associated with atypia. This change usually occurs at the end of the reproductive phase.

Treatment

— If excessive bleeding is secondary to psychosomatic, haematological, endocrine or genital tract disorder, treatment is directed to the primary cause.
— Obese women must be advised to lose weight.
— In the majority, bleeding is due to an anovulatory cycle which will usually respond to progestogen therapy from day 15 or earlier to day 25 of the cycle.
— If curettage is indicated, it could be diagnostic as well as therapeutic in some, hence it is worth while observing the patient for 2 to 4 months.
— If endometrial hyperplasia is found, it often responds to progestogen therapy.
— Norethisterone (10–40 mg) or Duphaston (10–30 mg) is given daily in divided doses for 10 to 14 days in the second half of the cycle.
— Larger doses of progestogens are given, when bleeding episodes are heavier, for 2 to 3 days, the dose being reduced after the initial period to complete a 21-day regime.
— Therapy is given for 3–6 cycles.
— A combined oestrogen/progestogen pill can be given to young women who need treatment as well as contraception.
— Excessive bleeding associated with ovulatory cycles is much more difficult to manage. Dicynene and Epsikapron may be useful.
— Prostaglandin synthetase inhibitors (e.g. mefenamic acid, flufenamic acid, naproxen sodium) will often reduce menstrual loss, but have little effect on cycle length.
— This group of drugs has fewer side-effects and is given at the time of flow.
— Clomiphene could be used for patients with heavy loss with anovulatory cycles and infertility.

— The disadvantage is that it is expensive and sometimes produces hyperstimulation.
— Danazol may be given if hysterectomy is contra-indicated or to stop bleeding and to correct anaemia while the patient is waiting to have a hysterectomy. It is also expensive.
— Uterine abnormality and fibromyoma will need surgical correction.
— Hysterectomy may be required if all medical treatments fail or the endometrium is hyperplastic with abnormal and atypical cells in irregular hyperplastic glands. The risk of adenocarcinoma is high in this group.

DYSMENORRHOEA

— Dysmenorrhoea or painful menstruation is the most common of all gynaecological disorders.
— Over half of all post-menarcheal women have some discomfort, and 10% are incapacitated for 1–3 days each month.
— The causes and pathophysiology of dysmenorrhoea remain poorly understood.

Definition and clinical features

Primary dysmenorrhoea *Painful periods for which no organic or psychological cause could be found*
— Is menstrual pain observed in the absence of any organic pelvic disease?
— It develops within a few years of the menarche.
— Pain begins with the onset of menstruation, lasts for a few hours, and has a spasmodic colickly nature.
— Pain is centred in the lower midline but may radiate to the lower back or down the thighs.
— Numerous symptoms may accompany the pelvic pain, including nausea, vomiting and/or anorexia, diarrhoea, headache, dizziness, tiredness and nervousness.
— Most women with primary dysmenorrhoea have a tendency towards spontaneous improvement.

Secondary dysmenorrhoea *Painful periods for which an organic or psychosexual cause could be demonstrated*
— This occurs later in life and is related to organic pelvic disorders, such as endometriosis, adenomyosis, pelvic inflammatory disease, fibromyoma, uterine anomalies.
— Acquired cervical stenosis following surgical procedures in the cervix is another cause.
— Pain begins several days before the menses and gradually increases in severity as menses approach.

— Pain may continue throughout the menses and may last longer.

Aetiology

Psychogenic
- This should never be overlooked.
- All factors which might accentuate or lessen the subjective element in the particular case must be considered.

Constitutional
- It is closely linked with the purely subjective group of causes.
- Anaemia, voluntary weight loss, diabetes, chronic illness and overwork may be associated with a lowering of the threshold of pain.
- Psychological problems predispose to pain, or in fact constitutional factors predetermine both psychological symptoms and menstrual pain.

Obstructive and anatomical
- Mechanical obstruction may have an aetiologic role in a small proportion of cases.
- Cervical stenosis, or acute uterine ante- or retroflexion could result in delayed passage of the menstrual discharge, formation of clots and distension of the uterine cavity.
- Dilatation of the internal os by the passage of clots causes discomfort.
- Pedunculated submucus fibroids or endometrial polyps also cause dysmenorrhoea, because the myometrium contracts in an effort to expel to expel the space-occupying lesions.
- The above mechanism is responsible for the dysmenorrhoea associated with an intra-uterine contraceptive device.
- Uterine malformations such as unicornuate uterus or unilateral horn of a bicornuate uterus.

Endocrine factors
- Dysmenorrhoea is almost always found with normal ovulatory cycles.
- Progesterone is thought to stimulate the production of prostaglandins, especially F2-alpha, which are found in high concentration in the uterus.
- The dependance of dysmenorrhoea on ovulation and progesterone production, as evidenced by the high cure rate when ovulation is suppressed.
- This suggests that the action of progesterone on the blood vessels and myometrium is important in causing the pain.
- Progesterone is known to cause narrowing of the cervical canal by an effect on local smooth muscle.

Prostaglandins

- These compounds are released just before and during menstruation.
- Their escape into the circulation is thought to cause some of the associated symptoms of severe dysmenorrhoea, e.g. nausea, fainting, headache, bowel and bladder disturbances.
- Subjects with primary dysmenorrhoea have significantly higher-than-normal concentrations of prostaglandins in the endometrium.
- These high concentrations of the prostaglandins may be due to increased synthesis, abnormal release, or decreased breakdown.
- That the prostaglandin synthetase inhibitors may relieve the symptomatology of dysmenorrhoea is further proof of the aetiologic role of prostaglandins.
- Prostaglandins increase the uterine contractility, the cause of dysmenorrhoea.

Associated factors

- Neither country of birth nor social class are related to prevalence of the disorder.
- This casts doubts on its relationship to such factors as poor health, sex education or lack of exercise.
- Dysmenorrhoea is more common in patients who smoke; this may cause the release of prostaglandins within the uterus.
- Alcohol drinkers and ex-drinkers have a high incidence of severe dysmenorrhoea.
- Many women have a retrograde flow of blood from the uterus through the fallopian tubes into the peritoneal cavity, and this causes peritoneal irritation with pelvic pain and tenderness.
- Dysmenorrhoea is more common in the age group of 15–24, who are single, separated or divorced, or who have borne only one child or are nulliparous.
- Those who suffer from migraine tend to suffer from dysmenorrhoea.

Treatment

- It is possible that variations in the pain threshold do occur and these may be susceptible to improvement by education and simple psychotherapy.
- Organic disease is responsible in a minority of patients and can usually be excluded by history, physical examination, dilatation of cervix and curettage, hysteroscopy and laparoscopy.
- It is important to exclude endometriosis and pelvic infection.

— Women with pelvic disease need appropriate treatment to deal with the primary disease.
— Women with no physical disease can be managed by one or more of the following measures.

Psychophysical

— Rest, relaxation, local heat, psychotherapy, breathing and general exercises may be useful.
— Reassurance and education are useful.
— Application of ice or cold spray are tried.
— Yoga, acupuncture and hypnosis are found useful.

Drugs

— Simple analgesics, sedatives, tranquillisers are to be tried initially.
— Antispasmodics have been found useful.

Endocrine therapy

— Steroid contraception has decreased the incidence of dysmenorrhoea because of the efficacy of inhibition of ovulation.
— Steroid contraceptive pills are particularly useful in women who have dysmenorrhoea and also need contraception.
— Progestational agents such as norethisterone and dydrogesterone from day 5 to 25 are useful in some women, especially in the younger age group.

Anti-prostaglandin

— Mefenamic acid, flufenamic acid and naproxen sodium are the drugs of choice.
— They are taken at the start of the menses, and repeated dosages are given until the pain subsides.
— This group of drugs relieves heavy periods in some patients.

Tocolytic agents

— The use of agents to inhibit muscular contraction and increase uterine blood flow is theoretically sound.
— The use of B-receptor stimulators has proved ineffective.
— The side-effects on cardiovascular system are undesirable — hence these agents are not widely used.

Calcium antagonists

— Nifedipine effectively decreases myometrial activity and intrauterine pressure.
— This group of drugs also has undesirable side-effects.
— They have no place in routine use.

Others

— Danol has been tried to stop the menstrual cycle to relieve dysmenorrhoea even in the absence of endometriosis.

Surgery

— Dilatation of the cervix may be useful in some women.

226 MANUAL OF GYNAECOLOGY

— Presacral neurectomy or sympathectomy is a rational and frequently effective procedure in intractable dysmenorrhoea.
— In 60–70% of cases, pain is relieved by surgery.
— In rare cases hysterectomy may be indicated, especially if there is pelvic pathology such as endometriosis, adenomyosis, fibromyoma and have completed their family.

Summary

— No therapy of such a subjective pain disorder as primary dysmenorrhoea can be based purely on prostaglandin synthetase inhibition, and endocrine, constitutional or psychogenic factors should not be overlooked.
— A general symptomatic approach, reassurance, with medical treatment and advice for the woman to try to remain up.
— When the dysmenorrhoea is more protracted and severe, drugs to inhibit ovulation or to counteract prostaglandins could be tried.
— In the younger age group, progestogens could be tried instead of ovulation suppression.
— Apart from usual analgesic and ergotamine preparations, propranolol has been found to be beneficial.
— Surgical treatment is advocated only when medical measures have failed, or patients have associated pathology and have completed the family.

PREMENSTRUAL SYNDROME (CYCLICAL OVARIAN SYNDROME)

— At least 30–40% of women suffer from premenstrual symptoms; only a small proportion (5%) experience severe incapacitating symptoms.
— Premenstrual syndrome is associated with symptoms experienced in the second half of the cycle.
— It can occur in the absence of menstruation or the uterus and is related to periodic changes produced by ovarian steroid hormone secretion, hence the name cyclical ovarian syndrome.
— The syndrome was not significantly appreciated until the early 1930s. It has been noted in many different cultures and ethnic groups.
— Women in the age group 18–35 are mainly affected.
— The basis of these cyclic changes may be hormonal, social or psychodynamic.

Clinical features

— Premenstrual tension in minor degrees is relatively common
  — extreme degrees are rare and may be very distressing.
— Symptoms may commence as early as day 15 of the cycle or
  as late as 2 or 3 days premenstrually.
— Amelioration is usually by the first or second day of the
  menses.
— Psychological symptoms which occur are nervous tension,
  irritability, anxiety, depression, fatigue, lack of confidence,
  memory and concentration.
— Physical symptoms are swelling of the fingers and legs,
  bloated feeling of abdomen and breasts, breast tenderness
  and/or nodularity, skin greasiness and acne, changes in bowel
  and bladder function, headache, dizziness and palpitation.
— Behaviour consequences of the physical and psychological
  symptoms are marital and/or sexual difficulties, school or
  work problems such as unpunctuality and forgetfulness,
  psychiatric relapse, and crime.
— Suicidal, homicidal tendencies, visits to emergency and
  psychiatric visits increase in the premenstrual period.
— Diseases such as hay-fever, asthma, migraine and epilepsy
  may get worse.
— Three out of four women are conscious of swelling of the
  body and report depression, tension or fatigue.
— Incapacitating headaches may be associated with the sensory
  or motor symptoms of cerebrovascular spasms.
— The syndrome is more common in women with menstrual
  irregularity, emotional difficulties, sex problems and in those
  who are separated or divorced and in non-users of oral
  contraceptives.

Aetiological factors

— The premenstrual tension syndrome is characterised by
  symptoms which increase in intensity 4–10 days prior to
  menstruation and disappear with its onset.
— Excessive tissue hydration is alleged to be responsible for the
  symptoms, and the intensity varies directly with the amount
  of water retained.
— Secondary aldosteronism due to extrinsic factors affecting the
  adrenal zona glomerulosa may be associated with increases in
  ACTH stimulation, potassium or progesterone, or to changes
  in body fluid volume, surgical trauma and anxiety states.
— It has been found, during the late luteal phase, the
  water/potassium ratio in litres/mol of potassium was

significantly higher in the patients with premenstrual symptoms.
— Another possibility is that there is no increase in weight but there may be redistribution of fluid causing disturbance in fluid balance.
— Patients who suffer from premenstrual oedema may have a shift of fluid from the intravascular to the extravascular space, with a predilection for abdomen and breasts.
— There is a possibility of disturbances in the renin–angiotensin system and aldosterone.
— The oestrogens are thought to be responsible for fluid retention.
— Progesterone, through its sodium-losing action, is believed to stimulate the renin–angiotensin system and to produce a luteal phase increase in aldosterone secretion leading to further fluid retention.
— Most studies have shown no difference in plasma progesterone and 17-β oestradiol.
— Aldosterone, by inducing sodium retention, may be the causative agent.
— Recently prolactin has been incriminated in the premenstrual syndrome. It has been found elevated in some women with symptoms in the luteal phase, which may decrease FSH/LH levels and impair gonadal steroidogenesis.
— It has been postulated that variation in levels of oestrogen and progesterone in the luteal phase causes a decrease in brain serotonin and dopamine, resulting in depression.

Treatment

— Clinical management of the premenstrual tension syndrome is a reminder that medicine is still an art and not an exact science; the therapy is by no means standardised.
— Discussion of symptoms, finding relaxing pursuits, avoiding conflicts may help to reduce psychological symptoms.
— Before therapy it is helpful for the patient to provide a chart indicating the symptoms experienced and the time in the cycle.
— Small doses of a minor tranquilliser (diazepam 2 mg twice daily) may reduce tension and irritability. Regular use of these drugs should not be encouraged.
— General nervous system stabilisers (Bellergal) may be helpful. Antidepressant drugs may be used for speciffic indication.
— In the milder cases, and in the younger group of patients when oedema is the predominating symptom, a low-salt diet may be helpful.
— Spironolactone given cyclically counteracts the tendency

towards secondary hyperaldosteronism. It crosses the blood–brain barrier and controls fluid accumulation in the brain, which may explain the beneficial effect in relieving the mental symptoms.

— The fall in progesterone in the premenstrual phase has been shown to decrease brain serotonin — at high levels it inhibits prolactin. The value of progesterone is not universally acceptable.

— Norethisterone (5–15 mg per day) or dydrogesterone (10 mg per day) or progesterone suppositories (Cyclogest 200–400 mg) from day 20 or earlier until day 26 to 28 was found useful.

— Pyridoxine (vitamin B_6) is required to produce pyridoxal-5 phosphate, a very important co-enzyme for the production of serotonin. Oestrogen is a competitive inhibitor of pyridoxine.

— A deficiency of serotonin due to depletion of pyridoxine may be responsible for the depression associated with oral contraceptives and the premenstrual syndrome.

— Recent evidence suggests that pyridoxine inhibits prolactin and hence may reduce salt and water retention.

— The dosage of pyridoxine is 25–50 mg b.d. commencing 2 to 3 days before expected onset of symptoms.

— A prolactin antagonist, bromocriptine (Parlodel) has been used as therapy for the syndrome. Results remain controversial; some patients appear to benefit. The dosage is 1.25–2.5 mg daily.

SUGGESTED READING

Dewhurst C J 1981 Integrated obstetrics and gynaecology, 3rd edn. Blackwell, London
Mackay E V, Beischer N A, Cox L W, Wood C (eds) 1983 Illustrated textbook of gynaecology. Saunders, Philadelphia, p 65
Magos A, Studd J 1984 Premenstrual syndrome. In: Studd J (ed) Progress in obstetrics and gynaecology, vol 4. Churchill Livingstone, Edinburgh, p 334
Scommegna A, Vorys N, Givens J R 1980 Menstrual dysfunction. In: Gold J J, Josimovich J B (eds) Gynecologic endocrinology. Harper & Row, New York, p 290
Speroff L, Glass R H, Kase N G (eds) 1984 Dysfunctional uterine bleeding. In: Clinical gynecologic endocrinology and infertility, 3rd edn. Williams & Wilkins, Baltimore, p 225
Vorys N, Scommegna A, Givens J R 1980 Therapy of menstrual dysfunction. In: Gold J J, Josimovich J B (eds) Gynecologic endocrinology. Harper & Row, New York, p 385

16. GESTATIONAL TROPHOBLASTIC DISEASE

INTRODUCTION

— Tumours of the trophoblast form a wide spectrum, from the partial hydatidiform mole at one end to the highly malignant choriocarcinoma at the other.
— Early diagnosis, prompt and adequate treatment will reduce the incidence of choriocarcinoma.

DEFINITION

— Gestational trophoblastic disease is the general term for a spectrum of proliferative abnormalities of the trophoblast.
— Hydatidiform mole represents a usually benign form of the disease.
— Choriocarcinoma is a very malignant and frequently a metastatic disease.
  These neoplasia arise from the trophoblatic elements of the developing blastocyst and retain certain characteristics of the normal chorionic villus such as invasive tendencies and the ability to make the polypeptide hormone human chorionic gonadotropin (HCG).
— The disease is always related to some pregnancy events and thus specifically differs from choriocarcinoma from germ cell tumours of the ovary or testis.

EPIDEMIOLOGY OF TROPHOBLASTIC DISEASE

Molar pregnancy

— Asian rates (Japan and Singapore) are 1.5–2.5 times higher than American rates.
— There is a significant difference in the rate between the

eastern half, especially Asia, and the developed western half of the world.

— There is a higher incidence in women aged 40 years or more.
— Geographic differences in incidence may be due to environmental, cultural, socio-economic or racial (genetic) factors.
— Japanese, Chinese, Filipino and Asian women from the Indian subcontinent tend to have a higher incidence than Caucasians.
— Incidence of recurrence of molar pregnancies is in the range 0.5–2%.
— Partial moles are commonly triploid or trisomic, while complete moles are usually 46XX with two identical paternal haplotypes and no maternal chromosomes.
— The ratio of partial to complete moles is about 2:1.

AETIOLOGY AND PATHOGENESIS

— The majority of trophoblastic tumours arise following pregnancy.
— The minority arise from germ cells of the gonad.
— Tumours are classified into two groups:
  • Hydatidiform mole, which may be totally localised, locally invasive or metastatic
  • Choriocarcinoma
— In hydatidiform mole there is oedema and decreased vascularity of hte core of the villi together with proliferation of the trophoblast.
— As malignant features develop:
  • There is loss of villus formation
Increasing proliferation of the trophoblastic epithelium
There is hyperplasia of both syncytial and cytotrophoblastic cells
Presence of haemorrhagic necrosis of invaded tissue by columns of hyperplastic cells
— Aetiology of mole is unknown
— Absence of blood vessels in the villus core or absence and death or stunting of the embryo may be either cause or effect.
— Abnormal epithelial proliferation may again be primary or related to anoxia or some other trigger.
— Alterations in the balance of trophoblastic invasiveness and host reaction account for the spread of these tumours beyond the normal site, i.e. the endometrium.
— The chromosomal complement of the classical mole is diploid (usually XX) and is considered to be entirely of paternal origin.

— Usually the ovum nucleus fails to persist and the sperm pronucleus duplicates.
— In partial mole (6% of the cases) the chromosomal complement is often triploid (69 chromosomes XXY and XXX, the extra set coming from the sperm).
— In most complete moles the chromosome complement is 46XX.
— They express only one pair of paternal HLA — A and B antigens.
— Findings suggest that complete moles usually result from fertilisation of the ovum by a haploid sperm which subsequently duplicates its own chromosomes by meiosis.
— Women who have a molar pregnancy have an increased incidence of balanced translocations.
— Partial mole is considered to be associated with severe pre-eclampsia, and the triploid fetus has characteristic malformations of the central nervous system.
— The disease is commoner at the extremes of the childbearing age.
— It is more prevalent among lower socioeconomic groups.
— It is more common among certain racial groups (South-East Asia, Mexico, Africa).
— It is higher among older women and carries the risk of malignant sequelae.
— There is some evidence to suggest that environmental factors and diet are also involved.
— Nutritional factors such as folic acid and iron deficiency are also incriminated; vascular agenesis as a result of folic acid deficiency as the cause of molar pregnancy.
— Protein deficiency is associated with molar pregnancy.
— Approximately 80% of patients initially diagnosed as having hydatidiform mole will follow a benign course following evacuation of the uterus.
— 12–15% subsequently develop locally invasive disease.
— 5–8% eventually prove to have metastatic lesions.

HYDATIDIFORM MOLE

There are two types
— Complete or classical mole — consists of hyperplastic hydropic villi and no fetus.
— Partial mole — focal hyperplasia of trophoblast with varying degree of hydropic villous degeneration with a fetus.
— Pathologically the hydatidiform mole is divided into benign mole, locally invasive mole and metastasising mole.

Incidence

— Ranges from 1 in 2,000 pregnancies in Western countries, 1 in 200 in some Asian countries and Nigeria, to 1 in 100 among Chinese races.
— Only about 1 in 30 develop into choriocarcinoma.
— The risk of developing choriocarcinoma is 1,000 times greater following molar pregnancy as compared with normal pregnancy.
— Incidence is higher among low socio-economic class.

Clinical features

— the mole is usually diagnosed as a threatened abortion.
— There is amenorrhoea combined with exaggerated pregnancy symptoms.
— Irregular vaginal bleeding occurs, and the loss may contain the classical vesicles.
— The diagnosis is often not made until the second trimester. $2^{4}/_{4}$
— The following features then become obvious:
  • Uterus is larger than expected (50–55%)
  • Uterus is sometimes tender
  • Uterus is doughy
  • No fetal heart is heard
  • No fetal parts are felt
  • Early onset of pre-eclampsia (15–20%)
  • Hyperemesis (25–30%)
  • Hyperthyroidism (5–10%) due to elevated TSH from placenta
  • Bilateral theca–lutein cyst felt in (10–20%)
  • Bilateral theca–lutein cyst seen on ultrasound examination (30–40%)
— Symptoms from metastatic spread, such as haemoptysis and/or pleuritic pain, spread to the lung.
— Sometimes the diagnosis is only made on histological examination of curetting from a suspected incomplete abortion.
— Histology shows a vascular stroma of the trophoblastic villi undergoing vesicular change:
  • Proliferation of the trophoblastic cells
  • Usually there is absence of the embryo/fetus
— Great diagnostic difficulty may arise if there is a mole with co-existent fetus (4%–6%).

Investigations

— Ultrasound examination shows typical 'snowstorm' appearance inside the uterus.

- No fetus or proper placenta usually seen
- Theca-lutein cysts may be visualised
- Multiple pregnancy will be excluded

— Urine pregnancy tests are positive in high dilution.

— Serum β subunit HCG levels are grossly elevated.

— Multiple pregnancy may cause confusion if HCG levels are high.

— HCG value above 100 000 IU in 24 hours urine or above 40 000 IU/ml in serum is suspicious of molar pregnancy which should be confirmed by ultrasound examination.

— In molar pregnancy the urinary products or blood levels of progesterone and oestrogen are usually below the tenth percentile for normal pregnancy.

— Radiography is seldom used nowadays.

— Arteriography, amniography are invasive procedures.

— Chest radiography is done to exclude metastasising lesions.

— Liver and renal fuction, haemoglobin, full blood count, blood group and cross-matching are done.

— Cervical smear and swab are done.

Management

— Patient is treated in close collaboration with a specialist in this disease.

— Once the diagnosis is confirmed, the mole needs to be removed.

— Suction evacuation and curettage are effective in experienced hands regardless of uterine size.

— Simultaneously intravenous infusion of oxytocin is given and at completion intramuscular Syntometrine may be given to reduce blood loss.

— Cervix may need preliminary dilatation using laminaria tent or prostaglandin pessary.

— Perforation is likely to occur unless procedure of emptying the uterus is done with care and gentleness.

— In some women, abortions may be in progress, and this should be augmented by intravenous oxytocin infusion or suction evacuation if bleeding is moderate.

— Extra-amniotic instillation of prostaglandin with intravenous oxytocin infusion is tried in some cases.

— After the uterus is evacuated, gentle but sharp curettage is done and all material is sent for histological examination.

— Size of the uterus and ovaries should be recorded.

— Blood transfusion may be necessary before, during or after the evacuation.

— Hysterotomy is very rarely needed.

— Hysterectomy is seldom needed at this stage.

— Hysterectomy may be of prophylactic value in the older patient with a completed family.
— The risk of malignant sequelae (invasive mole and choriocarcinoma) is significantly greater in women aged more than 40 years, especially if para 3 or more.

Subsequent care

— Careful follow-up is needed for at least 12 months after the HCG test becomes negative.
— Since cure is not achieved in 10–15% of patients, all patients need close follow-up.
— HCG estimation in urine and blood is carried out weekly until levels are showing a steady downward trend.
— HCG estimated once in two weeks until β subunit HCG is negative on two consecutive occasions (urine HCG 12 IU/l or serum HCG 0–4IU/l); this usually takes 3–10 weeks.
— Thereafter this is done monthly for 6 months and 3-monthly for further 6 months.
— Patients are registered with one of the regional centres.
— If β subunit HCG could not be assayed, initially ordinary pregnancy HCG assay with a switch, to the more sensitive β subunit HCG assay after levels have fallen, to save expenses.
— Radiography is used at regular intervals to check the presence/activity of chorionic tissue in the lungs.
— Patient should have her condition explained and be reassured regarding the importance of avoiding pregnancy in the ensuing 1–2 years, and regular follow-up examination, blood and urine tests for HCG levels are mandatory.
— A barrier method for contraception should be used until HCG levels are normal, then oral contraceptive pills (combined) can be used.
— There is some suggestion that the incidence of choriocarcinoma may be higher if the oral contraceptive pill is given before HCG levels are normal.
— Careful gynaecological assessment should be carried out every 2–4 weeks, and ultrasound examination is carried out at the same time to check the uterine size, contents if any inside the cavity and presence and size of the theca-lutein cysts.
— In 90% of patients, a negative HCG level is reached by 42 days.
— Ultrasound examination should be done if pregnancy is suspected due to contraceptive failure.

Persistent molar disease

— This may be due to locally invasive mole or metastasising mole.
— If the HCG levels fail to fall progressively, it is possible that

all the molar tissue may not have been removed at the previous curettage and this should be repeated after an ultrasonic examination of pelvis and chest radiography.
— If the level remains static or increasing, a diagnosis of persistent disease is made.
— In this situation the mole shows an aggressive behaviour, with tissue destruction and myometrial and blood vessel invasion, sometimes leading to perforation of the uterine wall.
— In some women metastatic spread may occur, usually to the lungs or vagina.
— Arteriography (invasive) or laparoscopy, chest radiography, ultrasound examination may be used to help diagnosis.
— Persistent molar disease occurs in 10–15% of patients with classical mole.
— Warning features of risk:
  • Age over 35
  • Uterus large for dates
  • Very high initial HCG levels
  • Small vesicles
  • Marked trophoblastic proliferation
  • Blood group AB or B and husband's O or A

Management
— This is similar to that described for choriocarcinoma.
— If mole has perforated the uterus, laparotomy and possibly hysterectomy will be needed as an emergency procedure because of haemorrhage.
— Morbidity and mortality of this disease result from penetration of the tumour through the myometrium and into the pelvic vessels with resultant haemorrhage.
— It is differentiated from choriocarcinoma by the persistence of villus pattern on histological examination.
— Local invasion of molar tissue into the myometrium is not easily removable by curetting and may need surgery or chemotherapy.
— Diagnosis is usually made after hysterectomy for haemorrhage.
— This group of patients will benefit from chemotherapy.
— Indication for chemotherapy following hydatidiform mole (Table 16.1):
  • Urinary HCG levels >40 00 I.U./day 4–6 weeks after evacuation or >25 000 I.U./day more than 10 weeks after evacuation
  • Elevation of HCG levels 5–7 months after evacuation
  • Intracranial, renal or gastro-intestinal tract metastasis
  • Pulmonary metastasis with high or increasing HCG levels

Table 16.1 Indications for chemotherapy

— Urinary HCG values 40 000 I.U./24 hr — Serum HCG values 25 000 I.U./l	4–6 weeks after evacuation of the mole

— Progressively rising HCG at any time after evacuation of mole
— Raised HCG values at 5–6 months after evacuation of mole
— Evidence of intracranial, hepatic, gastro-intestinal metastasis
— Pulmonary metastasis with persisting or rising HCG levels
— Persistent uterine haemorrhage with a raised HCG level
— Evidence of choriocarcinoma on histology

  (a few opacities on X-ray <2 cm in diameter may not require therapy if the HCG levels are falling)
- Persistent or recurrent uterine bleeding with raised urinary HCG levels
- Histological evidence of choriocarcinoma at curettage or hysterectomy

— There is no indication for routine prophylactic chemotherapy in molar pregnancy, since 95% of moles undergo spontaneous regression.

CHORIOCARCINOMA

Introduction

— This is a highly malignant tumour characterised by disordered growth of syncytio- and cyto-trophoblast and invasion of the myometrium causing tissue necrosis and haemorrhage.
— Metastasis is common.
— It is rare except following molar pregnancy (50%).
— Lateness in appearance of symptoms after preceding gestation, be it normal (20%), abortion or ectopic (30%).

Incidence

— Choriocarcinoma forms 3–6% of trophoblastic tumours.
— There are about 1 in 20 000–40 000 such pregnancies in Western countries, increasing to about 1 in 150 pregnancies in the Far East.
— One in 30 of hydatidiform moles progresses to choriocarcinoma.
— Prognosis is different from choriocarcinoma which occurs in germ-cell tumour of the gonads.

Clinical features

— Typically some 3–6 months after gestation the patient will notice symptoms related to the site of the tumour.
— Unfortunately, metastasis may signal their presence before the primary growth in the uterus declares itself.
— Uterus:
  • Bleeding, discharge and pain
  • Purplish tumour nodules may be noticed in the cervix and vagina
  • Uterus and adnexae may be irregularly enlarged
— Lungs (70%):
  • Pleuritic pain effusion
  • Dyspnoea, cough
  • Haemoptysis
  • Rounded opacities on chest radiography ('cannonball' or 'snowstorm' appearance)
— Central nervous system:
  • Headache
  • Evidence of increased intracranial pressure
  • Sudden intracranial or cerebrovascular haemorrhage
  • Localising signs such as hemiparesis
— Liver:
  • Enlarged and palpable
  • Jaundice and severe anaemia
  • Rupture and haemoperitoneum
  • Ascitis
— Gastro-intestinal tract:
  • Bleeding
  • Perforation
— Kidneys:
  • Pain
  • Haematuria
— Local extension is frequent.
— Lymphatic spread is rare, but blood spread is most common.

Diagnosis

— Microscopcally the features are as follows:
  • Disorderly growth of trophoblastic tissue
  • Affects both syncytio- and cyto-trophoblast
  • Invades muscle and blood vessels
  • Marked destruction and extensive coagulation necrosis and haemorrhage
  • Villus pattern is completely lost
  • Destruction of tissue by the infiltrating columns of trophoblastic tissue with tissue destruction, coagulation

necrosis and haemorrhage which are not seen in an
invasive mole.

Management

— Complete history and physical examination.
— First appropriate diagnostic investigations are made:
- Histology
- Chest X-ray
- Ultrasound examination of pelvis, liver, kidney, spleen
- Full blood count, differential and platelet count
- Isotopes
- CT scan to exclude brain metastasis
- Liver, renal function and full blood count
- Serum or urinary HCG levels, if possible β subunit
- Lumbar puncture if intracranial lesions are suspected
- Excretion urography and selective arteriography if
indicated
- Bacteriology screen is done to exclude infection

Prognostic factors in choriocarcinoma

— In general the patient is either cured of her disease or
succumbs within a few months.
— Low, medium or high risk can often be assigned (Table
16.2).
- The longer the interval between the disease and the
antecedent pregnancy, the higher the risk of drug
resistence

Table 16.2 Categorisation of patients with gestational trophoblastic tumours — risk factors

Risk factors	0	10	20	40
Age (years)	<39	>39	—	—
Parity	1,2	3 or 4		
Antecedent pregnancy	Mole	Abortion	Term	
Interval in months (AP-chemotherapy) HCG plasma/urine)	<4 10^3–10^4	4–7 10^4	7–12 10^4–10^5	>12 10^5
ABO female/male (Blood group)	A X A XB XAB	O X O A X O	BX ABX	
No. of metastases	Nil	1–4	4–8	>8
Site of metastasis	Not detected, lungs, vagina	Spleen, kidney	GI tract, liver	Brain
Size of tumour	<30 mm	30–50 mm	>50 mm	
Lymphocytic infiltration	Marked	Moderate	Slight	
Immune status	Reactive	Reactive	Unreactive	Unreactive
Previous chemotherapy	Nil	Nil	Single drug;	2 drugs or more

low risk ($\leqslant$50)
medium risk (55–95)
high risk (>95)

- There is usually a good response to treatment in all patients if the disease develops up to 6–7 months after molar pregnancy or 3–4 months after non-molar pregnancy
- Irreversible intracranial or pulmonary damage is a bad prognostic feature
- A well-developed mononuclear cell infiltration around the tumour is usually a favourable feature
- Masses of tumour >80 mm in diameter are less likely to respond to therapy
- If brain metastases develop after treatment has started, the prognosis is poor
- Women of blood group AB have a poor prognosis
- If patient is group A or B when her partner lacks these antigens, her tumours are liable to metastasise widely but respond well to treatment.

Surgical treatment

— Hysterectomy is usually avoided as initial treatment.
— The indications for hysterectomy:
  - Uterine perforation or intraperitoneal haemorrhage has occurred
  - Chemotherapy is not proving effective: residual disease in the uterus
  - High-risk patients (older and/or multiparous)
  - Full-dose chemotherapy must be deferred for at least 2 weeks post-operatively
  - Solitary pulmonary or vaginal metastasis resistant to drug therapy may be removed.

Chemotherapy

— For low-risk patients:
  - Methotrexate 1 mg/kg I.M. or 15–25 mg I.M. daily for 5 days every 48 hours for 4 doses
  - and folinic acid 6 mg I.M. every 48 hours for 4 doses
  - Repeated after 7 days; a total of 4 courses are given
  - If bone-marrow depression or other complications occur, the interval is lengthened
  - The side-effects of the above regimen are usually quite tolerable (gastro-intestinal upset and ulceration of mouth)
  - HCG levels fall to normal level within 4 weeks of starting treatment in most patients (urine HCG 12 I.U./l, serum 0–4 I.U./l)
  - 1 in 10 fails to respond even to 6 or 7 courses, or relapses after treatment is completed — falls into medium-risk group.

— For medium-risk patients:
  • The number of courses depend on the extent of the disease and the patients' response
— Combination of drugs used:
  • Hydroxyurea
  • Methotrexate
  • Actinomycin D
  • Mercaptopurin
  • Vincristine
  • Cyclophosphamide
  • along with folinic acid
— Side-effects are much more significant with such intensive chemotherapy, particularly to the bone marrow.
— High-risk patients:
  • Defined as those women in whom tumour masses are present >60 mm diameter or the antecedent pregnancy occurred 2 years or more ago
— The following combination of drugs is used:
  • Actinomycin D
  • Methotrexate
  • VP 16–213
  • Cyclophosphamide
  • Folinic acid
  • Constant check on WBC and platelet count should be done: if WBC is <1000, platelets are <50 000 or mucositis develops, then the interval is lengthened
  • For cranial metastasis or for prophylaxis, methotrexate 12.5 mg intrathecally may be given. Actinomycin D is more effective in penetrating the blood–brain barrier

Complications of therapy
— Marrow suppression
— Sepsis and other infections due to marrow suppression
— Haemorrhage from metastasis
— CNS complications
— Gastro-intestinal lesions
— Malnutrition
— Genito-urinary problems
— Serositis
— Dermatological complications.
— D.I. vas coagulation (D.I.V.C.)
— Pathological fractures

Radiotherapy

— Trophoblastic disease is not especially sensitive to radiation therapy.
— Patients with metastases in liver and brain may develop

haemorrhage into the metastatic lesions as they undergo necrosis from chemotherapy.

- In such cases external radiation with 20 Gy (2000 rad) per tumour dose is usually given for 10–14 days together with chemotherapy

Others

— Continuous intravenous or arterial infusion of chemotherapeutic agents is given to treat resistant liver or brain metastases

— Courses of treatment are continued until HCG levels have been normal for 3–4 weeks.

Post-treatment follow-up

— Close follow-up by HCG monitoring of samples sent to the centre.

— This allows early detection of a relapse which occurs in less than 5% of cases.

— Normal values reassure the patients.

— Regular chest X-ray, full blood count, liver and renal functions are helpful.

— Ultrasound examination of pelvis, uterus and ovaries, liver and kidneys is also useful to detect early problems.

— Patient must avoid pregnancy for at least one year after cessation of the chemotherapy.

— There is no contra-indication for pregnancy in cured patients.

— Patient needs good counselling, explanation and reassurance all the time.

— Long-term surveillance (up to 5 years) is necessary for these patients.

Prognosis

— With the advent of effective chemotherapy and tumour monitoring with beta HCG, there has been a dramatic improvement in prognosis.

— Survival is now usual unless extensive metastatic disease is present; cerebral and liver metastases carry a poor prognosis.

— Other bad features are choriocarcinoma arising after a normal pregnancy, a long history of delay, previous unsuccessful chemotherapy.

— A large tumour mass and very high HCG titres are unfavourable.

Conclusions

— In the majority of patients a hysterectomy is unnecessary.
— Chemotherapy cures the problems in the majority.
— Pregnancy should be avoided for one year following the cessation of chemotherapy.
— The effect of cytotoxic chemotherapy on ovarian function is relatively slight.
— In younger patients normal menstruation starts shortly after the HCG reaches the undetectable value by RIA.
— There is no increase in fetal abnormalities following chemotherapy.
— With chemotherapy almost 100% of patients with non-metastatic disease can be cured, and a high percentage of patients with metastatic lesions are also curable.
— Average cure rate varies in the range 80–90% in the high-risk group.
— Choriocarcinoma following a full-term pregnancy seems to have a poor prognosis. Survival rate is approximately 60%.
— Overall survival rate is 94%.

SUGGESTED READING

Bagshaw K D, Begent R H J 1981 Trophoblastic tumours: clinical features and management. In: Coplesion M (ed) Gynecologic oncology: fundamental principles and clinical practice, vol 2. Churchill Livingstone, Edinburgh, p 757

Elston C W 1984 The pathology of trophoblastic disease — current status. In: Fox H (ed) Clinics in obstetrics and gynaecology, vol II. Saunders, Philadelphia, p 135

Huddleston J F, Morrow C P 1984 Gestational trophoblastic neoplasia: surgical pathologic considerations with clinical emphasis, vol 27. Harper & Row, New York, p 160

Mackay C V, Beischer N A, Cox L W, Wood C (eds) 1983 Illustrated textbook of gynaecology. Saunders, Philadelphia, p 231

McDonald T W, Ruffolo G H 1983 Modern management of gestational trophoblastic disease. Obstetrical and gynaecological survey, vol 38. p 67

Morrow C P (ed) 1984 Trophoblastic disease in clinical obstetrics and gynecology, vol 27. Harper & Row, New York, p 151

Newlands E S 1983 Treatment of trophoblastic disease. In: Studd J (ed) Progress in obstetrics and gynaecology, vol 3. Churchill Livingstone, Edinburgh, p 158

Ratnam S S, Chew S C 1979 The modern management of trophoblastic disease. In: Stallworthy J, Bourne G (eds) Recent advances in obstetrics and gynaecology, vol 13, p. 237

17. AMENORRHOEA AND OLIGOMENORRHOEA

DEFINITION

— Amenorrhoea is not a disease but a symptom and may be arbitrarily defined as a failure of menses for 3 months or longer.
— Primary amenorrhoea is defined as the failure of menses to appear and should not be diagnosed before the patient has reached the age of 17 years.
— Secondary amenorrhoea implies the cessation of the menses after an initial menarche.
— Physiological amenorrhoea is the normal absence of menses before puberty, during pregnancy and lactation and after the menopause.
— Oligomenorrhoea is defined as a reduction in the frequency of menses; the interval must be longer than 38 days but less than 3 months.

Table 17.1 Common causes of primary amenorrhoea

A. Chromosomal
   Turner's syndrome
   Mixed gonadal dysgenesis
B. Gonadal
   True hermaphrodite
   True gonadal agenesis
   Virilising male intersex
C. End-organ resistance
   Testicular feminisation syndrome
D. Hypothalamic–pituitary disorder
   Panhypopituitarism
   Hypogonadotropic hypogonadism
   Laurence-Moon-Bardet-Biedl syndrome
   Olfactogenital syndrome
   Pre-pubertal polycystic ovary syndrome
E. Adrenal hyperplasia
F. Gynaetresia
   Congenital
   Cryptomenorrhoea
G. Delayed menarche

AETIOLOGY

    — See Table 17.1 and Figure 17.1.
    — If the amenorrhoea is not physiological, it may be due to:
- Disorders of the central nervous system
- Disorders of the anterior pituitary
- Disorders of the ovary
- Disorders of the outflow tract and/or uterus
- Disorders of intermediate metabolism and nutrition

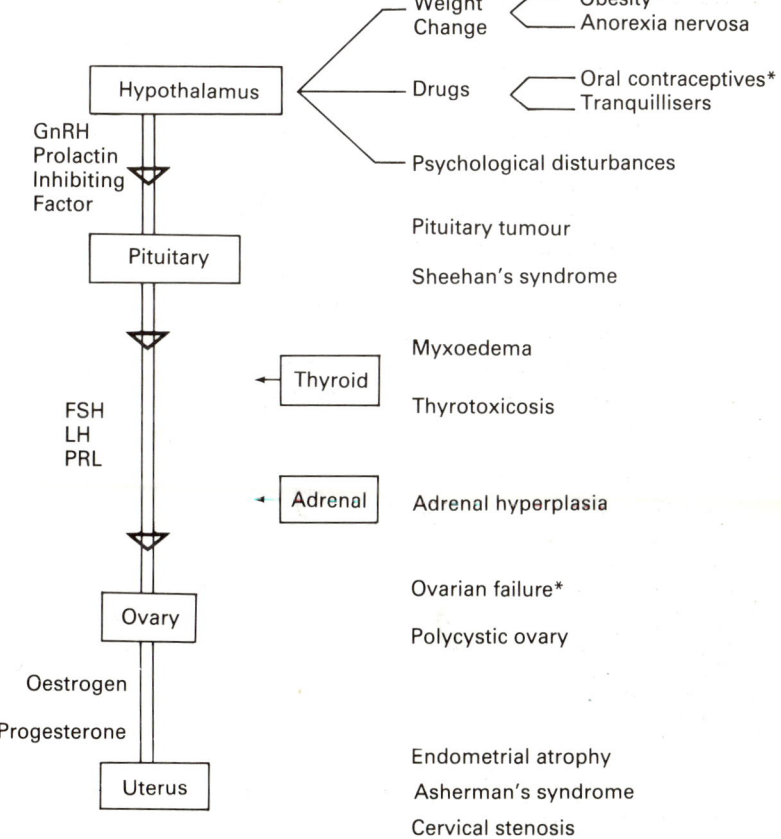

* Common causes of secondary amenorrhoea

Fig. 17.1

CENTRAL NERVOUS SYSTEM LESIONS

Neurogenic — hypothalamus and above

— Organic:
  - Destructive lesion
  - Tumours
  - Scars
— Insufficiency — hypothalamic dysfunction
  - Polycystic ovarian disease
  - Deficient prolactin inhibiting factor (hyperprolactinaemia, Chiarri-Frommel syndrome)
  - Iatrogenic due to drugs
  - Congenital defects (hypogonadotropic eunuchoidism, anosomic amenorrhoea, Kallmann's syndrome)

Psychogenic amenorrhoea — Functional

— Stress:
  - Psychiatric disease
  - Polycystic ovarian disease
  - Hyperprolactinaemia
  - Anorexia nervosa
  - Pseudocyesis

Pituitary disease

— Insufficiency:
  - Destructive processes (Sheehan's syndrome and Simmonds' disease)
— Tumours:
  - Chromophobe adenoma (non-functioning, partial gonadotropin- or TSH-secreting); prolactinomas (Forbes-Albright)
  - Acidophilic adenoma (aeromegaly)
  - Basophilic adenoma (Cushing's disease)
— Cogenital defects (hypogonadotropic eunuchoidism).

GONADAL LESIONS (OVARIAN AMENORRHOEA)

Insufficiency

— Cogenital developmental defects:
  - Gonadal dysgenesis (Turner's syndrome)
  - True hermaphroditism

- Male hermaphroditism (androgen insensitivity syndrome)
- Testicular feminisation syndrome (androgen insensitivity syndrome)
— Premature menopause:
  - Chromosomal
  - Destructive (iatrogenic — surgical, drugs, irradiation, neoplasia, infection)
  - Auto-immune disease
  - Constitutional

The insensitive ovary

Tumours

— Arrhenoblastoma, hiluscells, adrenal rest.
— Granulosa cell, thecoma.
— Non-specific with steroidogenic stroma.

END ORGAN LESIONS (DISORDERS OF OUTFLOW TRACT AND/OR UTERUS)

Congenital defects

— Imperforate hymen.
— Absence or atresia of vagina.
— Septum of vagina.
— Absence of uterus.

Traumatic

— Stenosis of vagina.
— Stenosis of cervix.
— Sclerosis of uterine cavity (Asherman's disease).

DISEASES OF INTERMEDIATE METABOLISM AND NUTRITION

Metabolic disease

— Thyroid (hypo- and hyperthyroidism).
— Pancreas (diabetes mellitus).
— Adrenal:
  - Cogenital adrenal hyperplasia
  - Adrenogenital syndrome and related disturbances
  - Cushing's disease and stress obesity
  - Tumours

Nutritional disturbances

> — Malnutrition:
> - Weight loss
> - Athlete's amenorrhoea
> — Exogenic obesity.

Excretory and metabolic organs

> — Liver — cirrhosis.
> — Kidney — chronic nephritis.

Chronic illness

PHYSIOLOGICAL AMENORRHOEA

> — Delayed puberty.
> — Pregnancy.
> — Post-partum amenorrhoea.
> — Menopause.

Clinical features

> — It is important to differentiate the condition of primary amenorrhoea from delayed puberty which requires only reassurance.
> — In true primary amenorrhoea significant structural and/or genetic conditions are often present, some of which may require early treatment (e.g. imperforate hymen).
> — A useful clue is the length of time that secondary sex characteristics have been present without menses starting.
> — If the length of time is 3 or more years, it is almost certain that there is absence of uterus or a vaginal septum causing blockage, or androgen insensitivity, or androgen excess.
> — Absence of secondary sex characteristics indicates absence or malfunction of the ovaries or a defect higher in the endocrine axis if the time limit for the onset of puberty has been exceeded.
> — In secondary amenorrhoea, there is far more likely to be either a physiological cause such as pregnancy, a direct failure of some part of the hypothalamic–pituitary–ovarian–uterine axis, or a metabolic disturbance in the body which secondarily affects the function of this axis.

Hypothalamic causes (psychological, drugs, organic lesion)
- — Psychological causes are relatively common.
- — Sometimes the stress involved may not be obvious to the patient.
- — Starting, changing or being dismissed from employment, changes or difficulties in interpersonal relationships, intrapersonal difficulties (non-acceptance of body image), fear, anxieties, phobias — may cause problems.
- — Psychiatric symptoms such as mood and behavioural changes may cause problem.
- — Examination reveals no significant general or gynaecological disturbance except possibly weight loss if patient is suffering from anorexia nervosa.
- — In some adolescents, the delayed development may be related to undernutrition and/or constitutional stress which is less pathological (the ballet dancer or athlete).
- — Anorexia nervosa is usually associated with a serious psychiatric upset.
  - • It occurs in 1/1000, usually in the age group 10–25
  - • The sufferer is brought to the doctor by a parent
  - • Theories of aetiology include: dieting gone out of control, attempting stave off sexual development
  - • Less frequently, the observed psychiatric symptoms may have occurred secondarily
  - • Symptoms include continual rejection of food, weight loss, amenorrhoea, constipation, hyperactivity and vomiting, usually self-induced
  - • The personality profile includes fear of adulthood, specifically sexual involvement, obedience and conformity, well-meaning domineering parents, deep fear of having no inner controls, lack of adolescent development of the capacity for self-evaluation and self-concept
  - • Increasing social isolation, self-imposed dieting, compulsive exercising; denial of the behaviour and its results are other features
  - • The syndrome is usually unmistakable and may produce primary or secondary amenorrhoea
  - • In doubtful cases exclude malignancy, tuberculosis and malabsorption
- — Drugs such as phenothiazines and oral contraceptives may produce amenorrhoea.
- — Organic lesions are rare — conditions such as craniopharyngioma, post-inflammatory conditions, extension of a pituitary tumour are to be considered.

Pituitary causes
- — Pituitary tumours such as basophiladenoma produce Cushing's disease.

— Acidophilademona produces gigantism and aeromegaly.

— Disturbances may occur as a result of function of the tumour or because of the pressure symptoms due to effects on the pituitary gland, or the optic chiasma or because of uninhibited prolactin release.

— Micro-adenoma causes very little distortion of the fossa.

— Post-partum pituitary necrosis (Sheehan's syndrome) is rather rare now. The amenorrhoea is preceded by marked asthenia, cold sensitivity, loss of libido, and mental torpor. There is significant reduction of secondary sex characteristics.

Ovarian disorders

— Failure of the ovary to develop (agenesis, dysgenesis) will cause primary amenorrhoea.

— Premature failure may occur at any time from the teens to age 35 years and will result in premature menopause.

— In gonadotropin-resistant ovary, follicles are present which are insensitive to gonadotropin.

— Ovaries may be removed or destroyed by cancer treatment such as surgery, irradiation, chemotherapy.

— Ovarian function may be destroyed by inflammatory disease, endometriosis and torsion and also by surgery for the same conditions.

Uterine disorders

— Uterine agenesis is rare and is usually associated with vaginal agenesis.

— Vigorous curettage to control heavy bleeding after abortion or delivery may remove the basal layer of the endometrium and produce obliteration of the uterine cavity (Asherman's syndrome).

— Diagnosis is made by hysterography or hysteroscopy.

Vaginal causes

— In virtually all cases there is a congenital malformation either of part of the vagina (septum, imperforate hymen) or its entirety (agenesis).

— Secondary sex characteristics are well developed in patients with imperforate hymen, as with menstrual molimina (tension, discomfort etc).

— Difficulty with voiding may be present.

• Examination will indicate the obstructing vaginal septum, and bimanual rectal examination will disclose a mass in the vagina or in the pelvis

Investigation

— History, examination (both general and pelvic examination) are important.

— When the disorder appears related to the hypothalamus or pituitary, FSH, LH and prolactin levels must be measured.
— High levels of FSH and LH indicate ovarian failure or absence.
— High levels of prolactin suggest pituitary adenoma (or micro-adenoma).
— If menstrual cycles are infrequent (oligomenorrhoea), weekly assays of ovarian steroids may identify the type of disorder, e.g. polycystic ovarian syndrome.
— Progesterone challenge test using medroxyprogesterone acetate (Provera) 5–10 mg daily for 5 days will assess the endogenous oestrogen level.
— If endogenous oestrogen level is adequate, patient will have bleeding following the course of progestational agent.
— If no bleeding occurs, the test can be repeated after a 20-day course of oestrogen (30 to 50 μg of ethinyl oestradiol orally per day), the progestin being given on the last 5 to 7 days to check the adequacy of uterine function.
— If hirsutism is the main clinical feature, androgenic hormones are measured.
— In congenital adrenal hyperplasia, 17-OH-progesterone levels are high.
— If androgenic tumour is present, 17-OXO and oxogenic steroids are higher.
— Thyroid function and carbohydrate metabolism should also be screened.
— Clinical changes of hypothyroidism are often subtle.
— In hypothyroidism, there is an increase in TSH level, which stimulates prolactin secretion, resulting in ovarian inhibition.
— Stimulation of the pituitary by GnRH and the ovaries by FSH and LH can be done as dynamic test and use GnRH or FSH/LH for treating amenorrhoea.
— Cytogenic analysis is necessary in patients with primary amenorrhoea (except those with anatomical anomalies of the uterus and the vagina) and also in those with secondary amenorrhoea when no other cause can be found.
— There may be mosaic patterns such as XO/XX where a hypoplastic ovary functions for a limited time.
— Pituitary fossa radiography is indicated in patients with primary and secondary amenorrhoea, hyperprolactinaemia, and oligomenorrhoea of long standing.
— Presence of double floor of the pituitary fossa indicates a need for tomography or CT scan.
— Visualisation of the ovaries and uterus using laparoscope may help in diagnosis and planning therapy.

Treatment

— See Table 17.2 and Figure 17.2 pp. 253–255.

— It is aimed at production of menses, restoration of coital function and/or fertility.

— Adequate explanation of the underlying problems, its management and prognosis should be included.

— Both physical and psychological stress can adversely affect menstrual function, and some insight is needed by the patient and by the doctor to appreciate this.

— In anorexia nervosa, the therapy is aimed to improve weight, standardised for the patient's height and build.

- The patient must be removed from the intense enmeshment with the family and encouraged in the attainment of self-acceptance and autonomy
- She must be encouraged to manage her social and sexual development

Table 17.2 Amenorrhoea — aetiology and management

	Aetiology	Management
Physiological	Pregnancy, lactation, menopause	Should be considered in differential diagnosis
Cerebral cortex	Stress, bereavement, disappointment	Remove the cause
Hypothalamus	Inhibition (psychiatric illness, stress, drugs)	Stop drugs, treat psychiatric illness, remove stress
	Tumour	Neurosurgery
	Delayed menarche	No action — reassurance
Pituitary gland	Congenital hypopituitarism	Replacement therapy
	Prolactinoma	Bromocriptine — sometimes surgery or irradiation
	Acidophil adenoma	Neurosurgery or irradiation
	Damage	Replacement therapy
Thyroid gland	Hypo- and hyperthyroidism	Medical and surgical treatment
Adrenal cortex	Congenital hyperplasia	Corticosteroids
	Hyperplasia (adult)	Corticosteroids
	Tumour	Surgery
Ovaries	Agenesis	Hormone replacement
	Damage or removal	Hormone replacement
	Premature failure	Hormone replacement
	Ovarian insensitivity	Hormone replacement
	Functioning tumour	Surgery
	Polycystic ovarian disease	Clomiphene, dexamethasone, surgery
Male intersex	Androgen insensitivity	Remove gonads + HRT after puberty
	Gonadal dysgenesis	Remove gonads + HRT after puberty
	Hermaphrodite	Remove gonads + HRT after puberty
Uterus	Absence or removal	No treatment available
	Asherman's syndrome	Surgery — IUD plus oestrogen
Cervix	Stenosis (surgery, irradiation)	Dilatation of cervix
Vagina	Imperforate hymen	Surgery — removal of membrane
	Atresia of vagina (congenital, trauma)	Creation of new vagina

Fig. 17.2 Investigations of amenorrhoea

Measure FSH
X-ray pituitary fossa
Measure prolactin
Exogenous progestogen test (Provera 5 mg × 5 days)
Clomiphene test

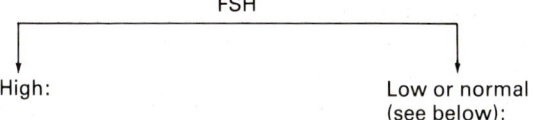

FSH

High: Low or normal
                                          (see below):

Assess oestrogen status:

Low (ovarian failure):   Normal (very unusual):

Replace oestrogen   Examination of ovaries
                                          by laparoscopy

Chromosomal   Open biopsy
analysis   (? resistant ovary syndrome)

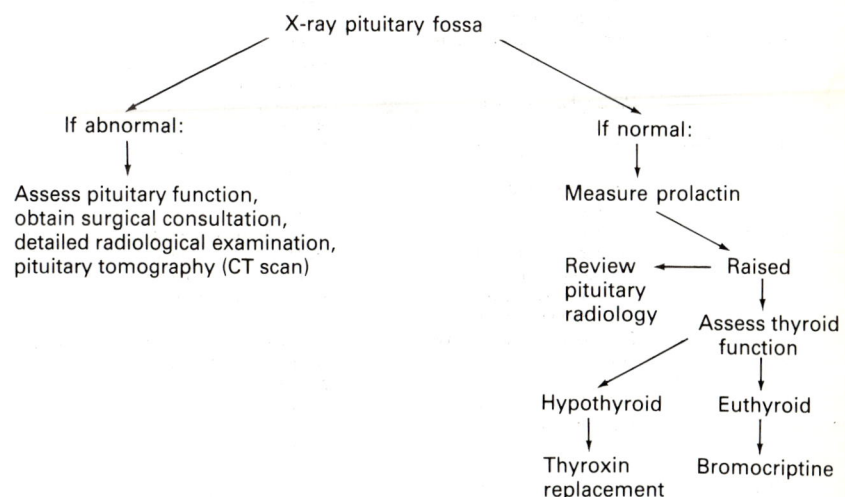

LOW OR NORMAL FSH

X-ray pituitary fossa

If abnormal: If normal:

Assess pituitary function,   Measure prolactin
obtain surgical consultation,
detailed radiological examination,
pituitary tomography (CT scan)   Review ◄──── Raised
                                          pituitary
                                          radiology   Assess thyroid
                                                              function

                                          Hypothyroid   Euthyroid

                                          Thyroxin   Bromocriptine
                                          replacement

Fig. 17.2 (*cont.*)

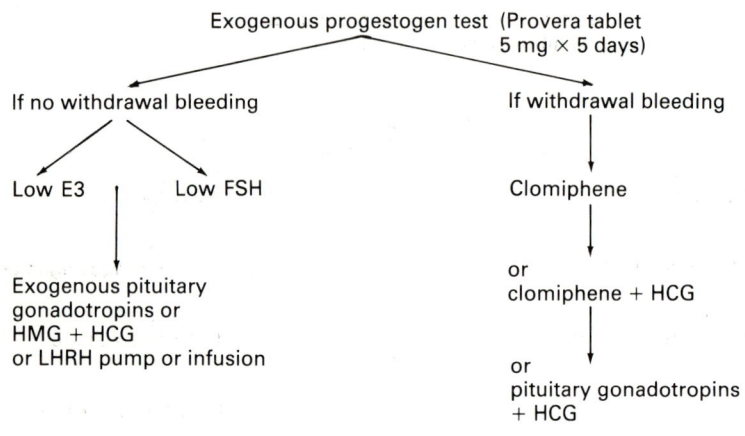

IF PROLACTIN IS NORMAL

Exogenous progestogen test (Provera tablet
                                          5 mg × 5 days)

If no withdrawal bleeding   If withdrawal bleeding

Low E3   Low FSH   Clomiphene

Exogenous pituitary   or
gonadotropins or   clomiphene + HCG
HMG + HCG
or LHRH pump or infusion   or
                                         pituitary gonadotropins
                                         + HCG

Weight-related amenorrhoea — Improve weight before therapy

COMMONEST CAUSE FOR AMENORRHOEA IS WEIGHT-RELATED

Hormone profile/Body weight
LHRH I.V. 100 µg
Normal weight — Average response
Heavy weight — Exaggerated response
Low body weight — Drop in LHRH response to 70–80%

Psychological aspects of weight-related amenorrhoea

Cosmetic over-dieting

Anorectic reaction: depressed first; bereavement; boyfriend disappointment
                       etc. — then develops anorexia. Often stops pills, then
                       develops amenorrhoea — mistaken diagnosis of post-pill
                       amenorrhoea; unhappy love affair; au-pair syndrome —
                       leaving home, nobody takes any notice of her

Physical causes: gut disorders, metabolic disorders, infectious diseases

Anorexia nervosa

Have good appetite but they suppress it; ballet dancers, athletes etc., usually
intellectual, well-educated

1. Avoidance of sexuality
2. Concern over body image
3. Physically and mentally very active
4. History often suppressed
5. Purging is common
6. Eating habits: abstinence, bingeing

Fig. 17.2 (*cont.*)

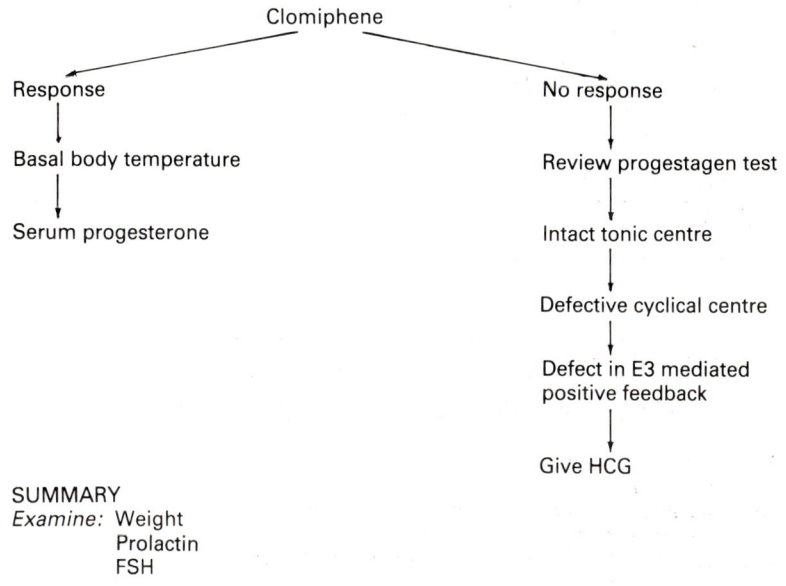

Bleed after progesterone

Indicates she is well-oestrogenised,
will respond to clomiphene

Clomiphene

Response   No response

Basal body temperature   Review progestagen test

Serum progesterone   Intact tonic centre

                                                            Defective cyclical centre

                                                            Defect in E3 mediated
                                                            positive feedback

                                                            Give HCG

SUMMARY
Examine: Weight
          Prolactin
          FSH

Give Provera — period + 5 days
100 mg of clomiphene 5 days one week after
PCT (day 22 of total cycle)

One week after progesterone assay
at 43 days — results of FSH/prolactin are available

- With a normal calorie intake there is rapid gain in weight
  and a return to normal function of the reproductive axis
- If prolactin levels are raised, bromocriptine is usually
  prescribed if the patient wishes to become pregnant or
  symptoms are present.
- Only extrasellar lesions need neurosurgery and/or irradiation.
- Premature ovarian failure or absence of ovaries requires
  hormonal replacement therapy.
- If secondary sexual characteristics are not present, oestrogen
  and progestin as in the contraceptive pill are necessary.
- Uterovaginal malformations in the presence of functional
  ovaries and uterus soon need to be treated surgically.

— If upper vagina is patent, surgical correction should be carried out.

— Androgen insensitivity syndrome (testicular feminisation syndrome) should be considered before therapy is decided.

— The gonads should be removed after puberty and then hormone replacement therapy started.

— When there is total absence of vagina, creation of artificial vagina should be considered.

— Treatment of Asherman's syndrome is usually dilatation of the cavity and separation of adhesion.

— This could be done under hysteroscope control.

— Insertion of a small bag or Foley catheter or IUD followed by cyclical oestrogen progestin therapy is useful.

Idiopathic

— Depending on the duration of symptoms and desire for fertility, the investigations and treatments are arranged.

— Exclude hyperprolactinaemia and hypothyroidism.

— If fertility is desired, ovulation induction is indicated.

— Otherwise no treatment is needed except follow-up at 6-monthly intervals.

— Cyclical oral oestrogen and progestogen therapy is indicated for those who have ovarian failure or absence of ovaries and absence of secondary sexual characteristics.

  • There are several general methods advocated for the production of ovulation when the amenorrhoea is due to factors located in the nervous system, either psychosomatic or neurogenic

— GnRH is used to stimulate the pituitary to release FSH and LH which in turn stimulate the ovary, induce follicular development, ovulation and formation of corpus luteum.

— GnRH is more physiological and seldom produces multiple ovulation.

— GnRH is given using a pump; ultrasound is used to assess ovarian follicular development.

— FSH and LH are given to induce ovulation, and are usually associated with multiple ovulation.

— GnRH, FSH/LH are used when endogenous oestrogen levels are low and progestogen does not produce bleeding.

— Clomiphene, tamoxifen, cyclofenil are used when progestogen produces bleeding. This group of drugs stimulates pituitary activity via the hypothalamus by blocking the oestrogen inhibitory effect.

Excessive adrogenic activity

— It is associated with adrenal hyperplasia or adrenal tumour or virilising tumour from the ovary or polycystic ovarian disease.

— If it is associated with tumour, it needs surgical treatment.

— If it is associated with adrenal hyperplasia, corticosteroids will restore the function and androgen levels to normal.
— In polycystic ovarian syndrome, there is a higher circulating androgen level which is treated by using clomiphene if fertility needs to be restored.
— If hirsutism is the predominant clinical feature, it could be treated using cyproterone acetate.

SPECIFIC CONSIDERATIONS

Lesions of the central nervous system

— Neurogenic.
— Psychogenic.
— Pituitary (trauma, tumour, abnormalities of gonadotropin production)

Neurogenic lesions
Organic brain disease

— Usually there is a history of encephalitis or related infections, accidents, injuries, or exposure to toxic substances such as lead or carbon monoxide.
— Gonadotropin levels are low or low/normal.
— Plasma oestradiol levels are low.
— There may be abnormalities in the function of thyroid, adrenal glands and pancreas, depending on the neurological lesion.
— Neurologic examination and electro-encephalogram are valuable diagnostic aids.
— Prognosis is usually poor except following trauma.
— Pituitary hormone replacement therapy will be necessary.

Hypothalamic dysfunction (insufficiency)

— This condition is rare.
— Menstrual problem starts from menarche.
— Usually there is a family history of menstrual problems.
— There is an absence of psychogenic factors and neurological abnormalities.
— FSH and LH levels are low.
— Patient may get pregnant without treatment, since patients do have infrequent ovulatory menstruation.
— If infertility is a problem, clomiphene may be given.

Polycystic ovarian disease

— A clinical syndrome of infertility, menstrual problems (mainly anovulatory cycle, hirsutism and obesity) found to be associated with enlarged polycystic ovaries.
— It is not a single entity but rather the end result of several conditions.
— Clinical features in order of frequency:
  ● Infertility
  ● Hirsutism
  ● Oligo-amenorrhoea
  ● Obesity
  ● Dysfunctional uterine bleeding
  ● Virilisation
  ● Vaginal epithelium looks normal
  ● Breasts are well developed
  ● There is no sign of oestrogen lack

Pathology

— Microscopically the ovaries are pearly white in appearance with multiple cysts beneath the capsule.
— There are numerous small follicular cysts lined by thin granulosal lining with a marked luteinisation of the theca interna.
— Ovarian capsule is thickened.
— There is a presence of theca cell hyperplasia and certain amount of atresia of granulosa cell.
— There is absence of corpora lutea.

Pathogenesis

— The exact pathogenesis is not clearly understood.
  It may be associated with, or a result of, a disease of the neuro-endocrine homeostasis control mechanism.
— The problem may be initiated by excessive androgen secretion by the adrenal gland.
— There seems to be extraglandular conversion of androstenedione to oestrogen.
— Possible mechanisms involved are:
  ● Androstenedione from ovary and adrenal is converted to oestrone, then oestradiol peripherally
  ● The rate of peripheral conversion is greater in obese women
  ● The excess oestrogen suppresses FSH secretion
  ● Hence follicular development is adversely affected
  ● LH secretion is stimulated by oestrogen, but LH surge does not occur, hence no ovulation
  ● Raised LH levels stimulate the theca cells, which produces androgen
  ● Excess androgen causes hirsutism, gradual defeminisation

and later virilisation, and also perpetuates the whole process
- Unopposed action of oestrogen sometimes leads to endometrial hyperplasia

Management
— Depends on the presenting symptoms.
— In general patient should be advised to lose weight, if she is overweight.

Infertility
— Induction of ovulation is necessary in most cases.
— Clomiphene; if LH is high, a small dosage of clomiphene is used; hyperstimulation is possible.
— Clomiphene plus HCG if clomiphene did not work. Tamoxifen may be an alternative to clomiphene.
— A corticosteroid may reduce the level of androgen, and this in turn may induce ovulation by allowing the hypothalamic-pituitary axis to work normally.
— Bromocriptine may be needed if there is associated hyperprolactinaemia.
— Finally, gonadotropins or LHRH may be tried.
— If medical treatment fails, wedge resection will be necessary.

Dysfunctional uterine bleeding
— Patients with PCO disease are in a high-risk category for the development of endometrial carcinoma.
— Hence endometrial biopsy should be done, or a full curettage in some patients.
— Dysfunctional uterine bleeding will respond to a oestrogen-progestogen pill or a progestogen one only.
— In the presence of hirsutism, it is better to avoid norethisterone and use other progestogens.
— In the presence of endometrial hyperplasia, it can be reversed by progestogens or by induction of ovulation.
— In the presence of atypical hyperplasia, progestin and induction of ovulation can be tried; if they fail to reverse the process, hysterectomy may be needed.

Hirsutism

— Defined as excessive facial and body hair.
— Frequently associated with menstrual problem.

Aetiology
— Physiological.
— Polycystic ovarian disease.
— Adrenal hyperplasia/Cushing's syndrome.
— Androgen-secreting tumours of adrenal or ovary.
— Idiopathic.

Investigation
- 17-hydroxyprogesterone level in the blood.
- 17-OXO and oxogenic steroid in the urine.
- If the above two investigations are normal, an adrenal problem is unlikely.
- If 17-hydroxyprogesterone in the blood and 17 OXO and oxogenic steroid in urine are higher, then ACTH stimulation and/or dexamethasone suppression tests should be done.
- If plasma testosterone is high, the possibility of an androgen-producing tumour is likely.
- If testosterone level is normal in a hirsute woman, it is important to test SHBG levels.

Treatment
- This depends on the cause.
- In PCO disease, induce ovulation if patient is infertile.
  - Combined oestrogen–progestogen pill to suppress androgen production and to raise SHBG to bind free testosterone
  - Cyproterone acetate is an anti-androgen with progestogenic activity
- In adrenal hyperplasia, the choice of treatment is a corticosteroid.
- Androgen-producing tumours need surgical removal.
- In idiopathic hirsutism, which may be due to an end-organ hypersensitivity, an oestrogen–progestogen pill may be useful. Electrolysis is useful cosmetically.

Hyperprolactinaemic amenorrhoea

- This may be due to excessive production of prolactin.
- Or it may be due to dopamine deficiency.
- FSH and LH levels are low normal or low.
- There is absence of positive oestrogen feedback.
- There is failure of LH surge.

Symptoms
- Amenorrhoea/oligomenorrhoea.
- Galactorrhoea.
- Infertility.
- Neurological and visual disturbance if tumour is big.

Treatment
- Exclude reasons of elevated prolactin levels:
  - Breastfeeding
  - Drugs
  - Hypothyroidism
  - Micro- and macro-adenoma of pituitary
- Treat the cause.
- Use bromocriptine.
- In rare cases use surgery and irradiation (seldom used now).

Congenital defects (CNS lesions, neurogenic)

— Anosmic amenorrhoea (Kallmann's syndrome).
— Hypogonadotrophic eunuchoidism.
— Isolated hypogonadotrophic hypogonadism can be caused by a familial LRH deficiency, usually associated with other abnormalities.
— Isolated gonadotropin deficiency related to defective LRH stimulation by defective neurotransmitters.
— Treatment is to use pituitary gonadotropin substitution therapy.
— LRH may also be found useful.

Psychogenic amenorrhoea

— Acute emotional and physical stress produces amenorrhoea; recovery usually is expected in a few weeks to 3 months.
— If spontaneous recovery does not occur, the patient needs further investigation, especially to exclude psychiatric illness.
— Anorexia nervosa is a disease of adolescence characterised by severe malnutrition.
  • Age distribution is usually 11–21
  • Most of the physical and laboratory findings are a result of the severe chronic malnutrition
  • Condition is secondary to severe emotional disturbance
  • Has a serious prognosis, since relapses are common
  • Treatment includes management of emotional stress, restoring weight to normality and then use of LRH or FSH/LH to induce ovulation if necessary
— Pseudocyesis is another condition associated with psychiatric aberration:
  • Basis of the problem is often the patient's desire to become pregnant and her inability to do so
— It is characterised by an obsession of pregnancy, weight gain, normal secondary sexual characteristics, lactation, absence of ovulation

Pituitary disease

Pituitary insufficiency (Sheehan's syndrome)

— Usually associated with anterior pituitary necrosis due to traumatic labour or delivery.
— Usually produces panhypopituitarism.
— Treatment requires total replacement therapy (corticosteroid, thyroxine and pituitary gonadotropins to restore wellbeing and fertility).

Pituitary tumours

— Headache, visual disturbances with amenorrhoea are suggestive of intracranial lesion.

— Investigation includes, X-ray of the skull, pituitary fossa, pituitary tomography, CT scan, visual field examination.

— Most common type of pituitary adenoma is the chromophobe adenoma; it has no specific endocrine symptoms, produces amenorrhoea through destruction of pituitary gland.

— Prolactinomas produce high levels of prolactin, and recently it has been thought that most chromophobe adenomas are prolactinoma.

— Basophilic, ACTH-producing adenoma produces Cushing's syndrome.

— Acidophilic adenoma is characterised by symptoms of aeromegaly due to excessive growth hormone.

— It is important to recognise these tumours before the occurrence of visual disturbance and other pressure symptoms.

— Treatment is usually surgery, irradiation and medical (bromocriptine for prolactinoma).

Gonadal lesions

Congenitally defective gonads

— Gonadal agenesis (Turner's syndrome).
  - Absence or streak ovaries
  - Normally developed but immature müllerian ducts
  - Chromosomal pattern is 45XO in most patients
  - Patients with pure gonadal agenesis have XX chromosome with normal growth
  - Turner's syndrome has characteristic clinical features
  - Gonadotropins are elevated
  - Treatment is replacement
  - Few may have XX/XO chromosomal pattern and may menstruate few times in their life

— True hermaphroditism is extremely rare:
  - Most of them are raised as men
  - The condition should be suspected in patients who show ambiguity of the external genitalia associated with breast development in the adult
  - Chromatin pattern can be positive or negative
  - 17-oxogenic steroid, androgen and gonadotropin levels are usually normal
  - Treatment is surgical correction

— Testicular feminisation (androgen insensitivity):
  - Normal female appearance with breast development and external genitalia

- There is always a short or absent vagina and no cervix
- Family history is important, as this syndrome is a sex-linked, dominant, heritable disease
- At laparotomy relatively normal testes are present and uterus is absent
- Karyotype is a normal 46XY, male pattern
- Treatment is removal of the testes after the age of puberty because of the fear of malignancy
- Vaginal plastic procedure
- Oestrogen replacement therapy after surgery

— Premature menopause:

- Disappearance of oocytes from the ovary
- Aetiology can be congenital or acquired
- Germ cell toxin can produce this end result
- Anomalies of the X chromosomes make the meiotic division of the germ cell impossible
- Cytotoxins, irradiation, viral infection can damage the germ cells
- Tuberculosis, certain rare tropical diseases, removal of ovaries, interruption of blood supply will produce premature menopause in the younger patient
- Patient develops climacteric symptoms
- Gonadotropins are elevated
- Treatment is replacement

— The insensitive ovary syndrome:

- There are apparently two forms: one associated with primary amenorrhoea and the other with secondary amenorrhoea
- It is characterised by well-developed breasts, axillary and pubic hair, but atrophic vagina and endometrial mucosa
- Gonadotropins are elevated and oestrogen is low
- The ovary grossly resembles a prepubertal organ and microscopically shows numerous primordial follicles, not developed beyond antrum stage
- Ovulation can occasionally be induced by excessive amounts of exogenous gonadotropins
- This syndrome may be due to lack of FSH receptor protein or an abnormality in the activator
- When the syndrome is associated with secondary amenorrhoea, the diagnosis of premature menopause is ruled out by ovarian biopsy
- Spontaneous recovery and subsequent pregnancy have been reported
- Replacement therapy may be needed

Ovarian tumours

— Androgen-producing tumours.
— Oestrogen-producing tumours.
— Treatment is surgery.

End-organ — uterine and vaginal cryptomenorrhoea

— Congenital absence of the müllerian duct.
— Imperforate hymen.
— Traumatic occlusion of the vagina.
— Congenital absence or atresia of the vagina.
— Vaginal septum.
— Traumatic occlusion of the cervix.
— Destruction of the endometrium.
— Treatment is usually surgery and some form of reconstruction.

Disease of the intermediate metabolism and nutrition

Metabolic disease

Thyroid

— Both hypo- and hyperthyroidism may be associated with menstrual irregularities and amenorrhoea.
— TSH assay is probably the most sensitive assay for the diagnosis of hypothyroidism.
— In hypothyroidism there is a reduced steroid hormone-binding globulin and a relative increase in unbound oestradiol and testosterone; there is also a shift towards increased production of oestriol instead of oestradiol, which influences the central feedback mechanism.
— In hyperthyroidism the associated amenorrhoea may be related to an associated auto-immune disease of the ovary.
— Treatment is correction of the primary lesion.

Pancreas

— Diabetes is more apt to be associated with dysfunctional bleeding; amenorrhoea is occasionally present.
— When diabetes is well controlled, menstrual problems are also cured.

Adrenal

— Congenital adrenal hyperplasia.
— Adolescent adrenal hyperplasia.
— Both need corticosteroid treatment.
— Adrenal tumour needs surgical removal.
— Cushing's syndrome needs surgery.

Nutritional disturbances

— Secondary amenorrhoea due to simple weight loss.
— Primary amenorrhoea due to constitutional weight/height disparity.
— The above two conditions have the same physical and laboratory findings as anorexia nervosa.
— History is one of nutritional weight loss with some goal in mind such as ballet dancing and modelling.
— The incidence of amenorrhoea among this category of women with all muscle and no subcutaneous fat is very high.
— Occurrence of amenorrhoea in patients with exogenous obesity is more difficult to explain; it may be due to psychogenic stress or excess conversion of androstenedione to oestrone.
— The treatment of malnutrition and obesity is directed towards improvement of general dietary habits.

Chronic illness

— Cirrhosis of the liver can produce an increase in circulating oestrogen which in turn can produce bleeding following periods of amenorrhoea.
  - Menstrual problems are related to the degree of renal failure
  - Amenorrhoea may be due to central disturbance or steroid clearance, or elevated prolactin levels

SUMMARY

— Amenorrhoea and oligmenorrhoea must be regarded as symptoms and not as diseases
— The decision as to whether or not these symptoms require investigation or treatment must be made on the basis of the individual case.
— Investigation is indicated if infertility is the predominant symptom or if the patient is anxious or disturbed about the absence of menstruation, or if there is an associated physical problem.
— When primary amenorrhoea is the symptom, it is important to determine if an anatomical abnormality of the genitalia exists.
— Effective treatment will depend on accurate diagnosis of the lesion.
— Human menopausal gonadotropin, chorionic gonadotropin,

human pituitary gonadotropin and GnRH (LRH) are useful when endogenous oestrogen levels are low.
— Clomiphene, tamoxifen and cyclofenil are useful if the endogenous oestrogen levels are adequate.
— If hyperprolactinaemia is the predominant feature, then bromocriptine is indicated if thyroid deficiency has been excluded.

SUGGESTED READING

Berger M J 1980 The polycystic ovary. In: Gold J J, Josimovich J B (eds) Gynecologic endocrinology, 3rd edn. Harper & Row, New York, p 610

Hull M G R 1982 Ovulation failure and induction. In: Studd J (ed) Progress in Obstetrics and gynaecology, vol 2. Churchill Livingstone, Edinburgh, p 207

Jacobs S (ed) 1978 Advances in gynaecological endocrinology. Proceedings of the Sixth Study Group of the R.C.O.G.

Lachelin G 1984 The polycystic ovary syndrome. In: Studd J (ed) Progress in obstetrics and gynaecology, vol 4. Churchill Livingstone, Edinburgh, p 290

Mackay E V, Beischer N A, Cox L W, Wood C (eds) 1983 Illustrated textbook of gynaecology. Saunders, Philadelphia, p 65

McDonough P G 1980 Diagnosis and therapy of primary amenorrhoea. In: Gold J J, Josimovich J B (eds) Gynecologic endocrinology, 3rd edn. Harper & Row, New York, p 271

Shearman R P 1979 The diagnosis and management of secondary amenorrhoea. In: Stallworthy J, Bourne G (eds) Recent advances in obstetrics and gynaecology, vol 13. Churchill Livingstone, Edinburgh, p 93

Speroff L, Glass R H, Kase N G (eds) 1984 Amenorrhoea. In: Clinical gynecologic endocrinology and infertility, 3rd edn. Williams & Wilkins, p 141

18. INFERTILITY

INTRODUCTION

— Involuntary infertility is a family problem.
— Affects the couple and any existing children.
— Investigation should include both partners.
— Condition and management may have a profound effect on the psychosexual aspects of the marriage.
— Ovulatory dysfunction is a common cause and the results of treatment are good if care is taken.
— Tubal occlusion should be prevented, and if it exists, prognosis is not good in spite of modern technological development.
— Male factors are responsible for about a third of fertility problems and prognosis in general is not good.
— Donor insemination is now widely practised.
— Extracorporeal fertilisation and embryo transfer is now offered to selected number of couples, and the success rate is increasing.
— The overall incidence is generally quoted as 10–15% of all couples.
— The following factors have increased the incidence:
  • Prolonged use of contraceptive measures
  • A later age at which conception is desired
  • Increased incidence of endometriosis
  • Increased incidence of sexually transmitted disease with subsequent damage to fallopian tubes
  • The use of intra-uterine contraceptive device may cause pelvic inflammatory disease (PID)
  • Increased incidence of termination of pregnancy may increase the incidence of PID
  • The use of oral contraceptive steroidal agents may cause endocrine problems and anovulation or amenorrhoea
  • The relative incidence of the different causes of infertility is not easy to arrive at

DEFINITION

— Sterility is a term applied when there is an absolute and irreversible factor preventing procreation.
— Infertility is the inability to achieve pregnancy within a stipulated period of time, usually 1 year.
— Primary infertility is a term used to define the condition when the patient has never conceived.
— Secondary infertility indicates that the patient has achieved a pregnancy.

AETIOLOGY

— Anovulation.
— Tubal factor.
— Uterine factor.
— Cervical factors.
— Male factor.
— Psychosomatic and psychosexual factors.
— Miscellaneous factors.

Influencing factors

— Fertility in women declines after the age of 35 years.
— Pregnancy is rare after the age of 45 years.
— Approximately 25% of women will be pregnant in the first month of unprotected intercourse.
— 63% become pregnant in 6 months, 75% in 9 months, 80–90% in a year.
— 3–5% will achieve pregnancy in the second year.
— 83% couples having intercourse 4 or more times a week achieve pregnancy in under 6 months of exposure.
— 16% of couples having intercourse less than once a week achieve pregnancy.

Initial interview

— Joint consultation is advisable.
— The age of the couple, the duration of the marriage, previous reproductive histories of both partners are important.
— Careful history and physical examination to exclude major medical or gynaecological condition should be documented.
— Results of previous examinations are important.
— A past and present medical history is essential.

— Chronic drug use and exposure to toxins are important.
— Normality of function of genital tract should be established.
— Socio-economic conditions may be of practical importance.
— Religion may be important in evaluating the infertility problem.
— Systemic examination and pelvic examinations are essential to exclude physical or mechanical problems.

Initial investigation

— See Table 18.1.
— Social, medical and reproductive history of couples are essential.
— Sexual history — frequency, timing and any problems should be elicited.
— Following a bimanual pelvic examination a pap smear from the cervix is taken.
— Cervical and vaginal swabs are taken to exclude infection.
— A flowchart for the infertility work is useful.
— Special investigations are done early if clinical features warrant.
— A chromosomal study is done if patient has primary amenorrhoea, or has only had a few periods.
— Or, if patient is short, eunuchoid, or has had recurrent early abortion or malformed fetus.

Table 18.1 Female infertility investigation

History
— Age
— Duration of infertility
— Menstrual history and ovulatory symptoms
— Sexual history — frequency, timing, pain lubricants
— Duration and type of contraception — problems
— Number of previous pregnancies, complications
— Sexually transmitted disease
— Drug and alcohol intake
— Medical and surgical illness
— Previous gynaecological problems and treatment
— Previous infertility investigations and treatment
— Symptoms of androgen excess — hirsutism, greasy hair and acne
— Galactorrhoea
— Genetic data

Examination
— General appearance, height and weight
— Hair distribution, acne
— Secondary sexual characteristics
— Breasts
— Thyroid and adrenal dysfunction
— Abdominal scars
— Bimanual pelvic examination, speculum examination
— Examination of the vulva — peri-anal region

Table 18.1 contd.

Investigation	
Routine	— Cervical smear and cervical swab, urethral swab
	— Basal body temperature chart
	— Post-coital test, cervical mucus study
	— Venereal disease study
	— Rubella antibody level
Special	— plasma progesterone and oestradiol
	— HSG and/or laparoscopy and dye test
	— Luteal phase endometrial biopsy
	— Plasma prolactin
	— Thyroid function test
Very special	— Plasma FSH, LH or urinary LH/FSH
	— Adrenal function test
	— Plasma testosterone, androstenedione, sex hormone binding globulin
	— Skull radiography, tomography, CAT scan
	— Visual fields
	— Cervical mucus study, sperm penetration study
	— Sperm antibody levels
	— Hysteroscopy
	— Psychiatric consultation
	— Sex chromatin and chromosomal analysis
	— Stimulation tests (LRH, clomiphene, HCG, HMG)

OVULATION

— Ovulation refers to the physical act of rupture of the follicle with extrusion of the oocyte.

— Definite evidence of ovulation is afforded only by diagnosing a pregnancy or by retrieving an oocyte from the peritoneal cavity or oviduct.

— Usually a presumptive diagnosis is made, which depends on the direct measurement of progesterone or indirectly on observations of its effect at end organs.

— Regular cycles, mid-cycle pain, premenstrual symptoms suggest an ovulatory cycle.

— Anovulation is suspected if there is a longstanding irregular menstrual cycle.

— If the weight of the patient is less than 45 kg, she will most likely have an anovulatory cycle.

— Anovulation usually results from failure of:
  • Adequate follicular maturation
  • Inadequate FSH stimulation
  • Failure of hypothalamic–pituitary positive feedback mechanism
  • Interference by excess prolactin or androgen secretion

Investigation to confirm ovulation

— Basal body temperature chart:
  • Simple but less reliable
  • In the first half of the cycle the temperature is low on the day before ovulation, a drop probably occurs, then a rise above the previous baseline and drops if conception has not taken place
  • Temperature drops to levels recorded in first half of the menstrual cycle 1–3 days prior to menstruation
  • The temperature chart usually indicates if the cycle is ovulatory
  • The possible time of ovulation is usually indicated in retrospect
  • It indicates the adequacy of the corpus luteum with certain reservations
  • It shows whether pregnancy has occurred
  • Entities such as follicular shortening, luteal shortening, late ovulation may be observed
  • Chart helps to time the intercourse, postcoital test and endometrial biopsy

Cervical mucus

— Quantity, quality and presence or absence of infection should be made at the first visit, or soon after.
— The quality of the cervical mucus is assessed by the viscosity and spinnbarkeit (ability to spin a thread), the number of epithelial cells, presence of bacteria and crystallisation.
— There is increased flow of clear mucus and when it is dried on a slide it shows ferning — due to oestrogen from the pre-ovulatory follicle.
— Good pre-ovulatory mucus is watery, copious, clear, acellular and has excellent spinbarkeit (80 mm or longer) and supports progressive motility of the sperm.
— A peak mucus flow is probably the most practical way of identifying imminent ovulation.
— In the luteal phase the mucus is scanty, thick, cloudy, highly cellular, does not allow sperm penetration and does not exhibit ferning.
— A cervical mucus score may be derived from a grading of the following: ferning (zero to complete), quantity (zero to cascade), spinnbarkeit (0–150 mm).

Endometrial biopsy

— In countries where the incidence of genital tract tuberculosis is low there is no need to do a full curettage.

— It is usually done late in the luteal phase.
— Criteria of ovulation are that there is basal subnuclear vacuolation in the cells lining the lumen of the endometrial glands, thus pushing the nuclei towards the surface.
— Glycogen is secreted into the lumen of the gland in the luteal phase.
— The glands become saw-toothed and there is associated oedema and hypertrophy.

Ultrasound

— The development and growth of the graafian follicle assessed by ultrasound usually indicate when ovulation is about to occur.
— Measurement of the graafian follicle is done from day 10 of the cycle using a high-resolution sector scanner.
— The follicle diameter reaches 18–20 mm prior to ovulation.
— Following ovulation the transonic graafian follicle becomes echogenic.

Other endocrine values

— Serial plasma oestradiol or urinary oestriol levels show a steep rise prior to ovulation.
— Serial plasma LH or urinary LH will also indicate the imminence of ovulation.

SPECIAL PROBLEMS ASSOCIATED WITH ANOVULATION AND DEFECTIVE OVULATION

Hyperprolactinaemia

— See Table 18.2.
— Prolactin is a hormone secreted by specialised cells in the pituitary gland.
— The mechanism of secretion is unusual.
— Secretion of prolactin follows release of inhibition) prolactin inhibiting factor).
— The main function of prolactin is in the production of milk from the mammary glands.
— It has a role in the events of puberty by stimulating adrenal androgen.
— It has a part to play in the control of the lifespan of corpus luteum.

Table 18.2 Causes of hyperprolactinaemia

Physiological — Pregnancy (high oestrogen levels)
      — Stimulation of nipple (breastfeeding, sex activity)
      — Sleep
      — Stress (physical and emotional)
Pathological — Interference with dopamine production
      — Interference with transport of dopamine to the pituitary (lesions involving hypothalamus, trauma, tumour).
      — Prolactinoma
      — Mixed pituitary gland tumour
      — Drugs depleting dopamine (methyldopa/reserpine)
      — Drugs blocking dopamine (phenothiazines, benzamides)
      — Hypothyroidism (TRH effect on lactotrophes)
      — Certain renal diseases
      — Chest well stimuli (surgery, skin disorder)

— It prevents ovulation during pregnancy and lactation.
— The major clinical importance of raised prolactin levels is in the disruption of the menstrual cycle and ovulation and thus fertility.
— Prolactinoma and certain drugs cause hyperprolactinaemia.
— Prolactin levels should be assayed in:
  • Anovulatory cycle
  • Deficient luteal phase
  • Menstrual irregularity
  • Galactorrhoea
  • Unexplained impotance and loss of libido in male

Physiology

— Prolactin is a polypeptide hormone.
— It is produced by specialised cells, lactotrophes, in the anterior lobe of the pituitary gland.
— Prolactin secretion is tonically inhibited by prolactin inhibiting factor (PIF).
— It is thought to be dopamine, which is released in the tubero-infundibular region of the hypothalamus, that passes via the portal system to the pituitary.
— Increased oestrogen levels raise prolactin levels.
— Nipple stimulation raises prolactin levels.
— There is significant diurnal variation; higher levels occur during sleep.
— Thyrotropin-releasing hormone (TRH) acts directly on lactotrophes and raises prolactin.
— Prolactin has a major role in breast development and milk production.

Aetiology

— Necropsy examination shows 5–10% have pituitary adenoma.
— Incidence is higher in women.
— Incidence is 15–30% in women with secondary amenorrhoea.
— 20–50% of those with galactorrhoea have adenoma.
— 3–5% of those with infertility have adenoma.

Clinical features

— Prolactin depresses the release of LRH, hence it diminishes the positive feedback responsible for mid-cycle LH surge, so no ovulation.
— It is associated with defective corpus luteum function and short luteal phase.
— Anovulatory cycle may produce dysfunctional uterine bleeding, and raised prolactin level eventually produce oligomenorrhoea and amenorrhoea.
— Galactorrhoea is another symptom.
— In the male, impotence, loss of libido, galactorrhoea and gynaecomastia are some of the symptoms.
— If the tumour is large, it produces pressure symptoms on optic chiasma, cranial nerves 3, 4, 6 and produces headache.
— If neoplasma are of mixed origin, there may be excess adrenocortical, thyroid and growth hormone activity.

Investigation

— Assay of serum prolactin level.
— If prolactin level is high, exclude adenoma.
— X-ray of pituitary fossa, tomography, CAT scan may be indicated.
— Exclude hypothyroidism.
— The patient may need neurosurgical consultation.
— Visual field assessment is carried out.
— Pneumo-encephalography, carotid angiography may be needed if macro-adenoma or extrapituitary space lesions are suspected.

Treatment

— This depends on the cause, the symptoms and the desire for a family.
— Options are just observation alone.
— Medical treatment by inhibition with a dopamine agonist such as bromocriptine or Lisuride.
— Surgery.
— Radiotherapy.
— Bromocriptine reduces the size of micro- and macro-adenoma.
— Dosage of bromocriptine is 2.5 mg — gradually increased to 7.5 mg per day.
— Side-effects are postural hypotension, dizziness, mood change, nausea, vomiting, headache, nasal congestion.
— These usually occur in the early part of treatment.
— Surgery is preferred if there is extrasellar extension, progressive enlargement or if there are troublesome symptoms.
— A transphenoidal approach is tried with the aid of an operation microscope.

— The problem with radiotherapy is late damage to other cells in the pituitary gland.

Polycystic ovary syndrome

— Stein and Leventhal in North America defined the syndrome in 1935.
— It is associated with multiple micro- or macrocysts in the ovary.
— The disorder is most commonly found in the first half of reproductive life.

Pathology

— Ovarian capsule (tunica albuginea) is thickened.
— Beneath the capsules many cysts 2–6 mm or more in diameter are found.
— A greater number of follicles in arrested maturation and arrested atretic process are found.
— Theca cell layer is often hyperplastic.
— In 5–10% of cases there is a discrete androgen-producing tumour.
— Ovaries look smooth, pearly white and usually twice the normal size.
— Endometrium is often hyperplastic.
— There is excessive peripheral production of oestrone, higher in obese women, from androgen.
— There are increased levels of circulating androgens — androstenedione, testosterone.
— There is usually no ovulation; progesterone level is low.

Incidence

— Polycystic ovaries are seen in 1 in 1000 laparotomies.
— They are more frequently seen at laparoscoy on patients with androgen excess, menstrual irregularity and infertility.
— They are present in 3–5% of young, infertile patients.

Pathophysiology

— The condition may be due to a primary defect in the ovary:
  • A fault in one of the steps leading to the production of oestrogen
  • Malfunction of one of the precursor enzymes
  • This leads to build-up of androstenedione or dehydra-epiandrosterone
  • Androstenedione may affect hypothalamic function
  • Androgen converted to oestrogen peripherally enhances the pituitary response to LRH.
  • This leads to higher LH levels and increased theca cell activity
  • It may be a defect in FSH receptors in the developing granulosa/theca interna cells

- Excess inhibin production
— It may be due to hypothalamic dysfunction.
  - This centre may be functioning more like that of the male, with tonic rather than cyclic LH release.
  - Hence there is increase in theca cells and increased androgen production.
— It may be associated with non-reproductive disturbance:
  - Androgen excess from adrenal gland or other source
  - High-level androgen affects unfavourably the cycling in the hypothalamus
  - High-level androgen affects the follicular development and atresia

Clinical features

— The condition presents in the second or third decade of life.
— Presenting symptoms are infertility, hirsutism, menstrual disorders, obesity.
— Menses may be scanty, infrequent, normal or heavy and prolonged.
— There may be a familial history.
— Patients are often obese, hirsute, with greasy hair and acne.
— Bimanual pelvic examinations may reveal enlarged ovaries.

Investigation

— There may be normal or elevated oestradiol.
— LH levels are high but there is no surge.
— FSH is low or normal.
— Excess of testosterone, androstenedione.
— Adrenal abnormality such as Cushing's disease, adrenal hyperplasia should be excluded.

Treatment

Medical

— Treat stress and obesity.
— Clomiphene is useful — smaller doses (25 mg) are chosen initially.
— If oestrodial levels are high, HCG 5000 I.U., i.m. on day 13 may be useful.
— In rare cases HMG/HPG and HCG may be tried.
— LHRH pump may be tried.
— Hyperstimulation is a problem and should be watched for.
— Corticosteroids (prednisone, dexamethasone) are useful if there is an enzyme defect or mild adrenal hyperplasia.
— With the reduction of circulating androgen, the hypothalamic–pituitary–ovarian axis resumes normal function.

Surgery

— Wedge resection of the ovary is recommended only if medical treatment has failed, if the woman is anxious to get pregnant, if she is worried by excess androgen.

— Wedge resection restores ovulatory function in 50–80% of patients.
— Possibly when the bulk of ovary is reduced, there is reduction in androgen level, which helps LH release and subsequent ovulation.
— Surgery should be done with meticulous care to avoid adhesions around the tube and ovary.

Progestin

— Progestin therapy is indicated when there are heavy periods and endometrial hypcrplasia.
— Medroxyprogesterone acetate or norethisterone acetate, or dydrogesterone may be given for 12 to 14 days to mimic the luteal phase.
— Progestin therapy suppresses the endometrial hyperplasia, LH is suppressed, and proper cycling may be re-established.

Inadequate corpus luteum

— Patients with borderline hormone values and short luteal phase charts require more detailed study.
— True luteal phase deficiency is comparatively rare (2–3% of primary infertility).
— Follicular development determines the quality of the corpus luteum.

Aetiology

— Inadequate follicular stimulus from the pituitary gland.
— The possible reasons are:
  • Inadequate response by the granulosa cells
  • A temporary or persistent increase in prolactin levels

Investigations

— Luteal phase lasting for 10 days or less.
— Poor thermal shift on basal body temperature chart.
— Low plasma progesterone levels.
— Inadequate secretory change on endometrial biopsy.
— In some women the poor secretory development may be due to a defect in the endometrial glands, lack of receptors for oestrogen and progesterone.

Treatment

— If oestrogen and progesterone are low, clomiphene is indicated.
— Bromocriptine is indicated if prolactin is high.
— If excess androgen is present, clomiphene or cortico steroids may be tried.

Primary and secondary amenorrhoea

— (See Chapter 17.)
— Investigation to assess hypothalamic–pituitary–ovarian axis.
— Exclude chromosomal abnormalities.
— Induce ovulation using HPG/HMG + HCG, LRH or clomiphene.

Treatment in general for induction of ovulation

Clomiphene citrate

— This acts on the hypothalamic–pituitary system.
— It increases the production of FSH and LH.
— Increased FSH and LH stimulate ovarian follicular development.
— It is given when anovulation is due to hypothalamic disturbances.
— It is given for 5 days early in the follicular phase of the cycle (e.g. days 1–5, or 5–9) in doses ranging from 25 mg to 150 mg.
— Primary ovarian failure (high FSH) and hyperprolactinaemia should be initially excluded if the problem is primary or secondary amenorrhoea.
— Ovulation occurs 8–10 days after the end of each course.
— Start with a lower dosage and monitor ovulation by methods already described.
— The main side-effects are hot flushes, palpitations, visual blurring and abdominal discomfort.
— The incidence of large follicular cyst and multiple pregnancy varies between 15% and 20%.
— There is a slightly increased rate of spontaneous abortion.
— If ovulation has not occurred, or if there is evidence of inadequate follicular and/or corpus luteum development, the dose of clomiphene is increased gradually in the next 2–3 cycles.
— Exclude pregnancy if the period is delayed.
— If 150–200 mg clomiphene is ineffective, HCG 5000–10 000 I.U. may be used on day 13 of the cycle.
— Cyclofenil (Rihibin) or tamoxifen may be used in place of clomiphene.

Gonadotropins

— Human pituitary gonadotropin (HPG), human menopausal gonadotropin (HMG) and human chorionic gonadotropin (HCG) are used.
— Gonadotropins are indicated when other methods are ineffective or inapplicable.
— HPG/HMG are given daily or on alternate days.

— Daily monitoring of ovarian follicle using ultrasound and plasma oestradiol levels should be done to avoid hyperstimulation and multiple pregnancy.
— Usually 5–7 injections are required to produce a suitable oestrogen rise (600–800 mol/l) and graafian follicle diameter of 18–20 mm.
— An ovulation-triggering injection of HCG is given (5000–10 000 I.U.).
— 80% of women ovulate on HPG/HMG and HCG regimen.
— 55–60% become pregnant.
— Incidence of multiple pregnancy is nearly 20% but may be as high as 50% if monitoring is not used.
— Treatment is usually given for 6 months.
— LHRH pump may be used instead of gonadotropins:
  • It produces more physiological status
  • No increase in multiple pregnancy
  • Disadvantage is the use of pump which needs close monitoring by the physicians
— Failure to conceive in 6 months should lead to a further assessment of other infertility factors.

Summary

— Investigation of the presence of anovulation and cause must be efficient.
— Treatment is time-consuming and expensive.
— Most women respond to clomiphene.
— Patients with hyperprolactinaemia respond to bromocriptine.
— Patients with primary amenorrhoea and those with secondary amenorrhoea not responding to clomiphene or bromocriptine may require gonadotropin therapy, or LHRH infusion or pump.

TUBAL FACTORS

Introduction

— Tubal factors are an important cause of infertility in approximately 20% of patients.
— Prognosis varies considerably according to the site of block.
— The amount of damage to the epithelial lining of the tube also determines the outcome.

Physiology

— Ovum pick-up is done by muscular contraction of the fimbriae which are the most important mechanism facilitating ovum pick-up.
— The transport of gametes through the tube depends upon muscular contraction, ciliary action and fluid flow.
— These mechanisms are controlled by the endocrine and neural systems.
— The spermatozoa and the developing embryo obtain nutrition from tubal secretion.

Aetiology

— Congenital anomalies are rare.
— Clinical or subclinical infection is by far the greater cause of tubal abnormality.
— This may result in tubal blockage.
— It may result in malfunction in terms of ovum pick-up, transport or nutrition.
— Dysfunction of the cilia may result from causes other than infection (e.g. cystic fibrosis).
— Endometriosis in and around the tube causes distortion, with resulting malfunction.
— Previous sterilisation is an increasing factor.

Investigation and diagnosis

— Tubal patency is demonstrated by Rubin test, hysterosalpingography (HSG), culdoscopy or laparoscopy with dye test.
— Laparoscopy is the preferred method.
— The next popular and reliable method is HSG.
— HSG provides information regarding anatomy or peritubal abnormalities.
— HSG has a significantly high false negative and false positive rate (30–40% : 20–25% respectively).
— Laparoscopy has revolutionised the management of infertility patients.
— It enables to assess tubal patency, to visualise the uterus, tubes, ovaries and pelvis.
— Laparoscopy will reveal silent endometriosis and pelvic inflammatory disease and adhesions.
— Early pyosalpinx or hydrosalpinx could be visualised.

Prevention

— Since treatment is unsatisfactory, prevention is important.
— Pelvic infection following abortion and confinement should be adequately treated following prompt diagnosis.
— Intra-uterine contraceptive devices produce pelvic infection in 4–10% of patients and should not be advocated for single nulliparous women.
— Prevention and early diagnosis and treatment of gonorrhoea are important.
— Early and adequate treatment of chlamydial infection is also a preventive measure.
— Routine screening of risk population, use of barrier method (condom) in casual sexual activities and education of young people are important.
— Approximately 0.1–1% of women seek reversal of sterilisation.
— Young couples requesting sterilisation need counselling.

Medical treatment

— Long-term appropriate antibiotic therapy is useful.
— Antibiotics against gram-positive and negative organisms, bacteroids, gonococcus and chlamydia, may be needed.
— Short-wave diathermy to the pelvis may be useful.
— Endometriosis may respond to progestin therapy or danazol therapy.

Surgical treatment

— The aim is to restore the normal anatomy of the tube and ovary.
— The aim is also to maintain effective musculociliary action, production of tubal secretion and ovum pick-up.
— Success following surgery varies between 5% and 70%.
— Incidence of ectopic pregnancies increases (10% or more).
— Indication for surgery:
  • Complete tubal block
  • Partial tubal block
  • Kinks and sacculation of the tube
  • Peritubal and peri-ovarian adhesions
— Contra-indications to surgery:
  • Severe male infertility (unless AID is chosen)
  • Anovulation has not responded to treatment
  • Conditions which contra-indicate pregnancy
  • Psychiatric illness such as schizophrenia
  • Severe degree of tubal damage

- Multiple tubal blocks
- Extensive pelvic adhesions
— Nature of surgery:
  - Adhesolysis
  - Salpingostomy
  - Tubal reimplantation
  - Uterotubal and tubal anastamosis
  - Ovario fimbryolysis
  - Extracorporeal fertilisation and embryo replacement
  - Tubal transplant

UTERINE FACTORS

— Uterine malformations.
— Scarring after curettage (Asherman's syndrome).
— Intrinsic lack of receptors to oestrogen and progesterone.
— Uterine myoma and polyp.
— Malformation and function related to mother taking diethylstilboestrol in early pregnancy.
— Adenomyosis.

Investigations

— Hysterogram.
— Hysteroscopy.
— Laparoscopy.
— Curettage.

Treatment

— Surgical treatment is myomectomy, ventrosuspension, utriculoplasty (Strassmann's operation).
— Uterine scarring needs breakdown of adhesions; may be using hysteroscope and keeping the cavity open with IUD temporarily.
— Uterine polyp needs removal.
— Adenomyosis seldom responds to progestin or danazol therapy.

CERVICAL FACTOR

— Cervical mucus is the first barrier that the spermatozoa have to overcome.
— Mucus is most receptive 12–36 hours before ovulation.

— Mucus favourable to sperm migration is thin, watery, clear and capable of drawing into long threads and exhibiting a good fern pattern when dried.
— Changes in cervical mucus depend on follicular phase oestrogen level.
— Progesterone makes the mucus thick, turbid and inhibitor to sperm passage.
— Major factor causing hostility in the normally favourable mucus are infection and antisperm antibodies.
— Previous conisation and diathermy to cervix and amputation of cervix affect the quality and quantity of cervical mucus.
— The compatibility of sperm in the mucus is usually assessed by the post-coital test (PCT).
— PCT is done as close as possible to the time of peak mucus production (day 12 or 13 of cycle).
— There should be at least five forward-migrating spermatozoa per high-power field in mucus taken from the internal os 2–3 hours after intercourse.
— If two PCTs are abnormal, sperm penetration test using donor mucus and sperm should be done to assess antibody problem.

Treatment

— Infection needs appropriate treatment.
— Ethinyl oestradiol 0.01–0.02 mg from day 4 to 12 of the cycle to improve the quality of cervical mucus may be given.
— If sperm penetration test suggests antibody in cervical mucus:
  • Barrier method 3–6 months
  • Barrier method except during ovulation time
  • Artificial insemination using husband's sperm higher up in the cervical canal

MALE FACTOR

Hypothalamic–pituitary disorders

— Testes are under the influence of the hypothalamus and pituitary.
— There is no evidence of cyclical activity.
— FSH is probably necessary for the acquisition of receptors for LH by Leydig's cells.
— Spermatogenesis requires both testosterone and FSH.
— Main site of action of FSH is on Sertoli's cells.
— Sertoli's cells play a supporting role in spermatogenesis.
— Inhibin suppresses FSH.

— Elevated FSH levels often signify a fault in inhibin production and often major damage to germ cells.
— Adrenal hyperplasia and elevated prolactin levels will cause gonadal dysfunction.
— Deficiency of hypothalamic gonadotropin releasing hormone results in failure of production of FSH and LH, which results in low androgen production.
— Androgen secretion by the testes is low and secondary sexual characteristics may not be well developed.

Investigation
— See Table 18.3.

Table 18.3 Male infertility investigation

History
— Age, age of puberty
— Previous children if known
— Maldescent of testes
— Mumps
— Trauma, surgery to testes, torsion, haematoma
— Sexual history — libido, erection
— Orgasmic ability
— History of sexually transmitted disease
— Medical and surgical illness
— Drug and alcohol intake
— Genetic data
— Occupation, exposure to heat and toxic agents
— Personal habits — clothes, hot-water baths

Examination
— Body habitus, weight and height
— Secondary sexual characteristics — hair, size and site of testes
— Evidence of other endocrine dysfunction
— Size of penis, circumcision, volume of testes
— Urethral orifice, discharge
— Testes — size, volume, consistency, position
— Vas — consistency, presence, granuloma
— Epididymis — consistency, cysts, granulomas
— Presence of varicocele (standing — Valsalva's manoeuvre)
— Presence of hernia
— Examination of prostate
— Systemic examination — blood pressure

Investigation
Routine   — Seminal analysis — culture
              — Venereal disease study
              — Urine analysis
Special   — Plasma testosterone, FSH and LH — prolactin
              — Stimulation tests (LRH, clomiphene, HMG, HCG, TRH)
Very special — thyroid and adrenal function
              — Testicular biopsy
              — Sex chromatin and chromosomal analysis
              — Skull radiography
              — Sperm antibody
              — Sperm penetration study
              — Vasography
              — Psychiatric consultations

SEMINAL FLUID

VOLUME — AVERAGE 4ml

liquefaction within 30 min

Count 20-200 million /ml

Motility at least 60%

Abnormal forms not more than 20%

Oligospermia < 20 million per ml

Treatment

— HPG or HMG will be required to stimulate spermatogenesis.
— HCG is added for interstitial cell development.
— Treatment is given for a minimum period of 3 months.
— If sperm count is improving, treatment should be continued as long as required.
— Results following clomiphene are disappointing.
— Synthetic male hormones such as mesterolone 100 mg/day are useful.
— Congenital adrenal hyperplasia is treated with corticosteroid therapy.

Testicular failure

— Spermatozoa are formed from spermatocytes in the seminiferous tubules.
— The maturation process takes about 70 days.
— Spermatozoa are then stored temporarily in the epididymis and the seminal vesicle.
— In some men there is a Sertoli's cell only in the seminiferous tubule; there are no spermatocytes.
— Gonadal dysgenesis (Klinefelter's syndrome) is a genetic anomaly (47 XXY).
— The Klinefelter individual is tall, eunuchoid, hairless, with small testes and elevated gonadotropins.
— Such men are usually sexually potent but azoospermic.
— Mumps virus impairs both spermatogenesis and Leydig's cell function.
— Gonorrhoea, syphilis, chlamydia, non-specific bacterial infection can also damage the testes and/or ducts.
— Testicular function will be affected by trauma, torsion, haematoma, maldescent, hydrocele or by general medical disorders such as liver, renal disease and diabetes.
— Exposure of male fetus to diethylstilboestrol intake during early pregnancy may result in testicular hypoplasia.
— The function of Leydig's cell will be affected in Klinefelter's syndrome and hypothalamic–pituitary disorders.
— Irradiation, chemotherapy usually has a harmful effect on spermatogenesis.
— Sperm-banking is worth while considering before irradiation and chemotherapy for cancer.
— Industrial chemicals, other drugs, high gonadal temperature have adverse effect.
— Elevated prolactin levels depress testicular function.
— Normal volume of testis is 15–20 ml (orchidometer).

Blockage of the vas/epididymis

— Blockage may be congenital.
— Infection, trauma, surgery may cause blockage.
— Microsurgery restores fertility in a selected group.
— Success of reversal of sterilisation is 50–70%.
— Success decreases after 10 years of occlusion (70–80% falling to 30–40%).
— Poor success is due to pressure effects, particularly on the epididymis, with rupture, granuloma formation and a rise in immobilising antibodies.

Varicocele

— Varicosities of the veins draining the testes will raise scrotal temperature and depress spermatogenesis.
— Faulty veins in the spermatic vein will also alter blood flow.
— Patient needs to be examined in a standing position and under Valsalva's manoeuvre to suppress venous return.
— Varicocele produces a mild to moderate degree of oligospermia.
— Motility is more affected than the numbers.
— Surgery is required to correct the problem.
— High ligation is the treatment.
— Pregnancy rate following ligation varies between 40% and 60%.

Infection of the genital tract

— Seminal plasma is an important component of the ejaculate.
— It is secreted by the prostate gland and seminal vesicles, and to a small extent by the urethral glands.
— It provides a medium in which the sperm can live and swim.
— It is slightly viscid, so that it tends to remain in a bolus near the cervix.
— Low volumes suggest inadequate levels of testosterone.
— Gonorrhoea, chlamydia and non-specific infections may cause infection of the male genital tract.
— Semen culture should be done if there are pus cells, and appropriate therapy should be advocated.

Miscellaneous

— Retrograde ejaculation into the bladder is a rare cause of infertility.
— This condition is treated by separation of the sperm from a urine sample obtained soon after ejaculation and an AIH is performed.

— Surgical correction of the bladder neck may cure the problem.
— Erectile failure will need appropriate treatment.
— Premature ejaculation will need psychosexual therapy.
— Hypospadias and other anatomical defects will need surgical treatment.

Artificial insemination by donor semen (AID)

— 3% of the population could be helped by AID.
— AID is indicated for:
  - Coital failure
  - Severe male infertility
  - Familial disease
  - Immunological disease
  - Severe rhesus disease
  - Positive hamster test (no penetration by the spermatozoa)
— Marriage should be stable and happy.
— Couple should have counselling.
— Legal status remains undefined.
— Child is registered as the child of the parents.
— Fresh or frozen semen is used

General considerations

— Screening of the donor:
  - No family or hereditary disorder
  - Ideal if he has already produced healthy children
  - Semen sample should be examined, microscopical and bacteriological
  - Total confidentiality should be maintained
  - Each specimen or donor should be used for five pregnancies

Treatment

— The recipient keeps a basal temperature chart to identify expected day of ovulation.
— One could check cervical mucus, serum oestradiol, and serum and urinary LH 2–3 days to possible ovulation time.
— Ultrasound could be used to check graafian follicle growth to time ovulation
— Semen is deposited against the external os and patient is asked to rest in dorsal position for 15 to 30 minutes.
— If cervical mucus shows strong fern pattern, she could receive AID the following day.
— Cervical mucus is examined the following day.
— Active sperms in the mucus exclude the hostility problem.
— Three cycles of treatment are necessary and 60% achieve pregnancy.

— Results are better if two inseminations are done per cycle and the ovulation time is monitored.
— Stress of this treatment should not be underestimated.

Artificial insemination by husband's semen (AIH).

— Indicated when there is failure to deposit ejaculate in the vagina.
— Results can be good as AID in a mechanical problem.
— If the count and motility of sperm are low, the result is poor.
— If immunological, inflammatory and biochemical abnormalities exist, the outcome is poor.
— Concentration and/or sperm washing and suspension in a different medium with intra-uterine insemination may sometimes be helpful.
— Sperm may be frozen from patients requiring surgery, radiotherapy and chemotherapy for cancer.

PSYCHOSOMATIC AND PSYCHOSEXUAL FACTORS

— These can be the cause of infertility or can develop during investigation and treatment.
— Hypothalamic–pituitary–ovarian axis is susceptible to stress, both physical and emotional.
— In addition to the usual anxiety and tension-producing factors, fears of coitus, pregnancy, mothering also compound the problem.
— Interpersonal conflicts, marital disharmony also produce menstrual problems and infertility.
— The couple should always be seen together and the investigation and treatment should be discussed.
— Ignorance of sexuality in which intercourse does not take place with penetration and ejaculation and insemination.
— Impotence and vaginismus may be present.
— Absence of sperms on post-coital tests may clinch the diagnosis.
— Appropriate treatment for sexual dysfunction should be achieved.

EXTRACORPOREAL FERTILISATION

— This most recent development has helped in certain types of refractory infertility.
— This method is offerred to people with gross tubal damage,

absence of tubes, unexplained prolonged infertility, immunological problems, certain male subfertility problems.
— Aspiration of one or more mature ova by a laparoscopic or ultrasonically guided perantaneous approach.
— Fertilisation of the ovum by exposure to a suitable number of sperms from the husband or donor if necessary.
— Culture of the conceptus (4–16 cell stage).
— Replacement into the uterine cavity.
— Four to six attempts at monthly intervals.
— Ovulation is usually induced using clomiphene, HMG and HCG regimen.
— There are considerable technical problems.
— The cost is high.
— Success rate varies between centres (6–15%).
— Legal problems abound, particularly if there is a move to donor ova, sperm or surrogate mothers in cases of ovarian or uterine absence or damage.

SUMMARY

— See Tables 18.4, 18.5
— If infertility has existed for 4 or more years, if woman is aged 35 years or more, the prognosis is not good.

Table 18.4 Summary of treatment in female

Incidence (70–75%)	
Uterine and tubal problems (15–20%)	— Appropriate surgery
Anovulation (occurs in 30–40%)	— Clomiphene ± HCG
	— HPG or HMG + HCG
	— LRH
	— Bromocriptine
	— Surgery — wedge resection of ovary, macro-adenoma of pituitary
Luteal phase defect (occurs in 2–4%)	— Clomiphene ± HCG
	— HCG alone
	— HPG or HMG + HCG
	— Progesterone i.m. luteal phase
	— Bromocriptine
Cervical factor (2–4%)	— Treat infection
	— Ethinyloestradiol 4–12 (0.01 mg)
	— AIH
Sperm antibodies in cervical mucus	— AIH
	— Barrier method
In male partner	— Corticosteroid therapy during first half of wife's cycle
	— Sperm washing
	— AIH
Androgen excess	— Clomiphene ± HCG
	— Prednisone/dexamethasone
Psychosexual and psychiatric disorders	— Referral
Extracorporeal fertilisation	— (0–15% success)
Embryo donation	
Surrogate mother	

Table 18.5 Summary of treatment in male

Incidence	
Epididymis, vas, obstruction	— Surge.y
Varicocele	— High ligation
Retrograde ejaculation	— Bladder neck surgery
	Collection of urine — sperm
	— AIH
Infection	— Antibodies
Hypothalamic–pituitary problem	— HPG or HMG ± HCG
	— Tamoxifen
	— Mesterolone
Testicular, excretory duct, genetic problem	— AID
Impotence	— Appropriate therapy
	— AID
	— AIH
Sperm antibodies	— Corticosteroid
	— Sperm washing
Psychiatric and psychosexual problems	— Referral

— If pregnancy does occur, morbidity may be increased because of such factors as age and basic abnormalities in the reproductive tract.

— Abortion, ectopic pregnancy, problems related to elderly primigravidity (pre-eclampsia, operative delivery, congenital malformation and perinatal mortality and morbidity) are often increased.

— In about 10% of infertile couples no cause can be found.

— These couples may eventually achieve pregnancy without therapy.

— Forty per cent conceive after 2 years.

— The remaining couples may need special methods such as IVF.

SUGGESTED READING

Barglow P, Peterson C M 1980 The psychological aspects of infertility. In: Gold J J, Josimovich J B (eds) Gynecologic endocrinology, 3rd edn. Pub. Harper & Row, New York, p 680

France J T 1982 The detection of ovulation for fertility and infertility. In: Bonnar J (ed) Recent advances in obstetrics and gynaecology, No 14. Churchill Livingstone, Edinburgh, p 215

Henderson S R 1982 The management of dysovulatory infertility. In: Bonnar J (ed) Recent advances in obstetrics and gynaecology, vol 14. Churchill Livingstone, Edinburgh, p 241

Hull, M G R 1982 Ovulation failure and induction. In: Studd J (ed) Progress in obstetrics and gynaecology, vol 2. Churchill Livingstone, Edinburgh, p 207

Lachelin G 1984 The polycystic ovary syndrome. In Studd J (ed) Progress in obstetrics and gynaecology. vol 4. Churchill Livingstone, Edinburgh, p 290

Menge A C, Behrman S J 1980 Immunologic problems of infertility. In: Gold J J, Josimovich J B (eds) Gynecologic endocrinology, 3rd edn. Harper & Row, New York, p 690

Pepperell R J, Hudson B, Wood C (eds) 1980 The infertile couple. Churchill Livingstone, Edinburgh

Pryor J P 1983 Treatment of male infertility. In Studd J (ed) Progress in obstetrics and gynaecology, vol 3. Churchill Livingstone, Edinburgh, p 334

St Michel P, Dizerega G S 1983 Hyperprolactinaemia and luteal phase dysfunction infertility. Obstetric and Gynecological Surveys 38: 248–254

Speroff, L, Glass R H, Kase N G Investigation of the infertile couple, 3rd edn., Williams & Wilkins, Baltimore, p 467

Steinberger E 1980 Male infertility. In: Gold J J, Josimovich J B (eds) Gynecologic endocrinology, 3rd edn. Harper & Row, New York, p 716

19. ABORTION

INTRODUCTION

— Abortion is the termination of pregnancy before the fetus is viable.
— It is a common complication of pregnancy and often passes unnoticed.
— In the majority of instances it occurs in week 2–4 of implantation.
— In many early spontaneous abortions there is a major defect present in the conceptus, usually of a chromosomal nature.

DEFINITION

— Abortion is the term now given to a pregnancy that terminates or is terminated at week 20 or less of pregnancy.
— In some countries an upper limit of 28 weeks is still used.
— The WHO uses the definition of a fetal weight less than 500 g or less than 22 weeks if the weight is not known.
— Habitual abortion is defined by the occurrence of three or more successive abortions.

INCIDENCE

— Approximately 10–15% of pregnancies end in spontaneous abortion.
— If one includes all implanted conceptuses, the figure will be nearer 45%.
— There is considerable wastage in the first 4–6 weeks of pregnancy.
— If a patient has a threatened abortion, the chances of the pregnancy continuing normally are about 50%.

AETIOLOGY

— No demonstrable cause — this is the commonest situation.
— Main cause is related to maldevelopment of the conceptus.
— Chromosomal anomalies may cause up to 25% of all spontaneous abortions, particularly trisomy, XO and triploidy.
— In a number of cases there is only an empty sac, or the sac contains amorphous tissue, or the sac contains a grossly malformed fetus.
— Abnormality of placental development.
— Multiple pregnancy.
— A deficiency of endocrine support.
— Uterine causes, both congenital and acquired abnormalities.
— Cervical trauma, cervical incompetence
— Chronic maternal diseases.
— Infections, e.g. rubella, cytomegalovirus, influenzal illness, any actue pyrexial illness, conditions causing peritonitis.
— Drugs.
— Pregnancy with IUD in situ.
— Commoner in older women (≥35 years), infertile women and women with poor reproductive history.

TYPES OF ABORTION AND MANAGEMENT

— It is important to distinguish the clinical type of abortion because management is different.
— Three clinical features are important:
  • History of passage of products of conception
  • An accurate size of the uterus in relation to the period of amenorrhoea
  • Whether the cervix is opened or closed
— The use of real-time ultrasound has enabled physicians to makes diagnoses more reliably and quickly.
— Introduction of ultrasound has served a considerable advantage to:
  • Reduce unnecessary hospitalisation
  • Reduce the anxiety of parents
  • Reassure the obstetrician
  • Avoid invasive or time-consuming investigations

DIFFERENTIAL DIAGNOSIS

- One of the types of abortion.
- Ectopic pregnancy.
- Delayed menstruation.

THREATENED ABORTION

- A period of amenorrhoea followed by slight vaginal bleeding.
- Pain is usually not a significant feature.
- Uterus is the correct size for dates.
- The cervix is closed.
- Real-time ultrasonic examination will show an intact sac with fetal echo compatible with the period of gestation, with fetal heart and movement activities.
- If date is uncertain, a weekly ultrasonic examination is important.
- β-HCG, oestrogen, progesterone, placental lactogen and other placental secretory products such as SP_1.
- If PAPP values in blood and/or urine are normal, 90% of pregnancies will continue.
- Speculum examination should be done to exclude extraplacental causes.

Treatment

- Advise regarding adequate rest, limitations of coitus.
- Adequate explanation and reassurance following ultrasound examination is helpful.
- If IUD is in situ and the thread is visible, it is advisable to remove it.
- Bedrest allowing the woman to get up for toilet purposes for a short period.
- Rest may be at home or in hospital, depending on the home surroundings and facilities.
- If bleeding continues or recurs, the ultrasonic examination should be repeated to check viability of fetus.
- Sedatives such as diazepam or similar compounds may be helpful for a tense, anxious and nervous patient.
- Mild analgesics have antiprostaglandin effects and may be used if pain is a worrying problem.
- Progesterone or HCG are not found to be very useful.
- If progesterone levels were low in the luteal phase and in very early pregnancy, then progesterone may be tried.

— Psychotherapy is essential for anxious patients.
— An adequate, simple explanation of the causes of bleeding, and reassurance for the patient that if the pregnancy continues, possibly all will be normal.
— Anxiety and guilt feelings should be assuaged.

INEVITABLE ABORTION

— The features are:
  • A period of amenorrhoea followed by heavy vaginal bleeding
  • Pain follows bleeding
  • Uterus may be small, large or correct size for dates
  • Cervix is dilating and the products of conception may be passing through the os.

Treatment

— Patient should be admitted to hospital.
— Give ergometrine i.m. or i.v. if bleeding is severe, or i.v. oxytocin should be set up.
— Evacuation of the uterus should be arranged.
— If uterus is larger than the size of 12 weeks cyesis, use oxytocin infusion first to cause reduction in uterine size by expelling part of the products, then evacuation of the uterus.
— On admission haemoglobin, blood group and cross-matching may have to be done.
— If condition of patient warrants transfusion, it should be given together with oxytocin in a separate infusion.
— All rhesus-negative mothers without antibodies must be given anti-D.

COMPLETE ABORTION

— A period of amenorrhoea followed by a variable amount of bleeding which has now stopped.
— Uterus is smaller than expected.
— The cervix is closed.
— Ultrasonic examination will help to confirm the diagnosis.

INCOMPLETE ABORTION

— Usually the outcome if abortion has occurred before week 16.
— Patient will have noticed the passage of products of conception.
— History of heavy bleeding associated with lower abdominal pain.
— Uterus is larger than normal but less for the period of amenorrhoea.
— Cervix is usually open.

Management

— Ultrasound examination will confirm the diagnosis.
— Curettage is indicated.
— If patient has lost blood, resuscitation may be necessary.
— Oxytocin (10 units i.v.) or Syntometrine i.m. is given if blood loss is continuing.
— Placenta caught in the cervix may produce shock; it should be removed gently.
— If only a small amount of curette was obtained, possibility of an ectopic pregnancy should be considered.

MISSED ABORTION

— Retention of the products of conception after death of the embryo or fetus.
— Gradual diminution of pregnancy symptoms and failure of the uterus to grow.
— A period of amenorrhoea during which an episode of slight vaginal bleeding may or may not have occurred.
— Uterus is usually smaller for dates.
— The cervix is firmer and closed.
— Pregnancy test may be negative or positive in less dilution.
— Ultrasound examination shows either a collapsed sac or failure of fetal heart activity and fetal movement.

Treatment

— If left alone, resorption or spontaneous expulsion may occur.
— There is a slight risk of coagulation defect developing if dead fetus is retained for more than a month.

— It is always advisable to evacuate the uterus if pregnancy is not continuing.

— If uterine size is 12 weeks or less, suction aspiration of uterus under general anaesthesia is possible.

— If uterus is greater than 12 weeks, vaginal prostaglandin E2 pessary, followed by oxytocin infusion, may expel the products. Evacuation may be necessary if it is incomplete.

SEPTIC ABORTION

— Incomplete abortion complicated by infection of the uterine contents.

— More common following criminal abortion.

— The features are as for incomplete abortion accompanied by:
  • Pyrexia ($\geq 38°C$)
  • Tachycardia
  • Marked lower abdominal pain and tenderness
  • Pelvic tenderness and purulent vaginal discharge
  • general malaise

— Other causes of an acute abdomen and generalised infection must be excluded.

— The common organisms are *E.Coli* and other gram-negative organisms, streptococci (haemolytic, non-haemolytic and anaerobic); bacteroides and staphylococcus.

— Infection with *Clostridium welchii* and *tetani* is now uncommon.

— Infection is usually mild in 80% (endometritis). It can spread to the myometrium and to the pelvis in 15%. In 5% it may be more generalised, and symptoms are due to release of endotoxins.

— In severe cases endotoxic shock and disseminated intravascular coagulation may develop.

Investigation

— Cervical, high vaginal and sometimes urethral swabs are taken for bacteriology.

— Blood cultures are taken if pyrexia is 38°C or higher.

— In severe cases, renal and coagulation status should be checked.

Management

— Antibiotic therapy using i.m. ampicillin or oral amoxicillin or alternative therapy if the patient is penicillin-sensitive, combined with oral or rectal metronidazole are given while awaiting results.

— In moderate to severe cases penicillin, gentamicin or the newer penicillins are given intravenously. Metronidazole is given rectally or intravenously.

— Evacuation of the uterus is done 12 hours after the antibiotic therapy is started, unless bleeding warrants early evacuation.

Endotoxic shock

— *E.Coli, Klebsiella, B. proteus, Ps. pyocyanae, Bacteroides* contain a lipoprotein–carbohydrate complex in the cell wall which, when released during a severe infection, causes cardiovascular collapse and other complications.

— Mortality rate ranges between 30% and 50%.

— Peripheral vasodilatation occurs due to direct effects of endotoxin and release of vasoactive amines.

— Venous pooling occurs and return of blood to the heart drops.

— Cardiac output and blood pressure fall.

— Due to hypoxia, capillary permeability increases and fluid escapes into extracellular space.

— Disseminated intravascular coagulation produces microthrombi which occlude vessels in the kidney, liver and lungs.

— Renal tubular and cortical necrosis and failure of pulmonary perfusion may follow.

Management

— To control infection, large doses of intravenous antibiotics such as penicillin and gentamicin, together with metronidazole, may be given.

— Evacuation of the uterus should be done as soon as the patient is fit.

— Sometimes a hysterectomy may be necessary.

— A central venous pressure line should be started to give fluid or plasma or blood to maintain circulatory volume.

— Fluid and electrolyte balance must be monitored.

— Vasodilator drugs and corticosteroids may be needed.

— Acidosis should be looked for and needs correction.

— DIC should be identified and treated.

— May need intensive care unit facility.

— Shock due to exotoxins should be treated vigorously with appropriate antibiotics.

RECURRENT ABORTION

— This is a sequence of three or more consecutive abortions.
— After two abortions, the risk of further abortions is 25%
and increases to 33% after three abortions.

Aetiology

— Genetic — hormonal or anatomic causes.

Genetic causes

— Approximately 50–60% of spontaneous first trimester
miscarriages are due to a chromosomal aberration.
— Trisomy accounts for 50–60%, monosomy X for 15–25% and
polyploidy for 20–25% of these.
— In the general population, a balanced translocation occurs
with an incidence of about 1.9/1000. In recurrent abortion
3% will have the problem.
— Karyotypic analysis should be done if possible on fetal tissue
following the second miscarriage, certainly following the third
miscarriage.

Hormonal causes

— Progesterone is essential both to implantation and to
maintain early pregnancy.
— An inadequate corpus luteum with a lower-than-normal
progesterone production may be responsible for recurrent
miscarriage.
— The incidence of luteal phase insufficiency is only about 3%
in the general population; in recurrent abortion the incidence
approaches 35–50%.
— Patients with low progesterone in the luteal phase may have
low levels in early pregnancy as well.
— However, the literature is full of contradicting opinions.
— At present there are no studies sufficiently controlled to
prove that progesterone therapy prevents subsequently
miscarriage.
— Progestational agents are contra-indicated.
— Hypothyroidism and abnormalities of carbohydrate
metabolism are occasional causes.

Uterine and cervical causes

— The incompetent cervical os is associated with sudden expulsion of a normal sac and fetus in the mid-trimester.
— It is prevalent in areas where abortion is practised.
— Excesive dilatation of the cervix, cone biopsy, amputation of the cervix may cause cervical incompetence.
— Easy passage of No. 8 Hegar or hysterogram will help to make the diagnosis.
— Ultrasound examination of cervix in pregnancy may be helpful in making an early diagnosis.
— Repair of the cervix prior to pregnancy or cervical cerclage inserted between 13 and 16 weeks may prevent the abortion.
— Uterine abnormality such as unicornuate, bicornuate or septate uterus may be associated with recurrent abortions.
— Submucous fibroid, endometrial polyp are other causes.
— Hysterosalpingogram, hysteroscopy and dilatation and curettage in non-pregnant state will diagnose the condition.
— Hereditary disorders of connective tissue (Ehlers-Danlos syndrome) might affect the fetal membrane resulting in premature rupture of membranes.

Infectious causes

— Listeria, toxoplasma, cytomegalovirus, brucella and T-mycoplasma have been implicated in causing recurrent miscarriage.

Metabolic and other causes

— Chronic disease, toxic environment exposure, metabolic and endocrine abnormality could cause recurrent abortions.
— Collagen vascular disease, particularly SLE, have been associated with recurrent abortions, especially if they have lupus antibodies.

Immunological causes

— Circulatory blocking antibody may protect the fetus against attack by maternal lymphocytes.
— Patients with problems of habitual abortion may lack in blocking antibody.
— HCG appears to be a suppressant of lymphocytes.
— If trophoblast were unable to produce sufficient HCG, a failure of immunological suppression may occur.

Iatrogenic causes

— Administration of a cytotoxic agent or other chemotherapeutic agents in the treatment of maternal diseases such as gout, and luteolytic agents such as progestational agents may cause problems.

Male factor

— Severe degree of oligoasthenospermia or hyperspermia are incriminated in causing recurrent abortion.

PRE-CONCEPTUNAL EVALUATION OF THE COUPLE

— Details of previous miscarriages.
— Operative procedure.
— Infections.
— A thorough physical and bimanual pelvic examination is necessary.
— Hysterosalpingogram and hysteroscopy.
— Karyotyping of husband and wife with banding studies.
— Full blood count, liver and renal function.
— Thyroid function.
— Blood group and Coombs' test.
— Torch screen.
— Endometrial biopsy late in the luteal phase to exclude tuberculosis.
— Culture of cervical swab for mycoplasma.
— Semen analysis.
— Drug history.
— Explanation and reassurance.

POST-CONCEPTUAL TREATMENT

— Treat the cause if possible before pregnancy.
— Coitus during early pregnancy is to be avoided.
— Bedrest is psychologically useful.
— Early ultrasound examination, reassurance of parents.
— Repeat the ultrasound examination.
— Progesterone is debatable, unless there is proven deficiency.
— HCG may also be useful in a few cases.
— Cervical cerclage after 13 weeks.
— Thyroid deficiency should be corrected.

SUGGESTED READING

Mackay E V, Beischer N A, Cox L W, Wood C (eds) 1983 Illustrated textbook of
    gynaecology. Saunders, Philadelphia, p 208
Poland B J, Miller J R, Harris M, Livingston J 1981 Spontaneous abortion — a study of 1961
    women and their conceptuses. Acta Obstetrica et Gynaecologica Scandinavica Suppl 102
Shearman R P 1980 Habitual abortion. In: Gold J J, Josimovich J B Gynecologic
    endocrinology, 3rd edn. Harper & Row, New York, p 751

20. MENOPAUSE AND CLIMACTERIC

Climacteric — the 'change' — from the reproductive to non reproductive phase of life

INTRODUCTION

— The menopause and climacteric are related to one another as are the menarche and puberty.
— Fifty per cent of women do not have any problems related to the cessation of periods.
— Twenty five per cent have some symptoms, but may be able to cope and their quality of life does not suffer much.
— The remaining 25% have disabling climacteric symptoms which adversely affect their life at home and at work to a significant extent.

DEFINITION

— The menopause is the physiological cessation of menstrual function.
— The cessation of periods for 6 months is required before a woman is considered menopausal.
— The average age of menopause is 50–52 (range 47–55).
— The menses may cease from the early forties to the mid-fifties in the absence of obvious pathology.
— The climacteric is the period (usually spanning several years) in which involution of the reproductive organs is occurring.

PHYSIOLOGY

— The menopause (cessation of menses) is due to failing ovarian function with associated decreased steroidogenesis.
— This in turn disturbs the pituitary hypothalamic feedback mechanism, causing elevation of FSH and LH and hypothalamic LRH. *Δ FSH > 40 IU/L*

— Despite normal hypothalamic pituitary function, the ovaries become progressively refractory.
— This may be due to diminished receptor function in the granulosa and theca cells and changes in the ovarian vessels.
— There is a gradual decline in ovulatory cycle and oestrogen levels.
— However, the menopausal ovary still continues to produce steroids, mainly androstenedione.
— Androstenedione is the preferential steroid synthesised by the ovarian stroma and adrenal cortex.
— Peripheral conversion of androstenedione to oestrone furnishes the major oestrogen source at this age.
— The level of oestrone is better in fat women who do not smoke.
— In some women the levels of oestrone are adequate to keep them symptom-free.
— The main oestrogen hormone is oestrone and not oestradiol.
— Smokers are more at risk of climacteric symptoms due to acidaemia consequent to lung emphysema.
— Thin women do not have the same peripheral conversion of ovarian and adrenal androstenedione to oestrone.
— Low oestrogen levels increase the sensitivity of bone to the resorbing effect of parathyroid hormone.
— This results in the loss of about 15% of skeletal calcium every decade, leading to osteoporosis in a significant number of women by the age of 65–70 years.

CLINICAL FEATURES

— Only 25% of all women experience climacteric symptoms severe enough to warrant treatment.
— Fifty per cent have no symptoms and the remaining 25% have mild symptoms which do not interfere with life in general.

Vasomotor symptoms

— The most common problem in the peri- and post- menopausal period are hot flushes.
— These consist of a subjective feeling of heat and flushing of the upper half of the body and face.
— Each episode lasts for 15–60 seconds.
— In approximately 80% of women hot flushes will persist for at least one year, and in 25% for at least 5 years.
— Experimentally, a flush has been seen to coincide with pulsatile bursts of LRH (GnRH) release from the hypothalamus.

— This is probably mediated by a temporary increase in sympathetic nervous system drive, perhaps mediated by such central neurotransmitters as serotonin and noradrenaline.
— A flush is usually followed by perspiration.
— Attacks are usually precipitated by an increase in ambient temperature such as in bed or crowded conditions, or at times of anxiety or after taking hot food or drink.
— Sleep is significantly interrupted by vasomotor episodes.

ATROPHIC SYMPTOMS

Reproductive system

— Breast atrophy is accentuated by decrease in parenchyma.
— Nipples become flatter and less erectile.
— The uterus and ovary become smaller.
— The weakness of fascial supports and loss of muscle tone increases the incidence of uterovaginal prolapse.
— The vagina becomes shorter and narrower.
— The vaginal wall (or skin) becomes thinner, less rugose and drier.
— Atrophic vaginitis is a common problem.
— Dyspareunia is a common symptom due to dryness and less distensibility of the vagina and associated atrophic vaginitis.
— The vulva also undergoes atrophic changes with reduction of fat tissues in the labia and mons pubis.
— There is diminished secretion from Bartholin's glands.
— Shrinkage and fragility may lead to pruritus vulvae.
— Loss of libido may be due to a combination of physical and psychological problems.

Urological system

— Senile or atrophic distal urethral syndrome produces frequency of micturation, dysuria and nocturia.
— The culture of the urine is invariably negative for infection.
— Patient then develops urgency and urge incontinence.
— The weakness of supporting muscles and ligaments may produce stress incontinence.
— Repeated senile or atrophic distal urethritis eventually produces stricture or narrowing.
— Urethral caruncle is related to atrophic change.
— Detrusor instability may develop as a result of distal urethral syndrome.

Skeletal system

— The skeletal system loses calcium phosphate relatively rapidly after the menopause, approximately 2.5% per year initially.
— This will lead to osteoporosis.
— Osteoporosis is most marked in thin, white, inactive, smoking females.
— It is worse when dietary intake of calcium and vitamin D is inadequate.
— Calcitonin was found to be deficient in most post-menopausal women with osteoporosis.
— Fracture of the neck of the femur, Colles' fracture involving tibia and fibula, and compression fracture of vertebrae are significantly higher in women as compared with men of similar age group.
— Compression fracture of vertebrae occurs in 25% of women by the age of 60.
— This produces reduction in height of some women and dorsal kyphosis.

— Changes occur in the jaws, particularly the alveolar bone in the mandible.
— Oestrogen will not overcome the ill effect of a poor dietary intake of calcium and lack of exercise and exposure to sunlight.
— On the basis of urinary-free cortisol studies, it is suggested that there are fast and slow calcium losers.
— Fast losers are at high risk — they have a fasting urinary hydroxyproline/creatinine ratio greater than 0:012.
— Arthralgia, locomotor instability are due to atrophic changes in muscles and joints.

PSYCHOLOGICAL SYMPTOMS

— These depend on basic personality, physiological changes, social and environmental changes.
— Psychological disturbances are more common among women with premenstrual symptoms, dysmenorrhoea, pregnancy problems, previous psychological disturbance and psychiatric illness.
— The more marked the climacteric symptoms, the more difficulty there will be in coping with the stress.
— Certain changes at home, such as the children leaving home, death of parents or husband, will produce changes in the woman's outlook.
— Patient becomes lonely and introvert.

— Patients who develop psychological and psychosomatic symptoms belong largely to a vulnerable group who are less likely to cope with stress.
— Insomnia may be largely the result of hot flushes and perspiration; when corrected with oestrogen, symptoms which are secondary to loss of sleep, such as fatigue and lack of concentration and memory, will improve.
— Oestrogen maintains the free tryptophan level in blood which controls the mood of a person.

CARDIOVASCULAR SYMPTOMS

— The levels of cholesterol, phospholipids, triglycerides increase after the menopause.
— The level of HDL gradually decreases and LDL increases.
— The alpha lipoprotein increases and β lipoprotein decreases.
— The above changes are supposed to increase the incidence of coronary artery disease.
— The incidence of ischaemic heart disease is thought to be increased in younger women who had oestrogen deficiency following surgical removal or irradiation to ovaries.

Diagnosis

— History and examination may reveal the climacteric status.
— Elevated serum or urinary FSH and LH are diagnostic features (FSH as high as 100 MIU/ml or above, LH values as high as 75 MIU/ml are not uncommon).
— Vaginal cytology will show mainly basal and parabasal cells.

PREMATURE MENOPAUSE

— Diagnosis of the premature menopause, especially in very young girls, is difficult.
— If the pituitary FSH levels are elevated and the patient complains of hot flushes, the diagnosis is almost certain.
— At least two assays of gonadotropins should show elevated levels.
— In some women it is useful to do an open ovarian biopsy.
— It is considered premature if women attain the menopause before the age of 40 years.

1) Iodiopathic
2) Surgical
3) Cytotoxic Drugs
4) Radiotherapy
5) Viral infection
   mumps
6) Autoimmune
7) Pituitary
8) Chromosomal
   29 times

Aetiology

— The most common cause is surgical removal of the ovaries or
  radiological destruction in the course of the management of
  pelvic malignancy.
— Cytotoxic chemotherapy may also damage the ovaries but
  rarely affects the endocrine function.
— Sex chromosomal disorders (Turner's mosaicism XX/XO),
  auto-immune disease and oophoritis are other causes of ovarian
  failure.
— Premature menopause should be differentiated from other
  causes of secondary amenorrhoea such as hyperprolactinaemia.

Clinical features

— Menstrual function (menarche) starts late.
— It ceases early by mid-twenties.
— Oestrogen levels are below the lower range of normal
  <0.1 pmol/ml of plasma oestradiol.
— Gonadotropins (FSH 5–12 times normal, LH 2–4 times
  normal) are markedly elevated.

Management

Assessment

— Careful appraisal of each patient is important, not only in
  relation to her symptomatology.
— Physical and psychological symptoms, her current domestic and
  social situation should be assessed.
— Evidence of oestrogen deprivation should be assessed on the
  basis of vaginal hormonal cytology, plasma oestrogen level and
  raised FSH level.
— The ratio of height to span will give an indication of vertebral
  compression.
— Androstenedione level is lower in women with osteoporosis.
— An elevated hydroxyproline/creatinine ratio, elevated serum
  calcium and alkaline phosphatase are seen in women with
  osteoporosis.
— Special attention should be paid to the conditions which may
  contra-indicate oestrogen therapy:
  • Previous thrombo-embolic disease
  • Past breast or ovarian or endometrial cancer
  • Active liver disease
  • Acute vascular disease
  • Central nervous system tumours
  • Melanoma
  • Neurophthalmic vascular disease
  • Severe hypertensive vascular disease

— Attention is paid to conditions requiring special supervision:
- Undiagnosed vaginal bleeding
- Gall bladder disease
- Mild hypertension
- Collagen disease
- Multiple sclerosis
- Diabetes
- Hyperlipidaemia
- Benign breast disease

— Strong family history of myocardial infarction, a cerebrovascular accident in the younger age group, familial hyperlipidaemia and cancer are considered to be a contra-indication for oestrogen therapy.
— Other endocrinological problems such as hypothyroidism should be excluded.

Treatment

— Findings from the history, examination and investigation should be explained to the patient.
— Explanation of the biological facts of the menopause and climacteric status is useful.
— Reassurance regarding the temporary nature of the symptoms is helpful.
— Consultations with psychiatrists are helpful if patients have psychiatric symptoms or previous history of psychiatric illness.

Non-hormonal therapy

— This is indicated when patients have contra-indication to oestrogen therapy.
— Patients do not desire to have oestrogen therapy.
— Clonidine hydrochloride (Dixarit) 0.25 mg one or two tablets 2 to 3 times daily can be given.
— Clonidine controls vasomotor symptoms.
— Bellegal 1 tablet 2 to 3 times is sometimes useful.
— Tranquillisers and sedatives are also useful for insomnia, depression and psychosomatic symptoms.
— Pyridoxin (B_6 50 mg) twice a day also is found useful in some cases.

Hormone replacement therapy

— This form of therapy is recommended for all symptomatic patients unless there is a specific contra-indication.
— Before starting treatment, the patient should have a complete general and pelvic examination, including breasts.
— Cervical smear, urine and blood examination to exclude diabetes, lipidaemia, liver dysfunction should be done.
— The aim should be to use the lowest dosage which will control the symptoms.
— Ideally a progestogen should always be added for 10 days or more, whether the patient has a uterus or not.

— Regular examination at 6-monthly intervals should be made.
— Ideally an endometrial biopsy or vabra aspiration or conventional curettage should be done prior to therapy.
— If there is a history of irregular bleeding, conventional endometrial curettage should be done to exclude malignant and premalignant conditions of the uterus.
— Endometrial lining should be examined using vabra aspiration once a year to exclude adverse effect.
— Oral preparations are usually preferred (equine oestrogen — Premarin, oestradiol valerate — Progynova, oestrone piperazine sulphate — Harmogen, together with norethisterone, medroxyprogesterone, dydrogesterone norgestrel or levonorgestrel).
— Oestrogen can be given continuously, and the progestogen is given from day 1 to 12 of each calender month.
— Oestrogen is also given on a cyclical regime for 21 days and progestogen is given for 10–12 days in the second half.
— Oestriol preparations are relatively much safer, since it has little end-organ effect on the endometrium and breast.
— Of the progestogens, medroxyprogesterone has the least adverse effect on HDL.
— Unopposed oestrogen therapy should never be given to a woman with an intact uterus.
— Combined preparations are ideal, even in hysterectomised patients.
— Subcutaneous implant (50–100 mg) of oestradiol is preferred by some women and by some physicians.
— The above regimen is supplemented by 10–12 days of oral progestogen.
— The addition of testosterone (100 mg) is useful to improve libido.
— The disadvantage of an implant is due to differences in absorption rate in different people and the inability to cease the treatment if required.
— Vaginal application of oestrogen cream (Premarin or dienoestrol) is useful if atrophic vaginitis and dyspareunia are the main symptoms.
— Vaginal application does promote systemic absorption, and one must be cautious in using this cream for a prolonged period.
— Norethisterone and medroxyprogesterone could be used if oestrogen is contra-indicated.

Disadvantages of HRT
— Endometrial hyperplasia and carcinoma are the real risks if the endometrium is exposed to prolonged unopposed oestrogen therapy.
— Addition of progestin to oestrogen therapy for 10–12 days almost abolishes the risk of hyperplasia and carcinoma.

— The incidence in that group is equal to the incidence in an untreated group.
— There are no obvious adverse effects on lipid and carbohydrate metabolism.
— Oestrogen therapy using natural oestrogen has not been found to alter clotting profile adversely.
— Patients may develop vaginal discharge, breast tenderness, dysmenorrhoea.
— They may also gain weight and sometimes develop premenstrual symptoms.

Duration of treatment
— This is a very debatable issue.
— Advantages of prolonged therapy are mainly the support provided for oestrogen-deprived tissues of the lower genital tract, to prevent osteoporosis and in the preventions of ischaemic heart disease in the young oophorectomised women.
— Adequate exercise and dietary calcium, perhaps supplemented by low doses of vitamin D (500–1000 u/day) will increase the beneficial effect of oestrogen in the prevention and treatment of osteoporosis.
— Oestrogen increases serum calcitonin effects, which may have a role in preventing bone resorption.
— Mortality associated with fracture of the neck of the femur is 20–40%, whereas that associated with endometrial cancer on oestrogen therapy is only 5–10%.
— For the above reasons one can make a case for prolonged therapy to prevent osteoporosis and the morbidity associated with it.
— The situation regarding prevention of atheroma and vascular thrombosis is still obscure and uncertain.
— There is the paradox that pre-menopausal women have relatively low rates for myocardial infarction, and this protection is removed if the patient is castrated.
— On the other hand, oestrogen/progestogen in the contraceptive pill increases the risk after the age of 38 years or more.
— The reason is probably the different effect of human versus synthetic oestrogens, differences in the balance of hormones in the pre-menopause with differential effects on lipids, the coagulation system and the vessel wall, and difference in the dose between contraceptive and replacement regimens.

SUGGESTED READING.

Greenblatt R B, Studd P (eds) 1977 The menopause. In: Clinics in obstetrics and gynaecology, vol 4. Saunders, Philadelphia
Hart D M 1982 The prevention of osteoporosis by oestrogen therapy in postmenopausal women.

In: Progress in obstetrics and gynaecology, vol 2. Studd J (ed) Churchill Livingstone, Edinburgh, p 241

Helgason S 1982 Estrogen replacement therapy after the menopause. Acta Obstetricia et Gynecologica Scandinavica Suppl 107

Mackay C V, Beischer N A, Cox L W, Wood C (eds) 1983 Menopause and climacteric. Saunders, Philadelphia, p 85

Notelovitz M, Ware M 1982. Coagulation risks with post-menopausal oestrogen therapy. In: Studd J (ed) Progress in obstetrics and gynaecology, vol 2. Churchill Livingstone, Edinburgh, p 228

Rakoff A E 1980 The female climacteric and the pros and cons of estrogen therapy. In: Gold J J. Josimovich J B (eds) Gynecologic endocrinology, 3rd edn. Harper & Row, p 482

Samsioe G (ed) 1981 Management of the female climacteric — benefits and risks. Symposium arranged by Schering. Acta Obstetrica et Gynecologica Scandinavica suppl 106

21. CONTRACEPTION, STERILISATION AND THERAPEUTIC ABORTION

INTRODUCTION

— A request for contraceptive advice is one of the commonest reasons for consultation in a gynaecology clinic.
— Major requirements of any contraceptive methods are:
  - Efficiency in pregnancy prevention
  - Minimal side-effects
  - Simplicity of use
  - Inexpensiveness
  - Easily reversible
— No perfect contraceptive method is yet available.
— Side-effects of some of the methods may be serious and life-threatening.
— The need for counselling, screening and follow-up examination should be stressed to the couple.

METHODS OF CONTRACEPTION

— See Table 21.1.
— These are described as four main groups:
— Coitus-dependent:
  - Barrier methods
  - Spermicidal agents
— Coitus-independent:
  - Steroids
  - Intra-uterine device (IUD)
— Coitus-inhibiting:
  - Abstinence
  - Withdrawal
— Surgical:
  - Sterilisation (male and female)
  - Hysterectomy
  - Abortion

Table 21.1 Available methods of fertility control

A. Contraception
  1. Coitus-dependent (traditional methods)
     • Condom ± spermicidal agents
     • Diaphragm ± spermicidal agents
     • Spermicidal agents
  2. Coitus-inhibiting
     • Rhythm (symptothermal)
     • Coitus interruptus
  3. Coitus-independent
     — Steroidal preparations
       • Combined oral oestrogen and progestogen (30–35 mg oestrogen combination)
         (incremental combinations)
       • Progestogen—only minidose
       • Injectable progestogen
       • Post-coital
     — Intra-uterine devices
       • Non-medicated
       • Copper-releasing
       • Progesterone-releasing
B. Sterilisation
  1. Female
     • Tubal occlusion by ligation, ring, clip, diathermy, thermal coagulation
     • Hysterectomy
  2. Male
     • Vasectomy
C. Abortion
  1. Menstrual regulation
  2. Vacuum aspiration and curettage
  3. Prostaglandins

Patient compliance

— This depends on the nurse and/or doctor who is friendly,
   sympathetic, non-judgemental, unbiased and prepared to take
   time.
— Adequate explanation of the available methods, advantages
   and disadvantages in relation to other methods is necessary.
— Discussion of failure rate and significant complications is also
   necessary.
— The need for follow-up examination should be discussed.

Factors affecting acceptance or rejection of a method

— Age of each partner.
— Frequency of intercourse.
— Religion and culture.
— Educational status.
— Marital status.
— Number of children.
— Menstrual cycle.
— Basic personality.
— Attitude to self-touching of genitalia.
— Medical disorders.

— Spacing or completion of family.
— Tolerance or otherwise of side-effects.

Assessment of efficacy

Methods available
— The pearl index gives the number of unwanted pregnancies per 100 woman-years.
— The life-table method is based on the failure rate in the first year of use per 100 married females aged 15–44 and takes this time factor into account.

COITUS-DEPENDENT (TRADITIONAL) METHODS

Barrier methods

— There are two methods commonly used.
— Vaginal diaphragm is used by the female.
— Condom is used by the male.
— Caps which fit over the cervix and sheaths which fit over the glans penis are also used, but are less efficient.
— Approximately 30 million couples use barrier methods.

Advantages

— Low cost.
— Protection from venereal disease.
— No side-effects — they are safe.
— Lower rates of cervical cancer.

Disadvantages

— Need medical help.
— Less reliable.
— Should be used together with spermicidal agents.
— Can be messy.
— Mechanistic and repetitive requirement of barrier methods is inhibiting to some.
— Some women find the genital exploration unacceptable.
— Methods need discipline and motivation.

Application of diaphragm

— Correct size is determined by the use of fitting rings.
— Commonly a size 70–80 mm is required.

— Correct initial placement by the patient is checked by the doctor.
— The upper rim is in the posterior fornix rather than in the anterior fornix.
— For the optimum efficiency 4–5 ml of spermicide is placed on the dome of the diaphragm.
— Diaphragm can be inserted at least 6 hours before intercourse.
— Difficulty in fitting may be due to:
  • Recent pregnancy
  • Significant change in weight ± 5–10 kg
  • Vaginal, cervical and pelvic surgery

Mode of action

— Prevents live sperm from entering the cervical canal:
  • By mechanical occlusion (caps and condoms)
  • By killing sperm by the spermicides used in conjunction with the barrier method.

Failure

— Common causes of failure include:
  • Size is wrong
  • Poorly fitted
  • Change is needed after childbirth
  • Badly inserted (poor instruction, too hasty, careless)
  • Spermicide not used
  • Spermicide not left in long enough after coitus

Condom

Failure

— Common causes of failure include:
  • Not applied before penetration
  • Entire penis is not covered
  • Inadequate vaginal lubrication
  • Inadequate room for the ejaculate and/or bursting
  • Lost in the vagina when the penis becomes flaccid before being withdrawn

Spermicides

— These create a chemical barrier.
— They comprise many forms — gels, creams, tablets, pessaries, sponges.
— Failure occurs because there is too short or too long a wait after insertion, or application is not repeated with the subsequent act of coitus.
— Material is placed too low in the vagina.

— It is omitted on safe days.
— Improved vehicles for chemical spermicides (sponges) can be inserted up to 24 hours before coitus and removed 8 hours later.
— They are immediately effective, less messy, cover repeated acts of coitus.
— Non-compliance rate of even 1 in 10 occasions will raise the pearl index 8 points.
— They are very easy to use and ideal for spacing the family.
— Recent collagen- or polythene-impregnated sponges are reported to have failure rates as low as 1–2%.
— Sperm enzyme inhibitors may be capable of successful development.

Efficacy of barrier methods

— Failure rates by the life-table method for the first year of use are as follows:
  • Condom 7; diaphragm 10; vaginal chemical 13; as compared with pill 2; IUD 3
— A really motivated person, using a barrier method correctly could have rates similar to those for the IUD (2/100 woman-years).

COITUS-INHIBITING METHODS

Coitus interruptus

— This is the oldest method used.
— It is still practised all over the world.
— It has little to recommend it except in an emergency situation.
— It is less reliable, likely to leave the female unsatisfied.
— This is the only method used in some cultures.

Safe-period method

— Among the methods used to detect the fertile and infertile phases in the cycle are:
  • The 'rhythm' or calendar method
  • Use of cyclical temperature changes
  • Use of cervical mucus changes
  • Combination of these

Rhythm method (safe-period)

— Only form of birth control practised by Roman Catholics.
— Used by those who find other contraceptive methods unacceptable or unsuitable.

— The method depends on:
  • The assumption that ovulation occurs only once in each cycle at about day 12–14 day of the 28- day cycle
  • Assuming that the ovum remains viable for 2–3 days
  • Spermatozoa remain viable for not more than 3–4 days
  • Ovulation is associated with phenomena detected by women
  • Willingness of the couple to practice abstinence

Basal body temperature

— This is more reliable than practising coitus in the second half for e.g. 17 to 28 days — coitus is avoided around the temperature change in the chart.
— Keeping a temperature chart discourages people.
— It is not good for less educated, less motivated people.
— Modification of the so-called natural method is termed the ovulation method.
— Temperature chart and cervical mucus together make the method more reliable.
— The woman examines her vagina daily and checks for cervical mucus.
— Mid-cycle pain suggests possible ovulation time, so intercourse can be abstained from.

Advantages

— No medication is required.
— Cheaper (thermometer and charts only).
— No adverse side-effects.

Disadvantages

— Coitus has to be abstained from. High motivation is needed.
— The method is less reliable.
— There are psychological problems.
— The need to examine the vagina daily does not appeal to some women.
— If cycle is irregular, the method is difficult to practise.

Efficiency

— Ideal for those who are educated and well motivated and whose libido is not above average.
— Pearl index rates 3.5 pregnancies/100 woman-years usual range (10–12/100 woman-years).

COITUS-INDEPENDENT

Steroidal agents

— Combined oral oestrogen and progestogen preparations.
— They were introduced in 1960.

— It is convenient to take pill.
— Unique efficacy of the method.
— Recently it has become less popular because of the side-effects.

Mechanism of action

— Prevention of ovulation by inhibiting the hypothalamic–pituitary system.
— Oestrogen inhibits release of FSH from pituitary gland by negative feedback inhibition and prevention of GnRH release from the hypothalamus.
— Lack of steroid production from ovary leads to less well developed endometrium.
— Progesterone-like compound inhibits LH in the same way as oestrogen-inhibiting FSH.
— Progestin-only pill acts mainly by changing the character of the mucus in the cervical canal.
— Cervical mucus becomes thicker and impermeable to sperms.
— Hence progestin has to be taken daily on a continuous basis.

Preparations

— There fall into two groups:
  • Combined oestrogen and progestin pill
  • Progestin-only (mini-pill)

Combined oestrogen/progestin pill

— The combined pill consists of an oestrogen, usually ethinyl oestradiol (0.02–0.150 mg) and norethisterone 0.5–2.0 mg.
— It seems that 0.03 mg of ethinyl oestradiol in combination with a progestin is the minimum dose which will suppress ovulation.
— In a sequential combination pill, the dosage of ethinyl oestradiol remains at 0.05 mg but the levonorgestrel increases from 0.05 mg for the initial 11 days to 0.125 mg for the last 10 days.
— More recently a three-phase formulation has been introduced (ethinyl oestradiol 0.03 mg × 6, 0.04 mg × 5, 0.03 mg × 10 days plus levonorgestrel 0.05 mg, 0.075 mg, 0.125 mg respectively).
— Triphasic formulation reduces the total norgestrel dose which has androgen-like effect on lipid metabolism.
— Triphasic preparation is relatively oestrogen dominant, with the associated side-effects and benefits.

Progestin-only pill

— There are two progestins commonly used: norethisterone 0.350 mg and levonorgestrel 0.030 mg.
— They are used continuously.

— They act mainly on the cervical mucus.
— They probably act on the secretion of the fallopian tubes.
— Changes in the mucus make it impermeable to the sperm.
— This pill does not usually inhibit ovulation.
— There is a smaller margin of error.
— The tablet is taken the same time every day.
— Factors which lower therapeutic levels are:
  - Forgetting to take the tablet
  - Poor absorption (diarrhoea, vomiting)
  - Increased liver enzyme activity (barbiturate, anti-epileptic treatment)
  - Marked obesity
— Since there is no oestrogen, cycle control is lost in approximately. 50% of patients.
— Some patients may have irregular bleeding.
— Ideal for those who breastfeed, when oestrogen is not suitable or contra-indicated.
— Failure rate is slightly higher as compared with the combined pill.

Long-acting injectable steroids
— Depo-Provera is the most commonly used intramuscular preparation.
— Dose is 150 mg every 3 months or 300 mg every 6 months.
— Pregnancy rate 0.02–1.2/100 woman-years.
— Disadvantages and advantages are similar to those described for the mini-pill.
— Less motivation is required by the patient.
— Oligomenorrhoea occurs significantly; occurs more often especially after 18–24 months.
— Reversibility of fertility is slower because of the persistence of activity in the microcrystals.
— Usually recommended for short-term use (post-vasectomy, post-partum, after rubella vaccination).
— Major problems reported (Breast nodules and cancer in the beagle).
— This drug acts on the anterior pituitary of the dog, causing increased secretion of both prolactin and growth hormone.
— Norethisterone enanthate (200 mg) is another long-acting progestin preparation.
— Progestin-only preparations cause minimal metabolic disturbance or morbidity.
— Other slow-release methods are silastic capsules with progestational steroids, inserted subcutaneously.
— Progestins are incorporated in vaginal rings which are easily removable.
— A special type of intra-uterine device also has a slow release progesterone.

— This group acts purely locally, and the main disadvantage is menstrual cycle disturbance.

Post-coital contraception

— This is largely an emergency measure.
— Stilboestrol was formerly used and then ethinyl oestradiol 2 mg/day for 4–5 days recently.
— Treatment is given within 24 to 36 hours of coitus.
— Combined preparation (ethinyl oestradiol 0.100 mg + norgestrel 0.5 mg is given, 2 doses 12 hours apart.
— This hormonal interception interferes with endocrine balance and disturbs endometrial development.
— Nausea, vomiting and breast tenderness are common.
— There is an added risk of thrombo-embolism.
— It is not recommended for routine use, but suitable in cases of rape.
— It is economical.
— Low-dose progestogens (norgestrel 0.35 mg) are effective with fewer side-effects, taken within 3 hours of coitus.

Trends

— Recently there has been a reduction in the dose of both oestrogen and progestin in the combined pill.
— The use of a sequential regimen containing phased doses of oestrogen and progestogen to mimic the normal cycle has been introduced.
— Alternative methods are advised for a woman over the age of 35 years who smokes, is slightly hypertensive and obese.
— No useful anti-oestrogen or anti-progestin preparations are yet available.
— Gonadotropin-releasing hormone antagonists are being investigated.
— Immunological methods, e.g. antibodies to reproductive hormones or compounds of the germ cells or conceptus are in the experimental stage.
— Hormonal contraception in the male is more difficult than in the female — agents suppressing spermatogenesis will probably suppress the libido as well.

Choice of contraception

— Consider the contra-indications — both absolute and relative (Table 21.2).
— Consider the degree of reliability required.
— Appropriate formulation can be decided following history and clinical examination.
— Preparation containing low oestrogen 0.03–0.35 mg ethinyl oestradiol) plus a progestin (0.150 mg or less levonorgestrel or 0.5 mg less norethisterone).

Table 21.2 Contra-indications to oral contraception

ABSOLUTE	Cardiovascular disease	— Cerebrovascular accident Coronary artery disease Thrombo-embolic disease
	Hypertensive vascular disease Acute and chronic liver disease History of cholelithiasis Oestrogen-dependent tumours	— Severe/moderate degree — Breast cancer Uterine cancer Liver hepatoma
	Otosclerosis	— (Showed deterioration in previous pregnancy or on the pill)
	Dubin-Johnson and Rotor syndromes Endogenous depression	
RELATIVE	Age over 35 years Epilepsy Moderate to severe smoking Gross overweight Migraine Diabetes Hyperlipidaemia Gall bladder disease Asthma Oligomenorrhoea Varicose veins—moderate and marked Sickle-cell anaemia	

- Levonorgestrel is a stronger progestin and cycle control is better, but progestational side-effects may occur.
- Progestional side-effects can be overcome by an increase in oestrogen and/or a reduction in progestin.
- In the combined sequential pill this is achieved by an increase in ethinyl oestradiol to 0.035–0.05 mg reduction in levonorgestrel to 0.050 mg for 11 days and 0.125 mg for the ensuing 10 days.
- A careful history and thorough systemic and pelvic examination are mandatory.
- Follow-up at regular 6-monthly intervals is advisable.
- Adequate counselling must be given to the couple.
- Special investigations such as blood lipids, glucose tolerance, liver function may be necessary if the history indicates.
- The possible interaction of other drugs with the pill should be discussed.
- Side-effects are prominent during the first 2 to 3 cycles and the patient should be reassured.

Special situations
- In the case of patients under the age of 16, moral and legal problems should be discussed.
- Contraception should not be prescribed to under 16s without the consent of the parents, if possible.
- It is safer to start from the first day of the cycle for the contraceptive to become immediately effective.

— Nulliparous oligomenorrhoeic women are offered other methods.
— The pill should be preferably stopped 4–6 weeks before the planned surgery, and other methods are advocated.
— If emergency surgery is needed, prophylactic anticoagulant therapy is offered until the patient is ambulant.
— There is no conclusive evidence of an association between pill use in early pregnancy and congenital abnormalities.
— Some association is found in smokers and pill users.
— A study of abortuses showed a preponderance of triploidy and XO monosomy in pill users.
— After termination of pregnancy of less than 12 weeks' gestation, oral contraceptives can be started immediately.
— After 12 weeks, a break of 3 weeks is advised in view of the possible risk of thrombo-embolism.
— Routine cessation after a few years' use is not necessary unless there are adverse clinical problems.
— Some form of contraception should be used for at least one year following the last spontaneous menstrual period in the menopausal age group.
— Women over 35 years who are obese, who smoke and are overweight with a positive family history for risk factors should be advised to use alternative method.

Advantages
— The pill is effective — it has a failure rate 1–4/200 woman-years. Among adolescents the failure rate is as high as 10%.
— The method is easy to apply.
— It is relatively trouble-free in the patient under 30 years of age.
— The method is not coitus-related.
— Reduction in premenstrual tension, menstrual pain and excessive menstrual loss.
— Benign breast conditions (cyst, adenomas) and ovarian retention cysts are less common.
— Incidence of all neoplasia is somewhat lower.
— Rheumatoid arthritis is reported to occur half as frequently in pill users.

Disadvantages and side-effects
— See table 21.3.
— Tablet should be taken every day without fail regardless of the frequency of intercourse.
— It is less suited to those who have infrequent coitus.
— Serious side-effects can occur in women who are older, overweight, who smoke and are hypertensive.

Gynaecological side-effects
— Erosion of the cervix, vaginal discharge.
— Recurrent moniliasis.

Table 21.3 Oestrogenic and progestogenic side-effects

Symptoms related to oestrogen excess:
— Menorrhagia
— Nausea, vomiting
— Breast enlargement, tenderness
— Fluid retention
— Leucorrhoea
— Headache — migraine
— Mood changes and irritability
— Chloasma
— Recurrent miniliasis — vaginitis

Symptoms related to progestogen excess:
— Weight gain
— Reduced menstrual flow
— Post-pill anovulation
— Depression, irritability, fatigue
— Androgenic symptoms — acne, hirsutism, greasy hair
— Loss of libido
— Dry vagina

— Menstrual changes are common with low-dose and progestogen-only pill.
— Spotting, breakthrough bleeding, scanty periods are some of the symptoms.
— Women with irregular, infrequent cycle may develop amenorrhoea — incidence is 0.4% (0.1–2.5% range).
— If breakthrough bleeding persists after 3 to 4 months, the oestrogen dose should be increased.
— If amenorrhoea develops, either stop the pill or use one with high oestrogen and low progestogen.
— Fibromyoma may increase in size and may cause menstrual symptoms and pain.

Thrombotic and cardiovascular effect
— The use of combined pill is associated with an incidence of:
  • Venous trhombosis
  • Pulmonary embolism
  • Myocardial infarction
  • Cerebral artery thrombosis
  • Mesenteric vascular ischaemia
  • Hypertension
— The oral contraceptive users in the UK have a mortality rate 2 to 10 times greater than that of women using non-hormonal contraception.
— The degree of risk varies with:
  • Age — women over 35 years are at greater risk
  • Number of cigarettes smoked — myocardial infarction is 3–4 times that of control groups when pill was used; in those who smoke as well, the risk increases to 40 times
  • Risk has been reduced since the dose of oestrogen was reduced from 0.05 mg to 0.03 mg

- The duration of pill-taking — some controversy exists
- A family history of cardiovascular disease
- Presence of sickle-cell disease (SS or SC)
- Diabetes mellitus, hypertension, renal disorders, Raynauds' syndrome, structural abnormalities of the vascular disease, tendency to abnormal fluid retention and abnormality of coagulation factors add to the risk factors of the pill

— Hypertension develops in about 5% of women within 5 years of commencing the combined pill.

- Rise in blood pressure is related to both oestrogen and progestogen compounds
- This problem is not age-related
- Women who developed hypertension in pregnancy, those with chronic renal disease, those with a family history of hypertension and women over 35 years are likely to develop hypertension on the combined pill
- Subarachnoid haemorrhage is not age-reated. Risk is low, but increases to 4 or more times in pill users
- Cerebral thrombosis and haemorrhagic strokes are rare, but the risk increases with pill use

Metabolic effects
— Glucose tolerance is reduced by the combined pill and to a lesser degree by the progestogen-only pill.
— Oral contraceptives in diabetic women may alter the diabetic regimen.
— Women with latent diabetes may develop overt disease.
— Hyperlipidaemia with contraceptive pill use was reported where a high steroid dose was used.
— With low-dose preparation there is elevation of lipids, mainly triglycerides, in some women and lowering of high-density cholesterol lipoprotein.
— Hyperlipidaemia may lead to pancreatitis.
— Strong family history of hyperlipidaemia add to the risk factor, serum lipids should be checked.

Hepatic effects
— These are rare:
— There is a slightly increased risk of developing the rare hepatocellular adenoma of the liver after prolonged use of the combined pill.
— Jaundice may arise in women taking the pill if they have had intrahepatic cholestasis during pregnancy, chronic idiopathic jaundice (Dubin-Johnson or Rotor syndrome), abnormal liver function as a residue of viral hepatitis.
— The combined pill may also facilitate the formation of gallstones in some patients.

Dermatological effects
- Chloasma.
- Sebaceous hyperactivity.
- Acne, rashes — discoid L.E.
- Purpura, granuloma, photosensitivity are some of the symptoms.

Infections
- Infections such as recurrent moniliasis and bacteriuria are increased on combined pills.

Tumourogenic effects
- None has been proved.
- There is increased incidence of focular nodular hyperplasia or adenoma of the liver. Patients with cirrhosis of the liver are more susceptible. Rupture of the nodule with intraperitoneal haemorrhage is often fatal.
- There is a suggestion that there may be a relapse or greater need for cytotoxic therapy in trophoblastic neoplasia if oral contraceptives are given before return of HCG value to normality.
- There is no conclusive evidence to suggest that the pill increases breast, uterine and ovarian neoplasia.
- Cervical intra-epithelial neoplasia may be indirectly associated in that it is related to sexual activity which may be facilitated by oral contraception.
- In breast cancer, melanoma treated within previous 5 years, another form of contraception is advisable.

Psychological effects
- May be due to progestogen and oestrogen.
- May produce loss of libido.
- Oral contraceptives interfere with serotonin levels in the brain and may produce or exacerbate depression; can be relieved by B_6.

Other side effects
- Breast tenderness, enlargement, fluid retention, migraine may get worse on pill.

Drug and hormonal interactions
- The contraceptive efficacy of low dose preparations is affected by antibiotics such as rifampicin, ampicillin, chloramphenicol and neomycin, by phenobarbitone, and to a lesser extent, phenytoin.
- Drugs that induce microsomal enzyme activity in the liver will accelerate the elimination of steroid hormones that comprise the oral contraceptive pill.
- Antibiotics affect micro-organisms in the gut which normally hydrolyse steroid conjugates excreted by the liver.

— Normal absorption of the freed steroid will not occur;
  enterohepatic circulation will be depressed.
— Similar effect will occur if absorption from the gut is depressed
  by intestinal hurry (diarrhoea).
— Conversely, the pill interferes with the action of warfarin and
  tricyclic drugs.

Situations in which current use of oral contraceptive pill must be reviewed
— Before elective surgery.
— Immobilisation in a plaster cast.
— When the patient complains of cramps, pain or oedema of the
  legs.
— Sudden migraine attacks or unusual headaches.
— Severe chest pain.
— Visual disturbance.
— Transient weakness of the extremities.
— Viral hepatitis.
— When hypertension develops.
— When depression develops.
— Gastro-intestinal upset.

INTRA-UTERINE DEVICES

Introduction

— These have still not reached a stage of development where
  widespread acceptance has been achieved.
— Ideally, they accommodate to change in the shape of the uterus.
— Their perimeters are composed of gentle curves to prevent
  penetration.
— They must have resistance to the expulsive force of the uterus
  and gravity without perforation of the lower segment or cervix.
— They must possess axial stiffness but transverse bend resilience.
— Their contraceptive effect is mainly the result of added
  non-harmful material.
— The ideal intra-uterine contraceptive device (IUD) should fulfil
  three criteria:
  • It must be an effective contraceptive
  • It must be easy to fit with minimal discomfort
  • It should remain in the uterine cavity until the woman wishes
    it removed

Types of iud

— The two main groups of device are the inert (Lippes loop and
  Saf-T-Coil) and the bioactive (Copper 7 and T and multiload)

which rely on the slow release of copper ions to provide a significant part of their effect. The Progestasert device containing progesterone has been withdrawn because of its association with ectopic pregnancy.

Lippes loop (1962)
— One of the most popular devices.
— Made of polyethylene; comes in four sizes (A, B, C and D).
— A recent innovation has been the application of a coat of ethylene vinyl acetate containing trasylol, a protease inhibitor, in order to lessen bleeding.

Saft-t-Coil (1965)
— Plastic device; comes in three sizes (25-S, 32-S, 33-S).
— The smallest size is useful for patients with a small uterine activity (50 mm–60 mm).

Copper T (1972)
— Originally there was a winding of fine copper wire around the stem.
— Copper wire is now present on both horizontal and vertical arms, and prolongs the effectiveness.
— Provides resistance to actinomycotic infection in the birth canal.

Copper 7 (1974)
— Similar to Copper T — shape is different.
— Has slightly reduced diameter (28 mm instead of 32 mm).
— Device with a further reduction in size (minigravigard) has been produced for women with a cavity less than 6.50 mm on sounding, especially in the nullipara.

Multiload (1974)
— There are two models (CU-250 and D.250).
— Plastic device has a copper winding on the vertical arm.
— Its characteristic features are the five serrated plastic fins on each transverse arms which secure the device in place.
— Has low pregnancy rate (<1%).
— Has low expulsion rate and removal rate.

Progestasert (1976)
— It is a basic plastic T device.
— Vertical arm contains a reservoir of 38 mg of progesterone which is released at a rate of 0.065 mg per day.
— The uterine therapeutic system was introduced by the same company.
— The latest device releases progesterone 0.025 mg per day or levonorgestrel 0.002–0.004 mg per day.
— Similar device from Finland utilises levonorgestrel; the release rate is higher; 0.02–0.03 mg.

Other devices

— Grafenberg ring and similar devices.
— Stainless steel wire ring used in People's Republic of China.
— OHT is a plastic ring used in Japan.

Mechanism of action

— This is not understood fully, and possibly more than one mechanism is involved.
— It may speed transport of the fertilised ovum in the tube.
— It may act directly on the uterine wall by abrasion or prevention of decidua formation.
— It may create an unfavourable environment because of its composition (zinc or copper).
— It may create a hostile response in the uterus phagocytic cells or lysozymes.
— Tubal pregnancies still occur.
— There are no major problems for the passage of spermatozoa upward through the uterus.
— Progesterone-releasing device may produce hostile mucus.
— The main effect is likely to depend on interference with events surrounding implantation.
— No one device is clearly superior to another, although the multiload copper appears to be the best of the copper devices.
— The skill of the operator in insertion of the device is certainly very important in determining efficacy and side-effects.

Clinical use

— Two factors are of major importance — counselling of the patient and proper insertion.

Pre-insertion counselling

— Information regarding the types of IUD available.
— Relative advantages and disadvantages, in relation to other forms of contraception.
— The risks of pregnancy and other complications.
— Nullipara is likely to have more pain and bleeding.
— Occurrence of ectopic pregnancy or infection is important problem in a nullipara, especially because of its effect on future fertility.
— Careful deliberation when IUD is inserted in nullipara.
— Patients with heavy and painful periods are not suitable for this method.
— History of PID (pelvic inflammatory disease) and multiple partners increase the risk of infection.

Insertion techniques

— Ideally the IUD is inserted towards the end of the menstrual flow.
— Post-abortal insertion seems safe and is recommended.
— Post-partum insertion suffers from problems of expulsion being 2–3 times higher than if the IUD is inserted 6 weeks after delivery.
— Following caesarean section, perforation is more likely and insertion should be careful.
— Post-coital insertion has been recommended for use in a manner similar to the post-coital pill.
— Proper insertion technique is vitally important.
— Most important considerations are an aseptic and antiseptic technique, and placement of the device high in the uterine cavity.
— Following principles should be applied:
  • No suspicion of pregnancy
  • No evidence of infection
  • No significant congenital or other abnormality of the uterus or its cavity
  • Uterine cavity should be 50 mm or more in length
  • Depth and direction of the uterus must be assessed carefully
  • If there is resistance, abandon the procedure
  • If there is significant persistent pain, the patient should not leave the clinic

Post-insertion counselling

— Patient should be counselled regarding possible complications and their early recognition.
— Slight cramping pain and heavier bleeding for the first 2–3 cycles are not uncommon and should be mentioned.
— Patient should be instructed to feel the nylon thread after each period.
— Amenorrhoea lasting 2 weeks or more longer than her usual cycle should be reported.
— Symptoms of pelvic infection (fever, pain, feeling unwell, discharge) should be reported.
— Six weeks after the insertion and at every six months, patient should be seen and examined to exclude problems.

Possible complications and side-effects of IUDs

Missing tail

— Missing tail may be due to:
  • Unnoticed expulsion (20–25%)
  • Tail drawn up into cervical canal or uterus (70–80%)
  • Translocation (4–6%)

- May coexist with pregnancy
- Diagnosis is made using ultrasound (preferred method), radiography, hysteroscopy
- Perforation of the uterus

Intra-uterine pregnancy
— Remove the IUD if the thread is visible; 15–25% abort following the removal.
— If the IUD remains in situ, spontaneous abortion occurs in 40–50%.
— If pregnancy continues, incidence of antepartum haemorrhage and premature labour increases.
— With certain IUDs (Dalkon shield) fatal sepsis is reported in pregnancy.

Ectopic pregnancy
— This condition should be always excluded especially if IUD is still in situ.
— The ratio of ectopic to intra-uterine pregnancies in IUD users is 1 in 30 compared to 1 in 3000 for non-IUD users.
— The incidence of intra-uterine pregnancy with IUD is 1 in 250 as compared with 1 in 25–30 of ectopic pregnancy.
— Ectopic pregnancy is 1–2/1000 users per year in IUD users.

Expulsion of IUDs
— This is most likely during the first month.
— About 50% of all expulsions take place within 3 months of insertion.
— After the first year very few IUDs are expelled.
— It is associated with young women of low parity, use of an inappropriate size or type of IUD and skill and experience of the person fitting the device.
— Expulsion rate is higher following late miscarriage, post-partum insertion.
— Lowest rate (2–3% /1 year) for Multiload Cu 250.
— For other devices the figures are in the range 3–15+%.

Bleeding problems
— May be a continued irregular loss or an increased bleeding with the menses (amount and/or duration).
— The incidence of irregular loss is 30–40%.
— Heavy and prolonged bleeding occurs with all devices other than the one containing progesterone.
— Bleeding may be due to abrasion of surface capillaries, increased prostaglandin formation, interference with haemostatic mechanism.
— Between 5% and 15% of users will request removal of the device because of bleeding.

Pain
— Some low abdominal pain or backache may follow insertion.
— Dysmenorrhoea can be worse if the woman is nulliparous.
— If pain is significant, suspect perforation, infection, ectopic pregnancy.

Vaginal discharge:
— May be temporary or may persist.
— Arises from the endometrium as it reacts to the presence of a foreign body.

Perforation and embedding
— Occurs in about 1 in 1000 insertions.
— May result in significant morbidity.
— Is more common with devices with sharp angles (CU7 and CUT).
— Usually occurs at insertion, due to operator error.
— More often with 'push-out' type of device.
— Embedded devices may require laparotomy and uterine incision, if difficult to remove from below.
— Extra-uterine devices may be removed through laparoscopy.
— Copper-containing devices produce marked reaction and form omental masses and adhesions, and laparotomy is often needed to remove these,

Infection
— Series of deaths due to infection in women becoming pregnant with the IUD insertion, especially the Dalkon shield.
— Pelvic infection is more common in IUD users, especially in a nullipara and in those with multiple partners.
— Infection is the most serious cause of morbidity.
— Approximately 2% of all users will develop pelvic infection within one year of insertion.
— If infection rate is higher, some increase in infertility is expected.

Contra-indications to the use of IUD

— Pregnancy known, or suspected.
— Pelvic infection.
— Recent septic abortions.
— Congenital abnormality of uterus, cervix, vagina.
— Abnormal menstrual bleeding.
— Suspected gynaecological malignancy.
— History of infertility or previous ectopic pregnancy.
— Previous problems with IUD.
— Need for greater degree of contraception.
— Uterine polyp or fibromyoma.
— Valvular heart disease.

— Chronic anaemia.
— Cervical dysplasia.
— Copper allergy.

Indications for IUD

— Best use of IUD is probably for family spacing after 1 or 2 children.
— While deciding on sterilisation.
— If reversibility and non-involvement by the patient are needed.
— Other methods are not ideal due to side-effects and complications.
— If surgical procedure is declined.

STERILISATION

Introduction

— Sterilisation of either partner is becoming an increasingly popular method of birth control.
— Peak age in women is between 30 and 34 years.
— Popularity of this irreversible approach is due to the limitations of other, reversible methods.
— Request is increasing because of the earlier completion of smaller families, dissatisfaction with a long period of other contraceptives and the development of safe and efficient sterilisation techniques.

Counselling of couples

— The procedure (in either male or female) must be considered to be irreversible.
— Alternative methods must have been fully considered.
— Sterilisation of either partner will not stabilise an insecure marriage.
— In general, sterilisation should not be done along with termination of pregnancy.
— Childbirth and abortion are stressful times, and extra care must be taken to ensure that sterilisation at these times is appropriate.
— The small failure rate of all methods must be explained.
— If post-partum sterilisation is requested, the couple should be advised to defer it for 3 months and have a planned procedure.
— Written consent must be obtained from the person undergoing the operation, and that of the partner is advisable, but not essential.

Female sterilisation

Laparoscopy

— Fallopian tubes are occluded by clips or bands.
— Diathermy is being used less and less because of its associated dangers.
— If diathermy must be used, the bipolar technique is safer than the unipolar method.
— Thermal technique can be used.
— Laparoscopy requires skill and experience, and there is an associated mortality of about 8/100 000 laparoscopies.
— It is not suitable for the post-partum period.

Complications

— The usual anaesthetic complications.
— Perforation of a viscus or blood vessel by the verres needle or trocar.
— Thermal injury to bowel if the diathermy method is used.
— Problems related to gas embolism.
— Minor complications occur in 2.5–3.0%, while major complications occur in about 0.5%.
— Cardiac arrhythmias, infection, pain and haemorrhage are some of the complications.

Culdoscopy

— Access through the posterior vaginal fornix.
— Technique is the same as in laparoscopy.
— It is less popular and has more complications.

Hysteroscopy

— Visualisation of the entrance of the fallopian tube into the uterus.
— Blockage is effected by chemicals, cautery or silicon plugs.
— This method needs to be perfected; it is not widely used yet.

Laparotomy

— Many techniques of tubal occlusion have been developed.
— Tubes should be divided and the ends are separated.
— Tubes may be removed partially or totally.
— Fimbrial ends may be buried in between the leaves of broad ligament.
— Clips and rings may still be applied.

Mini-laparotomy

— A small incision is usually made.
— Access to the tubes is by proctoscope or Cuscoe's speculum or similar instrument inserted through a small suprapubic incision.
— The fallopian tubes are divided and the ends are separated.
— Rings and clips can be applied.

Posterior colpotomy
— The tubes are approached through a small incision in the pouch of Douglas.
— This method is not popular.

Female sterilisation as part of another operation
— Caesarian section should not be used as a too-ready reason for sterilisation. It is ideal to wait for 3 months. Full discussion with patient is mandatory. Written consent beforehand is essential.
— Termination of pregnancy is best not combined with sterilisation.
— If patient has uterovaginal prolapse and requests sterilisation, she may benefit from a vaginal hysterectomy.
— Abdominal hysterectomy may be indicated if the woman has severe menorrhagia or in the presence of cervical intraepithelial neoplasia.

Efficacy of female sterilisation
— With modern techniques, failure rates should be less than 1% (0.1–0.5%).
— A significant number of pregnancies will be ectopic.
— Procedures carried out in the puerperium and following abortion and termination are more difficult, less reliable and have more complications.

Long-term effects of female sterilisation
— Mortality is 8 per 100 000 operations (Table 21.4).
— Heavier menstrual loss, pelvic pain, and dysmenorrhoea are reported.
— The excess loss may be due to cessation of oral contraceptive pill prior to sterilisation as the cycles revert back to original pattern.
— Abnormal ovarian function has been suspected if ovarian blood supply is damaged by the diathermy — this may also cause menstrual problems.
— Effect on sex is usually favourable.

Indications for female sterilisation
— Completion of family.
— Woman does not wish to use other methods.
— Cannot tolerate other methods.
— Health reasons which contra-indicate further pregnancy.
— Scarred uterus (more than 3 or 4 caesarean sections).
— Medical reasons (hypertension, cardiovascular, renal, neurological diseases).
— Psychiatric (schizophrenia, depression).
— Eugenic (hereditary disorders).

MALE STERILISATION

Introduction

— It is a relatively safer, simple, short procedure.
— Can be performed by one trained person.
— Training is relatively simple.
— It is quicker than female sterilisation.
— Local anaesthetic is adequate, there is usually no need for general anaesthesia.
— Very little equipment is required.
— Hence the method is cheaper and economic.

Complications

— It takes some time to be effective.
— Re-canalisation is more common.
— Mortality is nil when the operation is performed aseptically under local anaesthesia.
— Short-term morbidity includes local infection and haematomas, epididymo-orchitis.
— Long-term morbidity includes anto-immune problems, testicular damage and increase in atherosclerosis are also suggested, but not proven.
— Two sperm-free specimens should be obtained from a man who has undergone a vasectomy.
— Until the semen is free of spermatozoa one of the partners should use some form of contraception.
— There are newer methods of vas blockage, done using alcohol and formaldehyde per cutaneous injection and silastic plugs, but are still experimental.

THERAPEUTIC ABORTION

Introduction

— No form of family planning is more contentious than therapeutic abortion, largely because of moral, religious and legal overtones.
— Abortion laws concerning therapeutic abortion range from absolute prohibition, though being permissible only when there is a threat to the mother's life, mother's mental and physical well-being, eugenic, humanitarian and social considerations, and finally to 'on request'.

— Currently it is estimated that approximately 65 million abortions are performed annually worldwide.
— If abortion carried out in the first trimester, morbidity and mortality are low.
— Complications increase after 12 weeks' gestation.

Definition

— Termination of pregnancy before 20–24 weeks' gestation.
— WHO recommendation is 22 weeks and this has been adopted by most countries.

Indications

— The main indication is the risk to mental and physical health of the mother if pregnancy is continued.
— The other main reason is fetal anomalies not compatible with normal life.
— Abortion is often based on legal or cultural grounds rather than on strictly medical ones.
— Decision is arrived at between two physicians and the patient.
— All relevant facts have been evaluated in relation to the patients reproductive, psychological, medical, surgical, social history and status on examination.
— There is no consensus as to the relative rights of the mother and of the fetus (Right to life).
— Currently the majority consider that the mother's rights are paramount.
— Therapeutic abortion largely eliminates criminal abortion with all its attendant problems.
— There is often a mixture of psychological, eugenic and social indications.
— Chromosomal abnormalities, renal agenesis, neural tube defects, gross cardiac anomalies are some of the abnormalities that indicate termination of pregnancy.
— In a minority, there will be specific pregnancy disorders (hyperemesis gravidarum, molar pregnancy) or more often associated medical disorders of any system which may be aggravated by the stress of pregnancy, childbirth and childcare.

Methods of termination

— These depend largely on the duration of pregnancy.
— Procedure is seldom easy, and with the advance of pregnancy it becomes progressively more complicated and dangerous for the mother.

Menstrual induction

    — This method is used up to about week 6–7 of pregnancy.

    — Prostaglandins in the form of a pessary are placed in the upper vagina or even into the cervix.

    — An alternative procedure in early pregnancy is that of endometrial aspiration.

    — Karman catheter or vabra aspiration may be used and a suction is applied either from a 50 ml syringe or suction bottle.

Dilatation and evacuation (D and E)

    — This technique is similar to that for diagnostic curettage, except that it is practised beyond week 6–8.

    — Evacuation of the products of conception requires either a suction curette or sponge or ovum forceps.

    — Antisepsis and asepsis are essential.

    — Cervical dilatation is done gently and slowly.

    — Some damage to the cervical sphincter probably occurs at 10 mm or more of dilatation and may produce cervical incompetence.

    — Prostaglandin pessary 6 hours prior to dilatation of cervix facilitates easy cervical dilatation which may reduce the incidence of trauma to cervix.

    — Blood loss is minimised by giving 5–10 units of oxytocin intravenously with the largest dilator still in the cervix.

    — A few physicians have used a laminaria tent 12 hours before D and E when uterus is more than 12 weeks.

    — D and E after 12 weeks is psychologically more traumatic to the doctor compared with the alternative method, but is less so for the patient and nursing staff. It requires more skill on the operators' part.

    — The maternal death rate is lower (8–10/100 000) than that of other two commonly used methods, prostaglandin (10–12/100 000) and intra-amniotic saline (14–16/100 000).

Prostaglandins

    — Prostaglandins are used for menstrual induction.

    — Compounds of the F2-alpha and E2 type and their synthetic derivatives have been administered for termination of pregnancy.

    — They are given orally, by intramuscular and intravenous routes, into the vagina and uterine cavity using intra or extra amniotic approach.

    — Prostaglandins may cause cervical softening, but act mainly on uterine muscle.

    — Side-effects are mainly gastro-intestinal nausea, vomiting, diarrhoea and sometimes fever.

Intra-amniotic prostaglandin and urea

    — This is usually done after 15–16 weeks' pregnancy.

— Amniocentesis is performed, 200–250 ml of amniotic fluid is removed and replaced with equal amount containing 80 g of urea and 2.5 mg to 5 mg of PGE_2.

— 30–50 mg of prostaglandin F2-alpha or its equivalent, prostaglandin E2, may also be used on their own.

— Intravenous oxytocin supplementation is often helpful if the uterine action is inadequate 6 hours after the procedure.

— Intramuscular pethidine plus anti-emetic are given for pain relief.

— Usually removal of retained products is done under general anaesthesia after the expulsion of the fetus and placenta.

Extra-amniotic PGE_2.

— It is used when the duration of pregnancy is more than 13 weeks.

— Via a Foley's catheter which is inserted through the cervix into the extra-amniotic space PGE_2 is delivered 100 μg per hour via a special pump.

— Oxytocin infusion may be necessary if the method has not been effective after 6 hours.

— After expulsion of the fetus and placenta, the patient often needs removal of the remaining products under general anaesthesia.

Complications of the intra- and extra-amniotic PGE_2 termination

— Both procedures will need further evacuation of the uterus under general anaesthesia.

— Infection is more common in extra-amniotic procedure.

— Trauma to the cervix in the form of a tear is reported with intra-amniotic procedure.

Hysterotomy

— This is rarely indicated.

— There is a higher incidence of risks to the mother, particularly thrombo-embolic disease.

— Endometriosis of the abdominal scar is reported.

— Later scar problems may arise.

— It is rarely carried out now.

Complications of termination of pregnancy in general

Early termination

— Complications are related to the technique employed.

— Major complications are rare in first-trimester abortion (0.5–1% immediate; 1–10% delayed).

— Haemorrhage, both immediate and late, is a common problem.

— Trauma — perforation of uterus and tear of the cervix are not uncommon and may require laparotomy and in rare cases hysterectomy.

— Retained products of conception may occur before week 14–16 and this leads to haemorrhage, infection, particularly by anaerobic organisms.
— Intra-amniotic saline carries its own special risk of accidental intravascular injection with consequent hypernatraemia and coagulation problems.

Late complication

— Infertility arising mainly from infection.
— Recurrent abortion from cervical incompetence.
— Psychological disturbance (< 10%).
— Menstrual disorders, mainly menorrhagia.
— Amenorrhoea may reflect over-vigorous removal of the endometrium (Asherman's syndrome).
— Psychiatric disturbance.
— Pregnancy continuing; curette might have missed the pregnancy or one fetus may have been removed and one left in the uterus.
— Rhesus ISO immunisation — all Rh-negative patients must be given anti-D gammaglobulin.
— Pregnancy following previous late terminantions is associated with more problems.

Counselling

Pre-termination

— Patient's problem is adequately discussed with her, as well as the options available, termination or continuing with pregnancy.
— If termination is requested, the methods and complications should be explained fully.
— Future methods of contraception should be discussed.
— The following should be explored:
  • History of previous contraceptive use
  • Previous therapeutic abortion
  • Drug and tranquilliser use
  • Psychiatric disturbance
  • Mental retardation
  • Strength of moral and religious feeling
  • Feelings of guilt and depression
  • Psychological antecedents to the pregnancy
  • Fulfilment of a neurotic or sociocultural need
  • Maturity, physical and mental, of the patient
  • Family and social network
  • Stability of life in general and in marriage

Post-termination

— Further psychological counselling should be given.
— Possible referral for more specialised psychiatric help may be needed.

— Contraceptive intentions should be ascertained and appropriate advise given.
— Possible late complications should also be discussed, together with the need for follow-up.
— Adequate advice regarding future contraception should be discussed before termination and stressed after the termination to avoid further termination.

Immunological methods

— Immunisation programmes employing HCG coupled with tetanus toxoid have been tried.
— Antibodies are produced to HCG but the method is not reliable.
— Other tissues may be used for immunisation.
— Spermatozoa, zona pellucida and other trophoblastic enzymes or hormones.
— The hypothalamic hormone LRH is also a possibility.
— LRH antagonists — a promising method — is a daily nasal spray of a drug antagonising gonadotropin-releasing factor (LRH).
— Continuous administration of LHRH agonists for female contraception.

Table 21.4 Number of deaths per 100 000 expected from different methods of contraception and childbirth

Method	Number
One pregnancy	11
Oral contraceptives for 1 year	20
Laparoscopic sterilisation	3
Laparotomy sterilisation	28
Interval abdominal hysterectomy	165
Interval vaginal hysterectomy	253
Hysterectomy associated with pregnancy	295

Table 21.5 Effectiveness of various contraceptives

Average number of pregnancies in one year for every 100 women using the method concerned	
MOST RELIABLE	Less than 0.4
Combined pill	
LESS RELIABLE	
Intra-uterine devices	3.0
Mini-pill (progestogen-only pill)	3.0
Diaphragm plus spermicides	3.0
Condom plus spermicides	4.0
NOT RELIABLE	
No contraceptives at all	Up to 40.0
The "safe period"	18.0
Spermicide alone	15.0
Withdrawal	17.0

— Amenorrhoea occurs; genital atrophy does not occur.
— Major problems abound: cross reactivity with normal tissue, difficulty in accurately timing the duration of effect, reversibility and possible side-effects.
— Tables 21.4 and 21.5 show the mortality rate and effectiveness of various methods.

SUGGESTED READING

Alberman E, Dennis K J 1984 Late abortions in England and Wales. Report of a national confidential study. RCOG.

Astedt B, 1980 Contraception and its complications. In: Gold J J, Josimovich J B (eds) Gynecologic endocrinology, 3rd edn. Harper & Row, New York, p 475

Burkman R T, King T M 1984 Second trimester termination of pregnancy. In: Symonds E M. Zuspan F P (eds) Clinical and diagnostic procedures in obstetrics and gynaecology. Part B. Gynaecology. Dekker, New York, p 241

Connell E B (ed) 1979 Contraception in clinics in obstetrics and gynaecology. Saunders, Philadelphia

Elstein M, Nuttall I D 1982 Progestogen-only contraception. In: Studd J (ed) Progress in obstetrics and gynaecology, vol 2. Churchill Livingstone, Edinburgh, p 166

Filshie G M 1984 First-trimester termination of pregnancy. In: Symonds E M, Zuspan F P (eds) Clinical and diagnostic procedures in obstetrics and gynaecology. Part B. Gynaecology. Dekker, p 223

Haspels A A, Rolland O (eds) 1982 Benefits and risks of hormonal contraception. In: The proceedings of an international symposium, Amsterdam. MTP, Lancaster

Hefnawi F 1979 Advances in fertility control. In: Stallworthy J, Bourne G (eds) Recent advances in obstetrics and gynaecology, vol 13. Churchill Livingstone, Edinburgh, p 47

Jones W R 1982 Immunological approach to contraception. In: Studd J (ed) Progress in obstetrics and gynaecology, vol 2. Churchill Livingstone, Edinburgh, p 183

Newton R J (ed) 1984 Contraception update. Clinics in obstetrics and gynaecology, vol 11. Saunders, Philadelphia

Nillius S J 1982 The use of LHRH analogues. In: Studd J (ed) Progress in obstetrics an gynaecology, vol 2. Churchill Livingstone, Edinburgh

Speroff L, Glass R H, Kase N G (eds) 1984 Steroid contraception. In: Clinical gynecologic endocrinology and infertility. Williams & Wilkins, Baltimore, p 409

LH   (MALE 1·4 – 9·7)

          FEMALE   FOLLIC 0·21
                   MID   4.1 – 70
                   LUTEAL 1 – 12·8

FSH   (MALE 1–7)
          FEMALE   FOLLIC 1–10
                   MID   6 – 25

PROLACTIN   (Normal < 360)

PROGESTERONE   (FOLL   2–8
                 LUTEAL 8 – 66)

Index

(handwritten annotations) TSH (0.5 — 4.0 POST MENOPAUSAL 0.5—6.3) FREE T3 ADULT 2.9–8.6 <19y 4.4 —10.6 .

Candida albicans, 37, 180
Carcinoma
  basal cell, 59
  cervix, 73
    lymphatic drainage, 12
    staging, 75
  endometrium, 96
    staging, 98
  intraepithelial, 75
  ovary, 122
  urethra, 60
  vagina, 64
  vulva, 51
  see also specific types, sites, and cancer
Cardinal ligament, 8
Caruncle, 174
Carunculae myrtiformes, 2
Cervical
  dysplasia, 79
  hostility, 282
  incompetence, 300
  os — internal and external, 5
  pregnancy, 211
  smear, 75
  stenosis, 72
Cervicitis, 70, 193
Cervix
  anatomy, 5
  benign disorders, 68–73
  carcinoma, 73–95
  causing infertility, 282–283
  cone biopsy, 80
  dysplasia, 75
  ectropion, 62, 68
  incompetence, 300
  intraepithelial carcinoma, 75
  ligaments, 8
  micro-invasive carcinoma, 73, 89
  polyp, 72
  stenosis, 72
  transformation zone, 69
Chancre, 47, 190
Chancroid, 46, 90
Chemotherapy
  ovarian cancer, 131, 132, 134, 240
  choriocarcinoma, 240
  see also specific tumours
Childhood disorders, 23, 195
Chlamydial infection, 71, 179, 184, 201
Chocolate cysts of ovary, 138
Choriocarcinoma, 237–243
Chorionic gonadotrophins, 234, 236, 237, 242
Chromosome, 25
Chronic pelvic inflammatory disease, 204
Clear cell carcinoma, 63, 124
Climacteric, 303
Clitoris
  anatomy, 2
  carcinoma, 56
Clomiphene
  anovulation, 276, 277, 278
  menorrhagia, 221
Colpocleisis, 155
Colpoperineorrhaphy, 153

Colporrhaphy, 153
Colposcopy, 79
Complete abortion, 295
Condom, 316
Condylomata accuminate, 43, 183
Condylomata lata, 47, 191
Cone biopsy of cervix, 83
Congenital anomalies, 25–35
  adrenal hyperplasia, 32
Contraception, 313–342
  barrier method, 315
  cap, 315
  coitus interruptus, 317
  condom, 316
  immunological method, 341
  intra-uterine devices, 327
  long-acting injectable steroids, 320
  oral, 318
  post-coital, 321
  progestin-only pill, 319
  spermicides, 316
  vaginal diaphragm, 315
Copper intrauterine devices, 327, 328
Cornual pregnancy, 211
Corpus luteum, 18
  inadequate, 277
Cryocautery, 84
Cryptomenorrhoea, 244, 247, 264
Culdocentesis, 214
Cullen's sign, 213
Cushing's disease, 247
Cyproterone acetate, 260
Cystadenocarcinoma of ovary, 122
Cystadenoma, 119
Cystic glandular hyperplasia, 221
Cystic teratoma, 118
Cystocele, 151
Cystometry, 167
Cystourethrography, 167
Cysts
  chocolate cyst of ovary, 136
  dermoid, 118
  endometriotic cyst, 118
  follicular and luteal, 116
  Gartner duct, 63
  inclusion, 63
  lutein, 117
  ovarian, 118
  parovarian, 120
  theca-lutein, 117
  vulval cyst/swelling, 48
  see also individual organs
Cytology
  cervix, 75
  endometrial, 100

Danazol, 143
  menorrhagia, 222
Decidual cast, 210
Decidual reaction, 211
Decubitus ulceration, 152
Dehydroepiandrosterone, 17
Delayed puberty, 20, 21
Depo-Provera, 320

Paget's disease of vulva, 53
Papilloma, 51
Paraurethral glands, 2
Parovarian cyst, 120
Pearl index, 315
Pelvic inflammatory disease, 196, 254
  abscess, 203
  management, 199
Pemphigus of vulva, 41
Pessary, uterine prolapse, 153
Physiology of lower urinary tract, 159
Pill, contraceptive, 319
Polycystic ovary syndrome, 258, 275
Polyp — cervix, 72
Positive feedback, 15
Postcoital contraception, 321
Posterior colpoperineorrhaphy, 153
Posterior urethrovesical angle, 165, 167
Post-menopausal bleeding, 72, 88, 99
Precocious puberty, 20
Pre-invasive cancer
  cervix, 75
  vulva, 53
Premenstrual tension syndrome, 226
Progestastert, 328
Progestin-only pill, 319
Prolactinoma, 260
Prolapse, 148
Prostaglandins, 338, 339
Pruritus vulvae, 36
Puberty, 19
  delayed, 20
  precocious, 20
Pudendal nerve, 11
Pyridoxine (vitamin B6), 228

Radical vulvectomy, 57
Rectocele, 153
Red degeneration of fibroma, 112
Releasing factor, gonadotrophic, 13, 14, 15
Reproductive system
  anatomy, 1–12
  physiology, 13–24
Retrograde ejaculation, 286
Retroversion of the uterus, 155
Rhabdomyosarcoma, 108
Rhythm method, contraception, 317

Saf-T-coil, 328
Salpingectomy, tubal pregnancy, 209
Salpingitis, 186, 196, 199, 200
  isthmicanodosa, 204, 205
Sarcoma, 106
  botryoides, 94
Schiller test, 75, 80
Secondary amenorrhoea, 244–257
Senile atrophy, 49
Septic abortion, 297
Septic shock syndrome, 298
Serous cyst adenocarcinoma, 126
Serous cyst adenoma, 119
Sertoli-Leydig tumour, 125
Sexually transmitted diseases, 42, 179
Skene (paraurethral) ducts, 2

Spermicides, 316
Spinnbarkeit, 271
Stenosis, cervical, 72
Sterilisation, 333
Stilboestrol (DES), 85
Stress incontinence, 164
Syphilis, 46, 190

Tamoxifen, 278
Teeth in dermoid cyst, 118
Testes in male infertility, 238
Testosterone, 284, 310
  infertility, 284
  in menopause, 310
Theca-lutein cysts, 117, 233
Threatened abortion, 294
Thromboembolism, contraception, 324
Thyrotropin-releasing hormone, 273
Tinidazole, 42, 181
Toluidine blue, diagnosis of vulva cancer, 51
Transformation zone of cervix, 73, 74
Transverse cervical ligament, 5
Treponema pallidum, 43, 67, 191
Treponema pertenue, 191
Trichomonas vaginalis, 39, 43, 179, 180
Trophoblast tumours, 230–243
Tube, fallopian
  anatomy, 6
  infection, 196
  infertility, 279
  patency test, 280
  surgery, 281
Tuberculosis
  cervix, 71
  pelvis, 204
Tubo-ovarian abscess, 203
Tuboplasty, 281
Tumour associated antigens (markers), 129
Turner's syndrome, 29

Ulcer
  cervix, 71, 88
  decubitus, 151
  vulva, 36, 41
Ultrasound scan
  abscess pelvic, 203
  cervical incompetence, 300
  detection of ovulation, 272
  ectopic pregnancy, 214
  hydatidiform mole, 233
  ovarian cyst, 122, 129
  uterine fibromyoma, 114
Unstable bladder, 169
Upper genital tract infection, 196
Ureter
  anatomy, 9
  endometriosis, 139
Uretero-vaginal fistula, 161, 162
Urethra
  anatomy, 10
  carcinoma, 60
  caruncle, 305
  disorders, 173
  diverticulum, 174